Care of the Postoperative Surgical Patient

To my family, especially my daughter Elizabeth Anne Watkins, SRN, on the threshold of her career in nursing (J.W.)

To my wife and family for their continuing patience and long-suffering of these literary exercises (J.A.R.S.)

Care of the Postoperative Surgical Patient

Edited by
John A. R. Smith, PhD, FRCS, FRCS(Ed)
Consultant Surgeon, Northern General Hospital, Sheffield
(Previously: Senior Lecturer in Surgery, University of Sheffield, and Honorary Consultant Surgeon, Royal Hallamshire Hospital, Sheffield)

John Watkins, BSc, PhD
Non-medical Consultant Immunologist and Deputy Director, Supraregional Protein Reference Unit, Department of Immunology, Royal Hallamshire Hospital, Sheffield

Butterworths
London Boston Durban Singapore Sydney Toronto Wellington

First published, 1985

British Library Cataloguing in Publication Data

Care of the postoperative surgical patient.
1. Postoperative care 2. Hospital patients
I. Smith, J. A. R. II. Watkins, J. (John)
617'.919 RD51

ISBN 0-407-00286-3

Library of Congress Cataloging in Publication Data

Main entry under title:
Care of the postoperative surgical patient.
Includes bibliographies and index.
1. Postoperative care. I. Smith, John A. R.
II. Watkins, John. [DNLM: 1. Postoperative Care.
WO 183 C271]
RD51.C32 1985 617'.919 85-3811

ISBN 0-407-00286-3

Photoset by Butterworths Litho Preparation Department
Printed and bound by Robert Hartnoll (1985) Limited, Bodmin, Cornwall

Preface

Increasingly, postoperative care is becoming a multidisciplinary responsibility. Expertise in the fields of surgical care, anaesthesia and monitoring of patients has now increased to such an extent that no one individual can be expert in all aspects of postoperative management. The interrelationship between analgesic therapy, antimicrobial agents, nutritional support and the pharmacological regimens commonly used in the postoperative period are complex, and may be modified by the effects of surgery and anaesthesia.

A greater understanding of preoperative preparation combined with improvement in anaesthetic skill, which has allowed more and more intricate surgery to be performed, has moved emphasis for obtaining good results in surgical practice away from the areas of preoperative care and intraoperative skill to the postoperative period.

This book aims to provide all clinicians interested in postoperative care with the specialist information necessary to optimize the management of the individual patient, both in the normal and abnormal environment. The emphasis has been on clinical care but, where appropriate, a physiological basis has been provided.

Certain areas discussed must be considered experimental for the present, but are included as likely to be the norm of the future.

J. A. R. Smith
J. Watkins

Contributors

Asbury, A. J., MBChB, FFA RCS, PhD
Senior Lecturer in Anaesthesia and Honorary Consultant Anaesthetist, University of Glasgow, Western Infirmary, Dumbarton Road, Glasgow G11 6NT, Scotland

Bax, N. D. S., BSc, MRCP
Lecturer in Therapeutics, Royal Hallamshire Hospital, Sheffield S10 2JF

Catto, Graeme R. D., MD, FRCP, FRCP(G)
Senior Lecturer in Medicine, University of Aberdeen, Foresterhill, Aberdeen AB9 2ZB, Scotland; Honorary Consultant Physician/ Nephrologist, Grampian Health Board

Charlton, J. Edmond, FFA RCS
Consultant Anaesthetist, Anaesthesia/Pain Relief, Royal Victoria Infirmary, Newcastle upon Tyne NE1 4LP

Clark, Ronald G., MBChB, FRCS(Ed & Eng)
Professor of Surgery, University of Sheffield; Honorary Consultant Surgeon, Northern General Hospital, Sheffield S5 7AU

Ellis, F. R., PhD, MBChB, FFA RCS
Reader in Anaesthesia, St. James's University Hospital, Leeds LS9 7TF

Fleck, A., BSc, MB ChB, PhD, FRCPath, FRCPG, FRSC, FRSE
Professor of Chemical Pathology, University of London, Charing Cross and Westminster Medical School, Fulham Palace Road, London W6 8RF

Hull, Christopher J., MBBS, FFA RCS
Professor of Anaesthesia, University of Newcastle upon Tyne, and Honorary Consultant Anaesthetist, Royal Victoria Infirmary, Newcastle upon Tyne NE1 4LP

Ledingham, I. McA., MD, FRCS(Ed), MRCP(Glasg), FRSE
Professor of Surgery, University of Glasgow, Western Infirmary, Glasgow G11 6NT, Scotland

Nelson Norman, J., MD, DSc, PhD, FRCS(Glasg and Ed), FInstBiol
Professor, and Director, Centre for Offshore Health, Robert Gordon's Institute of Technology, Kepplestone Mansion, Viewfield Road, Aberdeen AB9 2PF, Scotland

Simpson, K. H., MBChB, FFA RCS
Lecturer in Anaesthesia, St. James's University Hospital, Leeds LS9 7TF

Smith, J. A. R., PhD, FRCS, FRCS(Ed)
Consultant Surgeon, Northern General Hospital, Sheffield S5 7AU. Previously: Senior Lecturer in Surgery, University of Sheffield, and Honorary Consultant Surgeon, Royal Hallamshire Hospital, Sheffield S10 2JF

Strachan, Colin J. L., MD, FRCSE
Consultant Surgeon, Royal Sussex County and Brighton General Hospitals; Honorary Research Fellow, University of Sussex, Falmer, Brighton BN2 3EW, Sussex

Symoens, J., DVM
Director of Clinical Research and Development, Janssen Pharmaceutica, B2340 Beerse, Belgium

Taylor, Ken, MD, FRCS, FRCSE, FSA
British Heart Foundation Professor of Cardiac Surgery, University of London; Professor of Cardiac Surgery, Royal Postgraduate Medical School, Hammersmith Hospital, Ducane Road, London W12 0HS

Thornton, J. A., MD, FFA RCS, FFARACS, DA
Professor and Chairman of the Department of Anaesthesia, and Director of Intensive Care, The Chinese University of Hong Kong, Shatin NT, Hong Kong

Vanhoutte, P. M., MD, AgES
Professor of Physiology and Pharmacology, Mayo Clinic and Mayo Foundation, Rochester, MN 55905, USA

Velasco, Nestor, MB, MRCP(UK)
Research Fellow in Medicine, University of Aberdeen, Foresterhill, Aberdeen AB9 2ZB, Scotland

Watkins, J., BSc, PhD
Non-medical Consultant Immunologist and Deputy Director, Supraregional Protein Reference Unit, Department of Immunology, Royal Hallamshire Hospital, Sheffield S10 2JF

Woodcock, T. E., MB BS, FFA RCS
Senior Registrar, Department of Anaesthesia, Bristol Royal Infirmary, Bristol BS2 8HW

Woods, H. F., DPhil, FRCP
Professor of Pharmacology and Therapeutics, University of Sheffield, Department of Therapeutics, Royal Hallamshire Hospital, Sheffield S10 2JF

Contents

Part I

Immediate problems

Chapter 1

The immediate recovery period

A. J. Asbury

Introduction

Thousands of patients undergo anaesthesia and surgery every year and their safe recovery tends to be taken for granted. The recovery period is, however, a dangerous time and complications can occur. Many of them are preventable.

Recovery period mortality

Difficulty of obtaining reliable mortality estimates

It is difficult to obtain reliable figures for the incidence of problems in the recovery period. Crude mortality rates, for example, usually underestimate the incidences because many potential disasters are anticipated and prevented by prompt treatment. DHSS figures are not very helpful because they only count cases where anaesthesia is specifically mentioned on the death certificate. Much of the useful information comes from local surveys. These can produce very reliable data, but unfortunately the conclusions may only be applicable locally. Bigger surveys are very helpful, but they can suffer from the difficulty in applying the definitions uniformly, and of course the effect of varying work patterns.

Recovery mortality

Clifton and Hotten, from the Royal Prince Albert Hospital in Sydney, Australia, analysed 162 deaths arising from 205 640 operations (Clifton and Hotten, 1963). The operations covered all surgical specialities, and post-neurosurgical and post-cardiothoracic deaths together accounted for 42.6% of the total. Approximately 40% of the deaths occurred in the recovery period, and the authors comment that 94.4% of these deaths occurred within the 4 h after the anaesthetic and 98.7% without return of consciousness.

In 1975, Bodlander continued the work of Clifton and Hotten in the same hospital and analysed a further 408 deaths which occurred during the subsequent 9-year period. The distribution of types of surgery was similar to Clifton and Hotten's report, but the number of patients dying in the postoperative period had risen to 62.1% (Bodlander, 1975).

In 1959, the Association of Anaesthetists appointed a committee to examine deaths related to anaesthesia. Deaths were reported on a voluntary basis for 5½ years and an analysis was undertaken when 1000 cases had been collected. The results showed that 42.6% of the patients died in the recovery period and 19.5% in the first half-hour (Edwards *et al.*, 1956).

In 1975, Wylie reported his investigation into 66 'anaesthesia related deaths' reported to the Medical Defence Union, and commented that the distribution of deaths during and after anaesthesia was approximately equal. Wylie (1975) commented that approximately 50% of the postoperative cardiac arrests could have been prevented had a proper preoperative assessment been made by the anaesthetist and had he been able to maintain direct responsibility in the immediate postoperative period.

The most recent information comes from a survey of mortality in five regions in the UK, conducted under the guidance of the Association of Anaesthetists. Information on deaths occurring within 6 days of anaesthesia was collected for one complete year starting in March 1979 (Lunn and Mushin, 1982).

Consideration of the 365 deaths for which detailed reports had been obtained showed that 37.5% of patients died on the same day as the operation, and a further 27.1% died on the first postoperative day (*Figure 1.1*). Of the 365 deaths, 16.1% of patients died in the operating theatre,

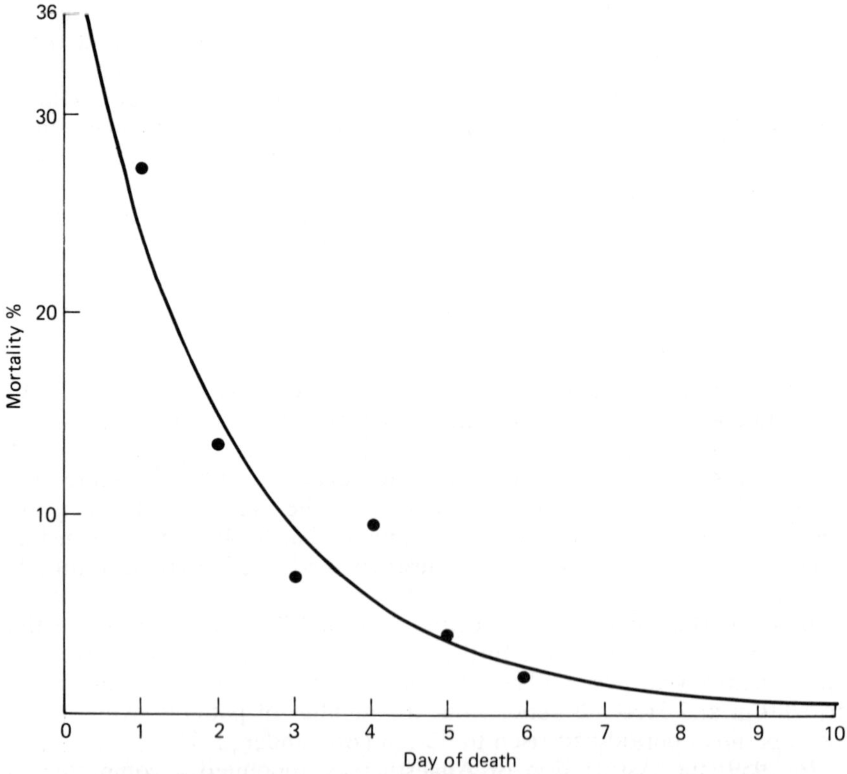

Figure 1.1. The relationship between mortality and the postoperative day in 365 patients for whom detailed records were available (From Lunn and Mushin, 1982, by permission of the publishers)

4.6% in 'recovery', 26.8% in an intensive care unit and 52.3% on the ward. This suggests that 83.7% of deaths occurred postoperatively, substantially more than the 62.1% quoted by Bodlander. The fact that Bodlander's survey only counted deaths in the first 24 h could account for this difference. Lunn and Mushin also noted the important fact that in 17.5% of cases where a death occurred, there was no recovery room, and that in 18% of cases where a recovery room was available, it was not used.

Subdivision of the recovery period

The recovery period can extend over many days and for descriptive purposes may be usefully subdivided into three phases – the immediate recovery phase, the intermediate recovery phase and the late recovery phase (Steward and Volgvesi, 1978).

Immediate recovery phase

At the beginning of this phase surgical anaesthesia is terminated and the patient is transferred to the recovery room. During this time the vital airway protecting reflexes become effective, consciousness returns and the patient exhibits spontaneous motor activity. This is a very dangerous phase because the patient's state changes at an unpredictable rate from surgical anaesthesia to a measure of independent safety, though still very sleepy. One major problem is that it is difficult to assess the patient's progress reliably in this changing situation. No observer, for example, looking at a patient breathing spontaneously, can determine whether he has adequate airway safety to cope with a vomit, and therefore from the viewpoint of practical patient care the nurse should always be within arm's reach of the patient during this phase. Only when the patient begins to talk rationally and move spontaneously can it be assumed that there is a measure of safety, and even then the patient may lapse back into unconsciousness when unstimulated.

Intermediate recovery phase

This phase commences when the patient has airway safety and can move spontaneously. During this phase the patient regains most of his power and co-ordination. Subjective feelings of dizziness and somnolence disappear and the patient begins to take an interest in his environment. Many day case patients are discharged toward the end of this phase, which may last up to 24 h.

Late recovery phase

This phase merges with the preceding phase and can continue for many days. During the late recovery phase the residual effects of the anaesthetic are only detectable by sensitive psychological tests. Henceforth in this chapter we consider only the immediate recovery phase.

General problems of the immediate recovery phase

Complexity of the recovery process

Recovery from general anaesthesia involves the diminishing effects of drugs used during the anaesthetic. It is the net effect of a drug that matters in this situation, rather than the dosage or the blood concentration.

In earlier days when only one drug, e.g. diethyl ether, was used for the anaesthetic, one saw the recovery process for just one drug. Nowadays, with modern anaesthesia, one sees the effects of several drugs and their inevitable interactions. A further problem of multiple drug use is attributable to the different time constants of the drugs. This may mean that when one drug is used to counteract an unwanted effect of a second, the effectiveness of the first may decrease, revealing the undesired effect of the second, e.g. the post-anaesthesia bradycardia following neostigmine and atropine. In addition to the pharmacological effects, the patient undergoes a series of physiological changes, e.g. fluid redistribution in body compartments, and these may be a consequence of the anaesthesia or surgery. These physiological changes, with those caused by the disease process itself, complicate the recovery pattern to such an extent that the assessment of recovery progress tends to be based simply on the degree of threat to life, rather than a consideration of the many factors involved, of which the threat to life is only one.

Problem of measuring progress in the immediate recovery phase

The measurement of progress in the immediate recovery phase (IRP) is difficult for two reasons. First, the recovery process is complex and, secondly, most measurement methods are relevant in the patient who is awake and capable of responding to the observer, but break down in the somnolent patient, and this applies to most of the patients in the IRP. It is the somnolent patient, however, who is at greatest risk and needs the greatest degree of supervision.

Subjective assessments by the patient

This technique relies upon the patient being able to hear and comprehend the question, and Aromaa (1977) suggests that this reveals little more than the fact that the patient is able to give some form of plausible answer. Herbert *et al.* (1983) found considerable discrepancies between subjective and objective recovery test results.

Simple observations

Most of these involve discrete observations at a given time, or a measurement of the time for one state to change to another. Some of the observations are: response to a painful stimulus, time to spontaneous opening of eyes, time to return of the eyelash reflex, presence of nystagmus, time to first verbal response, time to when the patient recognizes his name and location, and time to when the patient can stand up unaided. All these observations have problems, in that their applicability may depend upon the form of the anaesthetic, the environment and the type of surgery. These observations are useful in the IRP, but cannot reliably be used to compare patients for the reasons given above. One way of improving the value of these observations is to combine them to form a recovery progress score (RPS).

Scoring systems

One of the earliest systems was designed mainly to assess surgical recovery, rather than the IRP. The body was subdivided into systems and the extent of the progress of a system to normal function was given a score according to a prearranged scheme. The total score was used as the index of recovery. Assessments were made on the 2nd, 5th and 15th days, postoperatively (Carignan, Keéri-Szàntò and Lavellée, 1964).

Aldrete and Kroulik (1970) designed a useful RPS, which was independently evaluated by Figueroa (1972). The system, which was simple to apply, divided the body into its systems and scored the functional ability of each. As a result of the studies, normal ranges for recovery progress could be established – a useful starting point for detecting abnormal recovery. Steward (1975) introduced a 'simplified scoring system', which works well.

A very helpful RPS was invented by Robertson, MacGregor and Jones (1977). It was initially designed as a research tool to assess the effect of doxapram in hastening arousal from anaesthesia, and for this purpose measurements at 2-minute intervals were advocated. Although perhaps slightly impractical for routine recovery room measurements, the short measurement interval does emphasize the speed with which events occur in the IRP.

Robertson's scoring system has been modified to make it easier to use routinely and some of the criteria employed in the score have been further defined (Asbury, 1981). Asbury's RPS also attempts to give an appropriate weighting to the parts of the RPS, with airway safety for example being more important than blood pressure measurements (*Table 1.1*).

Measurement of physiological variables

The problem with most measurements is one of interpretation and relevance to the IRP. Many measurements are possible; for example, reaction time, flicker fusion testing, measurement of extra-ocular muscle balance, the electro-oculogram and the electroencephalogram (EEG). With the exception of the EEG, these tests require a degree of patient co-operation which makes them useless in the IRP. The problem of the EEG is one of practicality. One needs standardized conditions and a still patient to obtain reliable EEG recordings, and even then there is the problem of interpretation.

Behavioural and performance tests

There is a wide variety of such tests, from pencil and paper tests, verbal response tests and manipulative skill tests, to simulated driving. All are inappropriate in the IRP because the patients would not be able to co-operate.

Table 1.1. An improved recovery scoring system (Asbury, 1981) which incorporates an empirical weighting for some of the observations. The colour test refers to the patient's ability to identify two named colours from a chart held at arm's length

Observation	*Score*
No respiratory movement at all	0
Adequate breathing	1
Able to move all limbs to command	2
Able to lift head for 5 s	3
No response to pain at all	0
Non-specific response to pain	1
Verbal response to spoken word	3
Colour test negative	3
Colour test positive	4
Tolerates airway or ETT	0
Will *not* tolerate airway or ETT	4
Systolic blood pressure ± 30 mm preoperative level	2
Systolic blood pressure above 70 mm Hg, but less than preoperative value less 30 mm Hg	1
Systolic blood pressure less than 70 mm	0
Central cyanosis (tongue and in mouth)	0
Peripheral cyanosis/pallor/sweating	1
Pink/warm/well perfused	2

The transport problem

The objective of recovery care is to manage the difficult phase after the anaesthetic and present the patient fit and safe to the ward. The problem is that because the recovery progress is so difficult to evaluate, it is difficult to determine when a patient is fit to transport. The risks of the transport should not be underestimated, as the patient may have to go down corridors and travel in lifts and ambulances where the chance of resuscitating him is small. There may be inadequate equipment, space (especially in lifts), drugs or oxygen supplies. The staff transporting the patient may well be too inexperienced, since it is only with reluctance that experienced staff are spared from the wards to collect patients (Stephens and Boaler, 1977).

The only way to resolve this problem is to keep patients in the recovery room longer than necessary to ensure their safe transport and this has considerable financial implications in terms of space and staffing. Obviously, adequate staff numbers must be available on the wards so that the existing patients do not suffer while an experienced person goes to collect the theatre patient.

In the IRP we have a patient undergoing a change of state which is unpredictable in speed and difficult to measure. The transfer of the inadequately recovered patient to the ward can be dangerous. It is difficult to assess when the patient is adequately recovered.

Specific medical problems

Cardiorespiratory problems

Many postoperative problems are attributable to the cardiorespiratory system and can be described systematically by considering the progress of atmospheric oxygen to its destination in the patient's tissues. The first part of the process is the central initiation and maintenance of normal ventilation; if the lungs do not perform their pumping function, they cannot perform their gas exchange function (*Figure 1.2*).

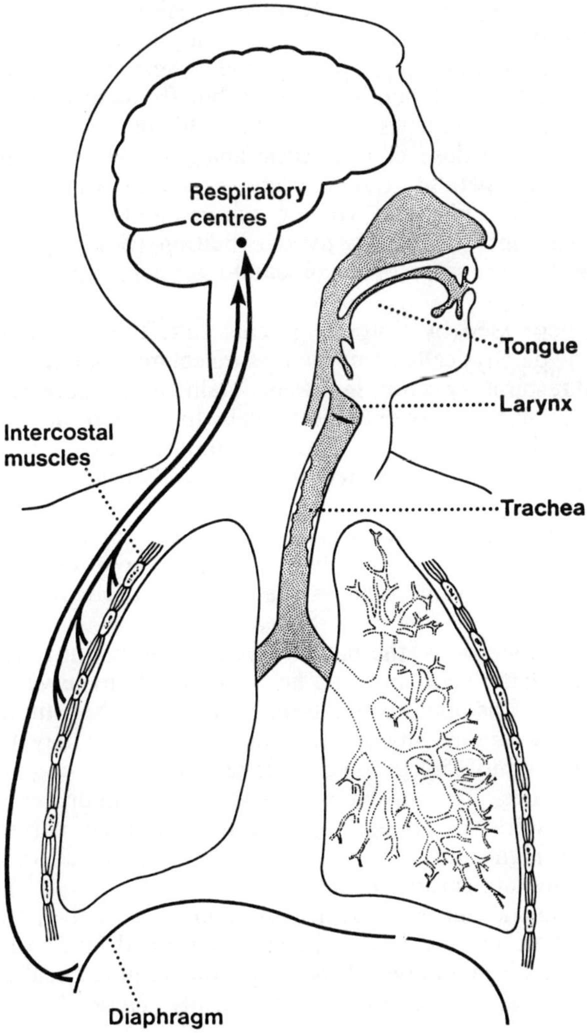

Figure 1.2. Some of the problem areas in the cardiorespiratory system

Failure of the central control of ventilation

Many general anaesthetics have some central depressant effect, and as the dose is increased this effect becomes evident. This is particularly well demonstrated by the classical signs of diethyl ether anaesthesia, which include progressive respiratory depression. Modern inhalation agents, however, do not show marked respiratory depression in clinical doses and this is rarely a problem in immediate recovery. Some intravenous hypnotic agents administered by continuous infusion, e.g. althesin, etomidate or thiopentone, may have a cumulative effect which lasts well into the recovery period.

The main danger of these general anaesthetic agents is synergism with other drugs, e.g. relaxants and narcotics, producing a confusing pharmacological picture during recovery. Narcotic analgesics are frequently used in modern anaesthesia, not only as a premedication but also alone and in combination with tranquillizers. Ideally, the anaesthetist should titrate the analgesic dose to the patient's response, but frequently this is impossible due to the surgical requests for paralysis. This means that the anaesthetist may give an overdose of a narcotic analgesic which in the recovery period leaves the patient conscious and hypoventilating. The patient can readily increase his tidal volume on demand, but when unstimulated lapses back into dangerous hypoventilation (Severinghaus and Mitchell, 1952) and on the ward this may lead to hypoxia and carbon dioxide narcosis.

Apart from being depressed by drugs, e.g. narcotics, the medullary centres in the brain may be physically damaged by surgical manipulation or trauma. The damaged respiratory centre fails to maintain an adequate tidal volume and the consequent hypoventilation leads to carbon dioxide accumulation and hypoxia. The carbon dioxide accumulation may then cause brain swelling, leading to further medullary centre damage and the vicious circle is completed.

Hypoxic medullary damage has occurred following cardiopulmonary bypass and is sometimes seen postoperatively in a patient whose return to consciousness and adequate ventilation is delayed or never occurs (Branthwaite, 1973).

During many surgical operations, the patient's ventilation is controlled mechanically by an automatic ventilator and he is frequently hyperventilated, causing hypocapnia. Postoperatively, in the absence of other stimuli (which may be blocked by residual anaesthetic drugs), the patient may not resume normal ventilation until the carbon dioxide tension rises enough to drive his respiratory centre. This problem is particularly important in patients with chronic respiratory disease, because their 'normal' carbon dioxide level may be high and the patient becomes hypoxic while hypoventilating to accumulate carbon dioxide.

Assuming that the central cerebral control mechanism is active, the efferent signals must be conducted to the diaphragmatic and intercostal muscles to actually pump air in and out of the lungs; this requires healthy muscles and an intact neural and neuromuscular pathway (*Figure 1.2*).

Failure of the neuromuscular junction and muscles of respiration

One of the commonest problems in the recovery period is the residual anaesthetic effects on the neuromuscular junction.

Non-depolarizing muscle relaxants. The muscles around the thoracic cavity are responsible for ventilation and, if they are partially paralysed, ventilation will be inadequate. For many operations requiring muscle relaxation, a long-acting non-depolarizing agent is used. Any residual effects are reversed at the motor end plate using an anticholinesterase drug such as neostigmine, which is given at the end of surgery. Their elimination from the body, however, is a much slower process and depends on renal and hepatic mechanisms. While still in the circulation, relaxants may reoccupy the motor end plate causing further paralysis, possibly on the ward.

Furthermore, the effectiveness of a given plasma level of relaxant depends on a further group of factors; for example, antibiotics (gentamicin, kanamycin), and hypokalaemia, the presence of synergistic agents (enflurane, halothane), and disturbances of acid–base balance (respiratory acidosis).

During surgery the anaesthetist will usually reduce the relaxant dosage towards the end of the operation to facilitate reversal and reduce the risks of re-paralysis, but in some cases this is not possible, e.g. in eye surgery, where good relaxation is required throughout. This may then lead to a high concentration of relaxant postoperatively and possibly hypoventilation in the IRP.

In recovery, the problem of residual peripheral paralysis should be detected because the patient is unable to breathe adequately on command, although obviously conscious and co-operative. The use of a nerve stimulator helps to confirm the diagnosis.

Depolarizing muscle relaxants. Depolarizing muscle relaxants are less of a problem in recovery because their duration of action is short. However, their effect may be prolonged when cholinesterase enzymes in the plasma are deficient or abnormal, when adjuvant drugs have been administered e.g. tacrine hydrochloride, or where a form of dual block has occurred with its depolarizing and non-depolarizing features. A patient may then have inadequate ventilation with the same dangers as for non-depolarizing relaxants, i.e. hypoxia, carbon dioxide accumulation and laryngeal incompetence.

Failure of muscles of respiration

Problems may arise further along the transmission pathway at the muscles (*Figure 1.2*). For muscles to act effectively they must be connected to a firm bony framework, and a defect in the bone structure of the thorax may cause problems. Such a situation occurs after thoracotomy or thoracoplasty, where the patient in the recovery period has to use an inefficient thorax to ventilate an alveolar surface reduced by surgical or accidental trauma.

The muscles in themselves must be efficient, and in some muscle wasting disorders the respiratory function may be impaired without any hindrance from anaesthetic drugs. The additional effect of the anaesthetic may well push such a compromised patient into respiratory failure and a period of elective postoperative ventilation may be advisable.

Having considered the failure of the lungs to function as a pump, the pathway of oxygen to the tissues can be followed, starting at the mouth (*Figures 1.2* and *1.3*).

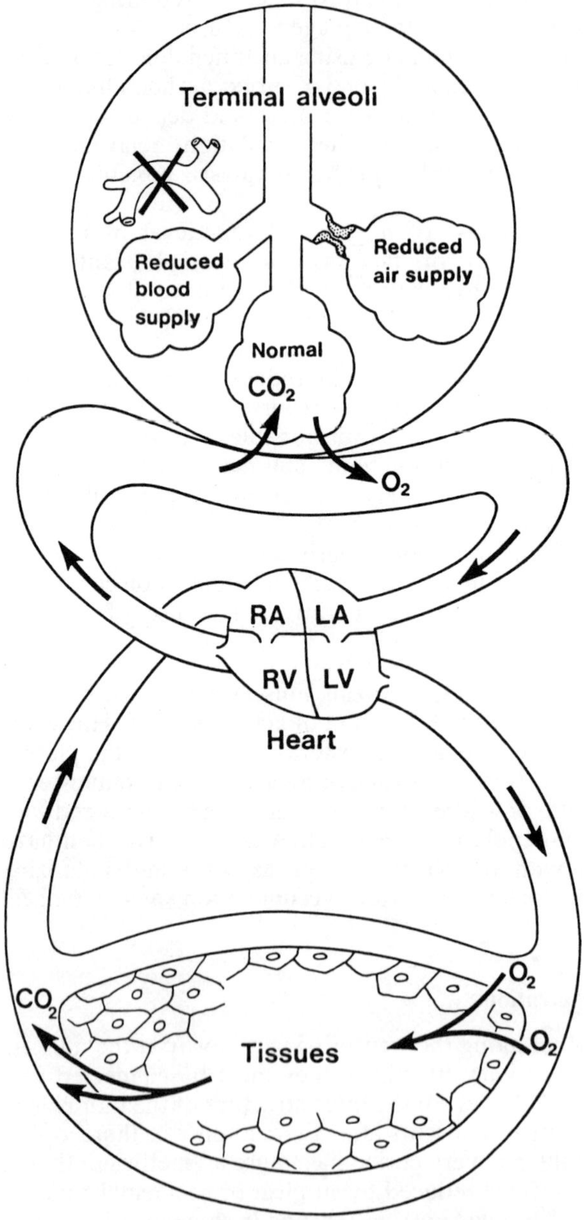

Figure 1.3. The path of oxygen beyond the major airways

Upper airway problems

The commonest problem in the recovery period is failure of airway patency, usually caused by the tongue falling back on to the posterior pharyngeal wall (*Figure 1.2*). This can be remedied simply by lifting the jaw forward and by inserting a pharyngeal airway, if necessary. The airway occlusion is similar to that observed during natural sleep when the tongue relaxes, but different in that the patient is unable to remedy the situation should obstruction occur (Remmers *et al.,* 1978).

The airway patency may also be endangered by extraneous material, e.g. blood, tooth fragments, vomit and foreign bodies. In the early recovery period, the patient may not be able to expel foreign bodies by coughing and may inhale them, thereby contaminating and obstructing the air passages.

Lower airway problems

During the anaesthetic the patient will accumulate airway secretions as the normal clearing mechanism, i.e. coughing, is inoperative. The task is made more difficult by dry anaesthetic gases which make secretions more viscous, and by the reduction of ciliary activity due to the anaesthetic agent itself. In the recovery period, the patient must clear these secretions, in spite of pain, to maintain a low resistance to air flow and an adequate oxygen supply (*Figure 1.3*).

An important cause of lower airway narrowing is bronchospasm. This frequently occurs with long-standing pulmonary infection, but it may be seen in the recovery period as an allergic response to anaesthetic drugs, e.g. pancuronium, or following mechanical trauma of the bronchi, e.g. by suction catheters.

Partial airway obstruction, by increasing the airway resistance, increases the work of breathing and the oxygen consumption, and may cause a lowering of the arterial oxygen tension. This may invoke further respiratory efforts which may lead to increasing hypoxia, hypercapnia and exhaustion.

During anaesthesia, the patient's normal gas exchange is disordered (Thornton, 1960; Gold and Helrich, 1965) and usually allowance is made for this in the anaesthetic technique. However, many of these changes persist into the recovery period, frequently manifesting themselves as arterial hypoxaemia (Thompson and Eason, 1970).

Distribution of inspired gases

During anaesthesia, the patient's functional residual capacity (FRC) may be reduced by up to 30% (Don *et al.,* 1970). This may persist into the immediate recovery period and is often made worse by the patient being in pain and unable to expand his chest. Consequently, the normal gas distribution pattern is disrupted. As the lung volume decreases, the dependent pleural pressure ceases to be sub-atmospheric and airway closure occurs in the dependent lung. Ventilation is consequently maintained, using mainly the non-dependent areas of the lung. In patients with normal respiratory health, the natural pulmonary elasticity causes the closing volume to be near the residual lung volume, but in elderly patients, the closing volume may approach the functional residual capacity (Morton and Baker, 1978) so that the patient's lung is exhibiting closure at normal tidal volumes.

Respiratory resistance in the postoperative period

Apart from the effects of secretions, normal respiratory resistance is composed of lung tissue resistance (20%) and airway resistance (80%) (Morton, 1977). In the postoperative period there is a marked increase in the total respiratory resistance, particularly in bronchitic patients, and this represents the sum of many of the obstructing factors listed above (Morton, 1977). The total effect is to increase the work of breathing.

Chest compliance

During anaesthesia, the patient's dynamic compliance decreases (Gold and Helrich, 1965) and this effect will persist into the postoperative phase, being aggravated by the low functional residual capacity (Morton and Baker, 1978). This results in an increased work of breathing and may lead to hypoxia.

Changes in alveolar oxygen tension caused by dilution (Fink effect)

During the recovery period, nitrous oxide leaves the blood faster than nitrogen (from the air) enters the blood. This is caused by the fact that nitrous oxide is 30 times more soluble in blood than nitrogen. The effect is to displace or dilute the inspired oxygen (Fink, 1955; Racklow, Salanitre and Frumin, 1961). This phenomenon is short lived (usually up to 5 min) and is frequently called 'diffusion hypoxia'. The path of oxygen to the tissues now leads through the alveolar membrane, into the pulmonary circulation (*Figure 1.3*).

Distribution of pulmonary blood flow

The matching of ventilation and perfusion is essential for effective oxygen transport. The distribution of the pulmonary blood flow should ideally adjust to the distribution of inspired gas. The pulmonary blood flow is, however, gravity dependent and hence, in a sitting patient in the upper zones of the lung, perfusion is poor and ventilation good, while the reverse applies to the lower zones. In the middle of the lung, pulmonary blood flow is controlled by the relation between pulmonary artery pressure and alveolar pressure (Morton and Baker, 1978).

In the recovery period, when the patient may have a low cardiac output, this gravitational effect becomes more important, possibly leading to hypoxia. There is, however, some evidence that the pulmonary circulation adjusts itself to the varying ventilation and perfusion conditions, tending to divert blood from poorly ventilated basal areas to better ventilated areas (Lloyd, 1966; Barer, Howard and McCurrie, 1967; Morton and Baker, 1978).

The ability to maintain a satisfactory balance between ventilation and perfusion depends on the blood being provided at a suitable pressure and flow. Although the pulmonary circulation is dependent on the right ventricle, it is not normal practice to measure right ventricular function in the recovery period. The function of the left side of the heart, however, is routinely assessed by standard sphygmomanometry. Any failure on the left side of the heart will lead eventually to problems in the lungs, e.g. pulmonary oedema, and possibly right-sided heart failure. The total effect of reducing the cardiac output may be to reduce oxygen flux and possibly arterial oxygen tension.

Reduced cardiac output in the recovery period

Blood volume deficit

This problem is most commonly recognized as a fall in blood pressure, tachycardia or bradycardia, or even an irregular pulse (Lappas, Powell and Daggett, 1977). In many cases the patient manages to compensate for a change in his blood volume with few outward signs. Thc commonest cause of postoperative hypotension is probably inadequate management of the patient's blood volume during surgery. When a patient comes to theatre, he may be partially dehydrated from the effects of the disease, e.g. vomiting, polyuria. Further fluid loss may occur with increased sweating in a pyrexial starving patient, and with pathological internal fluid shifts, e.g. ascites. Inadequate intraoperative replacement may lead to hypotension solely due to a relative reduction in blood volume (Roth, Lax and Maloney, 1969).

A further cause of postoperative hypotension is rapid bleeding. A normal individual uninfluenced by anaesthetic drugs would compensate by a tachycardia and peripheral vasoconstriction, but a patient in the recovery period with residual anaesthetic effects may be unable to compensate, and hypotension will occur.

Myocardial depression

Many anaesthetic drugs, e.g. halothane, cause myocardial depression, which decreases contractility, and this effect may persist into the recovery period, reducing the patient's ability to compensate for changes in blood volume.

If the heart has required positive inotropic drugs during anaesthesia, postoperative hypotension may occur when these are discontinued. There is a danger that with decreased contractility and a consequent poor cardiac output, myocardial hypoxia could occur which could lead to a further reduction in contractility and to arrhythmias. This effect would be increased in elderly patients with pre-existing myocardial and valvular disease.

Abnormal rhythms and rates

To maintain a cardiac output the heart needs to contract at an adequate rate, but allowing time to fill during diastole. In the immediate postoperative phase, when the atropine wears off, the effect of neostigmine, causing a bradycardia and possibly hypotension, may be revealed. Other causes of bradycardia in the immediate postoperative phase are: halothane, myxoedema, hypothermia, raised cerebrospinal fluid pressure and inadvertent pressure on the carotid sinus.

Tachycardia in the immediate postoperative phase is less common, and can also relate to residual effects of anaesthetic drugs, e.g. gallamine and trimetaphan. As would be expected, a tachycardia is seen in anxious patients and those with pyrexia due to infection. Certain endocrine abnormalities produce a tachycardia, particularly thyrotoxicosis if it is not adequately controlled. Adrenal insufficiency can also produce tachycardia. Arrhythmias seen for the first time in the recovery period are unusual and possibly indicate a new cardiac pathology. Frequently, their presence is suggested by a lowered blood pressure with an irregular pulse; full investigation, however, requires an electrocardiogram and relevant biochemical tests (Boba, 1978). In recovery, an innocuous arrhythmia may be converted to something more dangerous by hypoxia carbon dioxide accumulation and synergistic effects of residual anaesthetic drugs.

Delayed return to consciousness in the postoperative period

With the trend to run anaesthesia in lighter planes, patients are expected to wake up rapidly after surgery (Eltringham, Coates and Hudson, 1978) and failure to return to consciousness may be attributable to some of the problems outlined above. Further causes include the effects of micro-emboli, hypothermia and fluid shifts across cerebrovascular membranes.

Emboli may be released during surgery, particularly neurosurgery, and heart surgery where air is easily admitted. In neurosurgery, particularly posterior fossa work, air may be drawn into open cerebral veins, while in cardiopulmonary bypass, air may be admitted on cannulation, or even released from the bypass pump. Frequently micro-emboli will be trapped in the lungs, but persistent arteriovenous connections may allow emboli to reach the brain. This may produce a variety of clinical pictures from the patient who is slow to awake in the recovery period, to the patient with obvious neurological damage.

Fat micro-emboli, produced in association with bony injury or surgical manipulation, cause a diffuse form of cerebral damage. This may lead to postoperative coma, presenting in the recovery area as a patient who is slow in returning to consciousness. With embolization there is not only the danger to the brain, but also damage to the lung which may have trapped most of the emboli until now. As the lung traps more emboli, one could imagine that a further ventilation–perfusion inequality could occur, potentially leading to hypoxia.

In some forms of neurosurgery, the patient is deliberately cooled to allow occlusion of the brain's blood supply and reduce the damage to the brain during that occlusion. When the body is rewarmed, each area of the body warms at a different rate and the brain may lag behind, with consequent prolonged unconsciousness.

Prolonged unconsciousness may also occur when a patient's chronic fluid deficit is rapidly corrected. A similar situation is seen in diabetic ketoacidosis, where marked fluid and electrolyte shifts occur across cerebrovascular membranes. Prolonged unconsciousness can also occur in myxoedematous patients following surgery.

Post-anaesthesia nausea

The incidence of nausea varies considerably in published studies. A figure of 15.5% was suggested by Brindle and Soliman (1975) following a survey of 500 patients undergoing laparoscopic tubal diathermy. They noted that 20% of patients felt nauseated for 5 d after the anaesthetic. These observations, although on a very specific group of patients, are important because these patients are probably some of the fittest to receive anaesthesia.

Aromaa (1977) demonstrated that after varicose vein surgery the incidence of nausea was 9% and 30% at 30 and 180 min after anaesthesia. She also showed that nausea was less frequent after an alcuronium, N_2O, hyperventilation anaesthetic, in which the patient's $PaCO_2$ had been maintained in the range 20–25 mm Hg, than in a technique using halothane and spontaneous ventilation.

Winning, Brock-Utne and Downing (1977), in a study of the effects of droperidol and diphenidol, showed that an incidence of 28.6% could be expected and that droperidol significantly reduced the incidence of post-anaesthesia nausea.

A further relevant fact is the linkage between nausea and pain. Anderson and Krogh (1976) administered narcotic analgesics to nauseated recovering patients who were in pain, and discovered that in 80% of the cases the nausea subsided as the pain was relieved.

One problem with studies of nausea is that they tend to be retrospective and patients may forget or not notice the nausea in the 'haze' of the IRP. Many patients may not even be able to relate the nausea to the IRP.

Post-anaesthesia vomiting

The danger of vomiting in the immediate postoperative period is that during the IRP the patient will have laryngeal incompetence and be unable to protect his bronchial tree from foreign material.

It is difficult to obtain widely applicable figures for postoperative vomiting, as medical practices are so diverse. Furthermore, some studies have been retrospective and others have considered only very specific groups of patients (e.g. early discharge outpatients who are on the move quickly) and the results may have limited general relevance. There are also many ways in which a vomit can be defined (e.g. vomit in the mouth, vomit on the pillow, vomit must have an acid pH, etc.) and it is not clear in many studies, some quoted below, in which phases of recovery the vomiting was observed.

Aromaa (1977) reported an incidence of 2–20% after outpatient varicose vein surgery. Brindle and Soliman (1975), on the other hand, studying outpatient laparoscopic sterilizations, calculated an incidence of 8%. These figures should be contrasted with the wider range for female inpatients, where an incidence of 3–67% was reported by Riding (1960) in his investigation of the effects of different premedications. Winning, Brock-Utne and Downing (1977) reported an incidence of 24.3% for urological and gynaecological patients, and Gold (1969) reported an incidence of 29% in his series of gynaecological outpatients.

There are many reasons why a patient might vomit in the recovery period. The patient may react to disturbance of his airway by coughing, which may provoke vomiting. In addition, he will probably have some degree of abdominal distension from the diffusion of nitrous oxide in the gut lumen, and this will increase the risk of vomiting. Further factors are the movement of the patient, e.g. transfer to and from theatre trolleys, and any residual drugs that have an emetic effect (Riding, 1960).

Certain types of surgery are particularly associated with postoperative nausea and vomiting, particularly gynaecological surgery (Riding, 1960; Gold, 1969).

Post-anaesthetic shivering

In a period when the patient's oxygen balance may be precarious, shivering or excessive demand may lead to hypoxia (Bay, Nunn and Prys-Roberts, 1968). Postoperative shivering has been related to the use of halothane (Jones and McLaren, 1965) and also to the fact that the patient is just cold (Soliman and Gillies, 1972). Soliman and Gillies further commented that spasticity was a frequent response and that the incidence after a halothane anaesthetic could be as high as 52%, compared with 39% for a non-halothane group.

Pflug *et al.* (1978), in a study of the prevention of shivering by directly warming the patients, reported that 50% of his unwarmed controls shivered and that there was a marked difference in the incidence between men and women.

Postoperative excessive movement

Postoperative excessive movement (Smessaert, Schehr and Artusio, 1960) is probably mainly related to the patient being in pain or emotionally distressed. Eckenhoff, Kneale and Dripps (1961) suggested that operations with a high emotional component, e.g. 'breast biopsy possibly proceed to mastectomy', result in a higher incidence of excessive movement. The use of hyoscine, cyclopropane, ether and barbiturates increases the incidence of excessive movement in the immediate recovery period.

Postoperative pain

As would be expected, postoperative pain is a common feature of recovery work, but less relevant in the immediate recovery period when the residual anaesthetic drugs have an analgesic effect (Eltringham, Coates and Hudson, 1978).

Apart from the humanitarian aspects of pain relief, it is important that a patient has adequate analgesia because this directly affects his physiological state. A patient in pain may be difficult to manage, as he is excitable and restless. This may increase his oxygen consumption, leading to hypoxia.

Furthermore, pain may be a contributory factor in causing nausea and vomiting (Anderson and Krogh, 1976).

There is some argument that the presence of pain, which is a powerful stimulus, contributes to the patient's awakening, and under these circumstances the administration of an analgesic could be expected to make the patient go back to sleep. This, however, cannot be separated from the inevitable hypnotic effect of the analgesic.

Psychiatric aspects of recovery care

A patient coming to hospital always worries and the strange hospital environment only adds to this (Carruthers and Taggart, 1973). These reactions are important in the recovery period, because anxiety and stress directly affect the patient's physical state, e.g. an anxious patient with a high sympathetic tone releasing adrenaline may have a tachycardia with peripheral vasoconstriction which could be mistaken for, or be actually masking, hypovolaemia.

Preoperative preparation paves the way for a calm and quiet recovery. The patient should be told to expect bandages, dressings and catheters, so that these do not come as an unpleasant surprise in the recovery period (Kornfeld, 1969). During the recovery period the false assumption is frequently made that the patient is asleep because he has his eyes closed. In fact, he may be hearing all sounds going on around him and may recall derogatory comments and remarks relating to clinical matters (Lambrechts and Parkhouse, 1961; Levinson, 1965).

An important psychiatric consideration is the memory of the recovery area retained by the patient on departure. This is particularly relevant in children, who may resist further hospital treatment on the basis of the memories of their recovery period. Fortunately, postoperative amnesia is common (Lambrechts and Parkhouse, 1961).

References

ALDRETE, J. A. and KROULIK, D. (1970). A post anesthesia recovery score. *Anesthesia and Analgesia Current Researches,* **49,** 924–934

ANDERSON, R. and KROGH, K. (1976). Pain as a major cause of postoperative nausea. *Canadian Anaesthetists' Society Journal,* **23,** 366–369

AROMAA, U. (1977). Anaesthesia for short stay varicose vein surgery with special reference to recovery. *Acta Anaesthesiologica Scandinavica (Supplement),* **21,** 5–43

ASBURY, A. J. (1981). Measuring immediate recovery from general anaesthesia using a scoring system. *Canadian Anaesthetists' Society Journal,* **28,** 567–574

BARER, G. R., HOWARD, P. and MCCURRIE, J. R. (1967). The effect of carbon dioxide and changes in blood pH on the pulmonary vascular resistance in cats. *Clinical Science,* **32,** 361–375

BAY, J., NUNN, J. F. and PRYS-ROBERTS, C. (1968). Factors influencing arterial PO_2 during recovery from anaesthesia. *British Journal of Anaesthesia,* **40,** 398–406

BOBA, A. (1978). Significant effects on the blood pressure of an apparently trivial atrial dysrhythmia. *Anesthesiology,* **48,** 282–283

BODLANDER, F. M. S. (1975). Deaths associated with anaesthesia. *British Journal of Anaesthesia,* **47,** 36–40

BRANTHWAITE, M. A. (1973). Detection of neurological damage during open heart surgery. *Thorax,* **28,** 464–472

BRINDLE, G. F. and SOLIMAN, M. G. (1975). Anaesthetic complications in surgical outpatients. *Canadian Anaesthetists' Society Journal,* **22,** 613–619

CARIGNAN, G., KEERI-SZANTO, M. and LAVELLÉE, J. (1964). Post anaesthetic scoring system. *Anesthesiology,* **25,** 396–397

CARRUTHERS, M. and TAGGART, P. (1973). Vagotonicity of violence. Biochemical and cardiac responses to violent films and television programmes. *British Medical Journal,* **3,** 384–389

CLIFTON, B. S. and HOTTEN, W. I. T. (1963). Deaths associated with anaesthesia. *British Journal of Anaesthesia,* **35,** 250–259

DON, H. F., WAHBA, M., CUADRADO, L. and KELKAR, K. (1970). The effects of anesthesia and 100 per cent oxygen on the functional residual capacity of the lungs. *Anesthesiology,* **32,** 521–529

ECKENHOFF, J. E., KNEALE, D. H. and DRIPPS, R. D. (1961). The incidence and etiology of postanaesthetic excitement – a clinical survey. *Anesthesiology,* **22,** 667–673

EDWARDS, G., MORTON, H. J. V., PASK, E. A. and WYLIE, W. D. (1956). Deaths associated with anaesthesia. *Anaesthesia,* **11,** 194–220

ELTRINGHAM, R. J., COATES, M. B. and HUDSON, R. B. S. (1978). Observations on 10 000 patients in the immediate postoperative period. *Resuscitation,* **6,** 45–52

FIGUEROA, M. (1972). The post anaesthesia recovery score. A second look. *Southern Medical Journal,* **65,** 791–795

FINK, B. R. (1955). Diffusion anoxia. *Anesthesiology,* **16,** 511–519

GOLD, M. I. (1969). Post anaesthetic vomiting in the recovery room. *British Journal of Anaesthesia,* **41,** 143–149

GOLD, M. I. and HELRICH, M. (1965). Pulmonary compliance during anaesthesia. *Anesthesiology,* **26,** 281–288

HERBERT, M., HEALY, T. E. J., BOURKE, J. B., FLETCHER, I. R. and ROSE, J. M. (1983). Profile of recovery after general anaesthesia. *British Medical Journal,* **286,** 1539–1542

JONES, H. D. and MCLAREN, C. A. B. (1965). Postoperative shivering and hypoxaemia after halothane, nitrous oxide and oxygen anaesthesia. *British Journal of Anaesthesia,* **37,** 35–41

KORNFELD, D. S. (1969). Psychiatric aspects of patient care in the operating suite and special areas. *Anesthesiology,* **31,** 166–171

LAMBRECHTS, W. and PARKHOUSE, J. (1961). Post-operative amnesia. *British Journal of Anaesthesia,* **33,** 397–404

LAPPAS, D. G., POWELL, W. M. J. and DAGGETT, W. M. (1977). Cardiac dysfunction in the perioperative period. *Anesthesiology,* **47,** 117–137

LEVINSON, B. W. (1965). States of awareness during general anaesthesia. *British Journal of Anaesthesia,* **37,** 544–546

LLOYD, T. C. (1966). The influence of blood pH on hypoxic pulmonary vasoconstriction. *Journal of Applied Physiology,* **21,** 358–364

LUNN, J. N. and MUSHIN, W. W. (1982). Results all data. In *Mortality Associated with Anaesthesia.* London; Nuffield Provincial Hospitals Trust

MORTON, A. (1977). Post operative respiratory resistance. *Anaesthesia and Intensive Care,* **5,** 378–380

MORTON, A. and BAKER, A. B. (1978). Clinical review: post operative respiratory dysfunction. *Anaesthesia and Intensive Care,* **6,** 56–61

PFLUG, E. A., AASHEIM, G. M., FOSTER, C. and MARTIN, R. W. (1978). Prevention of post anaesthesia shivering. *Canadian Anaesthetists' Society Journal,* **25,** 43–49

RACKLOW, H., SALANITRE, E. and FRUMIN, M. J. (1961). Dilution of alveolar gases during nitrous oxide excretion in man. *Journal of Applied Physiology,* **16,** 723–728

REMMERS, J. E., DEGROOT, W. J., SAUERLAND, E. K. and ANCH, A. M. (1978). Pathogenesis of upper airway occlusion during sleep. *Journal of Applied Physiology,* **44,** 931–938

RIDING, J. E. (1960). Post operative vomiting. *Proceedings of the Royal Society of Medicine,* **53,** 671–675

ROBERTSON, G. S., MACGREGOR, D. M. and JONES, C. J. (1977). Evaluation of doxapram for arousal from general anaesthesia in outpatients. *British Journal of Anaesthesia,* **49,** 133–139

ROTH, E., LAX, L. C. and MALONEY, J. V. (1969). Ringers lactate solution and extracellular fluid volume in the surgical patient. A critical analysis. *Annals of Surgery,* **169,** 149–164

SEVERINGHAUS, J. W. and MITCHELL, R. A. (1952). 'Ondines Curse': failure of respiratory centre automaticity while awake. *Clinical Research,* **10,** 122–128

SMESSAERT, A., SCHEHR, C. A. and ARTUSIO, J. F. (1960). Observations in the immediate postanaesthesia period; II Mode of recovery. *British Journal of Anaesthesia,* **32,** 181–185

SOLIMAN, M. G. and GILLIES, D. M. M. (1972). Muscular hyperactivity after general anaesthesia. *Canadian Anaesthetists' Society Journal,* **19,** 529–535

STEPHENS, D. S. B. and BOALER, J. (1977). The nurse's role in immediate postoperative care. *British Medical Journal,* **1,** 1199–1202

STEWARD, D. J. (1975). A simplified scoring system for the postoperative recovery room. *Canadian Anaesthetists' Society Journal,* **22,** 111–113

STEWARD, D. J. and VOLGVESI, G. (1978). Stabilometry: a new tool for the measuring of recovery following general anaesthesia for outpatients. *Canadian Anaesthetists' Society Journal,* **25,** 4–6

THOMPSON, D. S. and EASON, C. N. (1970). Hypoxemia immediately after operation. *American Journal of Surgery,* **120,** 649–651

THORNTON, J. A. (1960). Physiological dead space. Changes during general anaesthesia. *Anaesthesia,* **15,** 381–393

WINNING, T. J., BROCK-UTNE, J. G. and DOWNING, J. W. (1977). Nausea and vomiting after anaesthesia and minor surgery. *Anesthesia and Analgesia Current Researches,* **56,** 674–677

WYLIE, W. D. (1975). 'There, but for the grace of God. . . .'. *Annals of the Royal College of Surgeons of England,* **56,** 171–180

Chapter 2

The case for patient-controlled analgesia

C. J. Hull

Introduction

The phenomenon of postoperative pain and the means by which it may be controlled or abolished now occupies a significant share of the surgical literature. Unfortunately, the incidence and severity of pain suffered by large numbers of patients has not diminished significantly. Keeri-Szanto and Heaman (1972) found that 20% of patients undergoing extensive surgery received inadequate analgesia, while 23% of cholecystectomy patients (Nayman, 1979) suffered severe postoperative pain. In another well-known study, it was found that 56% of patients undergoing upper abdominal surgery categorized their pain as 'very unpleasant indeed; I would be most upset if I had to go through that again' (Cronin, Redfern and Utting, 1973).

To a great extent this unchanging pattern is due to a sharp divergence in knowledge, experience and attitudes between those who have campaigned for higher standards and those who are responsible for pain management at bedside level. Too often, the control of severe pain is delegated to the most junior and inexperienced member of the surgical team, whose grasp of practical therapeutics and appreciation of the range of techniques available is incomplete. Moreover, he is likely to be influenced by long-standing ward 'routines' and popular perceptions of drug characteristics. Despite undergraduate teaching to the contrary, he is led to believe that while opioids should be given when required, at least 4 h should elapse between doses of morphine.

The actual timing of analgesic doses is often left to the discretion of nursing staff, and therefore subject to displacement by the rituals of ward routine, calls to the theatre suite, meal breaks, handover-reporting and the demands of other patients. The patient who can express his pain vocally is treated, while the pain of the patient who suffers in silence (either for fear of causing trouble or simply because he is physically incapable of calling for help) may be allowed to continue. The fallacy that liberal prescribing of opioids leads to tolerance, addiction and then abuse is still widely accepted, as is the belief that life-threatening respiratory depression follows any but the most niggardly dosage schedule.

It is no surprise that heavily ritualized prescribing of poorly understood drugs leads to the persistence of pain as a major problem. Complacency is a formidable obstacle to progress, and every clinician concerned with the management of patients in pain should reflect upon McInnes' bitter commentary on 'the nonchalant attitude of the medical profession towards quite unnecessary suffering' (McInnes, 1976).

Variation in response to parenterally administered opioids

Although Lasagna and Beecher (1954) claimed that the optimal intramuscular dose of morphine is 10 mg per 70 kg body weight, close adherence to this schedule will yield a significant proportion of patients who are either over- or under-dosed. This wide variation in response is due to a number of factors.

Variation in both muscle-depot pH and perfusion will influence the rate of absorption, and bioavailability may be less than 100%. Evans *et al.* (1975) showed that blood flow in the vastus lateralis muscle varied with a coefficient of 25% in healthy volunteers. Furthermore, these authors pointed out that in several experiments the washout of Xe-133 was very slow indeed, and they attributed this to extramuscular injection (presumably into fat, despite a high degree of care). It is not unreasonable to speculate that postoperative patients might show even greater fluctuations in blood flow and perhaps a higher incidence of extramuscular injections! These observations were confirmed in a study by Rigg *et al.* (1978) of plasma morphine concentrations after intramuscular injection, in which the peak concentrations were found to range between 30 and 160 ng/ml after a dose of 0.15 mg/kg. Similarly, the time taken to reach peak concentration (C_{max}) varies between 4 and 60 min.

There is wide variation in the rate-processes governing the distribution of opioids, and also in the apparent volumes of distribution. The distribution volumes for most opioids are very large (more than 300 l in the case of morphine) and variation is poorly related to age, sex or body weight.

Eliminational processes are also subject to wide variation. Although the eliminational half-time for the decaying plasma concentration is often cited, clearance is the preferred index, since it expresses the efficiency of drug elimination (i.e. the rate of elimination per unit plasma concentration). Morphine clearance has been found to be fairly consistent in healthy subjects, but that of methadone in patients (ASA I–II) undergoing major surgery has been found to vary between 39 and 307 ml/min (Gourlay, Wilson and Glynn, 1982). Nilsson, Meresaar and Anggard (1982) found that methadone elimination is sensitive to variation in urinary pH, so that (as would be expected in the case of a basic drug) clearance is increased by some 40% when urinary pH is lowered by the oral administration of ammonium chloride. In some studies, the variation in opioid clearance has been shown to correlate with factors such as age and pre-existing disease (Chan *et al.*, 1975; Klotz *et al.*, 1975; Mather *et al.*, 1975).

Pharmacodynamic factors are also important. Austin, Stapleton and Mather (1980) showed that the minimum effective analgesic concentration in plasma (MEAC) for pethidine was consistent for individual subjects in the very short term, but differed widely between subjects. They commented that both perception and appreciation of pain are highly subjective phenomena and cannot readily be quantified by a simple pain : drug relationship. Gourlay, Wilson and Glynn (1982) confirmed that the analgesic effects of methadone were closely related to plasma concentration, and that patients with long-lasting analgesia were those with long eliminational half-times for this agent.

However, Rigg *et al.* (1978) could show no relationship between the plasma concentration of morphine and the intensity of respiratory depression. This may reflect a substantially greater equilibration time between plasma and the CNS sites of action for morphine as compared with pethidine or methadone. This is to be expected, since morphine is much less lipid-soluble; heptane : water partition coefficients for morphine, pethidine and methadone have been estimated as 0.000 01, 3.4 and 44.9, respectively (Von Cube *et al.*, 1970). In the case of buprenorphine, the rate of drug : receptor association and dissociation has been found to be slow (despite high affinity), so that poor correlation between plasma concentration and effect would be expected despite very high lipid solubility (Hambrook and Rance, 1976).

Boyle and Parbrook (1977) showed that pain severity in postoperative patients is related to personality factors, as assessed by the Eysenck personality inventory (Eysenck and Eysenck, 1969). In common with other authors (Austin, Stapleton and Mather, 1980; Gourlay, Wilson and Glynn, 1982), they found a positive correlation between pain severity and the neuroticism (*N*) score.

Simpson and Parkhouse (1961) commented that 'There is no more certain way of reducing the pain threshold than by fear'. In many institutions the mixing of pre- and postoperative patients in a surgical ward does little to minimize anxiety, especially when the postoperative patients are seen to suffer unrelieved pain. In the minds of many patients awaiting surgery, fear of death or mutilation and fear of overwhelming postoperative pain compete for supremacy. However, in the early postoperative period pain becomes the major (if not sole) preoccupation, and the intensity of 'pain-present' intensifies the dread of 'pain-future'. Those who dispute this assertion have not undergone cholecystectomy!

The surgical site has great influence upon the severity of pain, with upper abdominal procedures resulting in mugh higher needs for opioid analgesia than lower abdominal or superficial operations (Loan and Morrison, 1967). It is also widely held that the care and gentleness with which tissues are handled during operation has an influence on the severity of postoperative pain.

A pharmacokinetic approach to dosing strategy

Given some assumptions based upon the above discussion, it is now possible to formulate a general strategy: *For any level of pain suffered by an individual patient, there is a corresponding minimal effective plasma concentration of any high efficacy, lipid-soluble opioid having rapid receptor kinetics. Drugs in this category include: pethidine, methadone, phenoperidine, fentanyl and alfentanil. Accordingly, an effective regimen will rapidly attain and then maintain that concentration, without reaching levels associated with unacceptable respiratory depression.*

Now the problem has resolved to that of first achieving and then sustaining the 'target concentration' (symbolized as C^{ss}). This is not quite as simple as it may seem, since variation in pain 'input' may necessitate revision of the target itself. If we could assume that following an

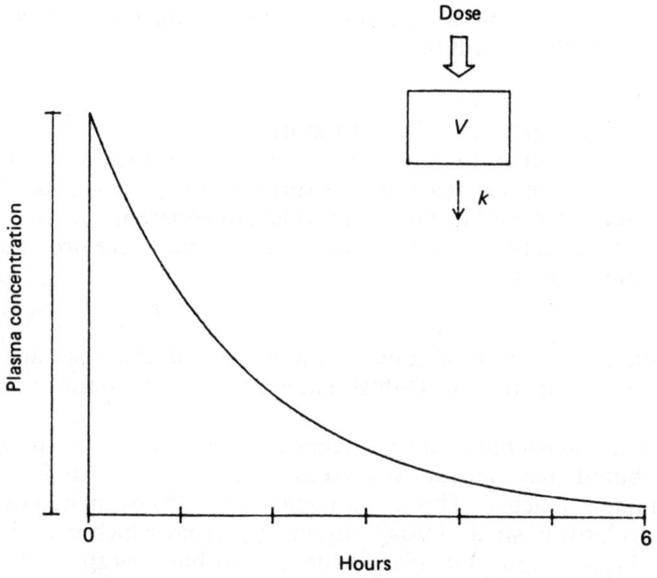

Figure 2.1. The one-compartment 'open model' in diagrammatic form, and a typical concentration decay curve after a bolus dose

intravenous bolus dose the agent would be dispersed immediately and homogeneously throughout a distributional 'space', from which it would be eliminated by a first-order process, then disposition would follow that of a simple 'one-compartment' model (*Figure 2.1*). Here, the plasma concentration would decline exponentially according to

$$C = C^0 \cdot e^{-kt} \qquad (1)$$

where C^0 is the plasma concentration at time zero (i.e. immediately following injection); C is the concentration at any time t; e is the base of the natural logarithm (2.718...); and k is the rate constant. As in any simple exponential function, the rate constant expresses the proportion by which the variable C changes per unit time. Alternatively, this may be expressed in the time domain as the time taken for the variable to decline to half its present value. This is known as the half-time or half-life, and is a simple function of the rate constant:

$$T_{1/2} = 0.693/k \qquad (2)$$

The apparent volume of the model can be determined as the dilutional space for drug, and is calculated from the dose Xd and initial concentration C^0:

$$V = Xd/C^0 \qquad (3)$$

Now the model can be solved in terms of any desired strategy. Clearly, a single intravenous injection can produce but not sustain the target concentration, while a constant-rate infusion can sustain C^{ss}, but takes a long time to reach it (in practice, at least five half-times) and is equally unsatisfactory. The correct strategy is to combine the two.

By rearrangement of equation (3), the dose required to 'fill' the model to a concentration of exactly C^{ss} will be

$$Xd = C^{ss} \cdot V \tag{4}$$

The rate at which drug must be added to the model in order to exactly balance losses will be equal to the elimination rate at the specified concentration (C^{ss}). Since the clearance expresses the rate of drug elimination per unit concentration and is the product of apparent volume V and eliminational rate constant k, the rate of loss (and therefore the desired infusion rate (k') will be

$$k' = C^{ss} \cdot V \cdot k \tag{5}$$

Thus a very simple combination of bolus and infusion will both load and maintain the desired concentration. Unfortunately, no opioids conform to this model!

When a drug is administered as an intravenous bolus, the 'space' into which it is distributed may appear to increase with time until a final 'steady-state' volume is reached. This phenomenon is readily explained by the concept of a relatively small 'initial' volume V_1, from which drug is further distributed (more slowly) to a larger 'deep' distributional space V_2. Pharmacokinetic studies of fentanyl, alfentanil, pethidine and methadone have established 'two-compartment' dispositional profiles of this type in a majority of subjects (Mather *et al.*, 1975; Bower and Hull, 1982; Gourlay, Wilson and Glynn, 1982; Tamsen *et al.*, 1982a), but in some cases a more complex (three-compartment) model containing two 'deep' compartments may be needed to satisfy the data. Tamsen *et al.* (1982a) derived two-compartment models (*Figure 2.2*) from a series of postoperative patients receiving pethidine, and their data is taken as the basis for an 'average model' which will be used here for illustrative purposes.

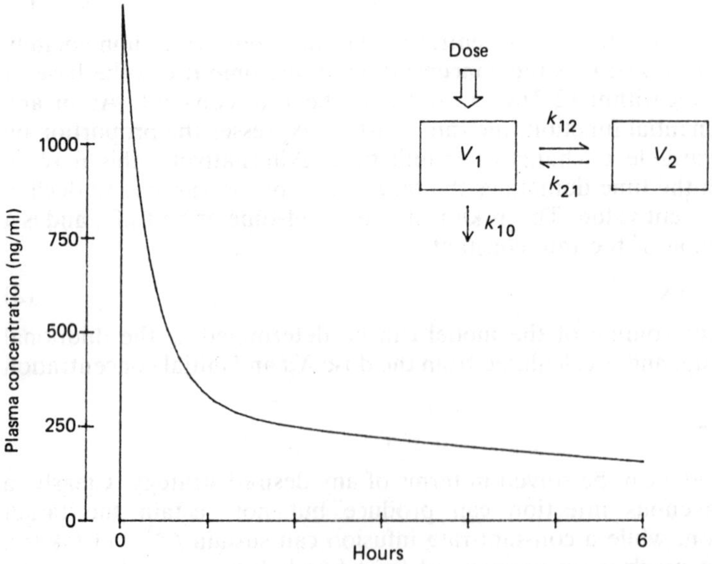

Figure 2.2. The two-compartment 'open model' diagram, with a concentration decay curve illustrating the model's response to a bolue dose

It must be emphasized that the kinetic model does not claim to predict the behaviour of any individual subject, since its parameters are drawn from a *sample* with considerable intrinsic variation.

Following a bolus dose, the plasma concentration in a two-compartment system declines in a more complex manner, with the expression for C amounting to the sum of two exponential terms:

$$C = A \cdot e^{-\alpha t} + B \cdot e^{-\beta t} \tag{6}$$

The exponents α and β are rate constants which characterize the fast and slow components of the decay function and do not directly correspond with any of the model constants. The constants A and B are each the product of a model-characteristic term and the initial concentration (X^0/V_1) (*see* Hull, 1979).

Here, devising a dosing scheme for constant concentration presents considerable difficulties, which will be summarized in an empirical manner in order to minimize mathematical complexity. As before, the maintenance infusion is easily determined since it simply balances drug elimination at the infusional equilibrium. As in the one-compartment system, the desired rate is C^{ss} × clearance, where clearance is now $k_{10} \times V_1$. Although the equation is not shown here, it should be remembered that if such an infusion were given alone (*Figure 2.3*), the approach to infusional equilibrium would be a complex function comprising the sum of the final concentration C^{ss} and two exponential terms.

The choice of a suitable bolus dose with which to load the model presents several options. If the bolus is calculated (Mitenko and Ogilvie, 1972) on the basis of the entire distributional volume, then the *initial* concentration will be much greater than desired, and may reach levels associated with major side effects. On the other hand, a dose which loads

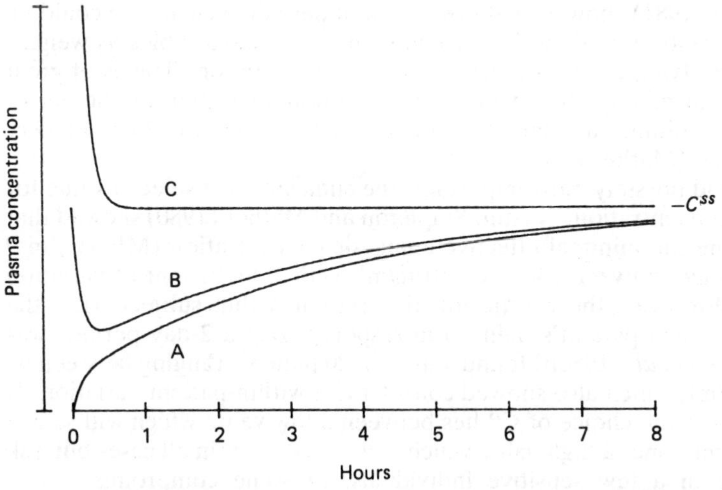

Figure 2.3. Dosing strategies for constant plasma concentration in a two-compartment system: A, infusion only; B, bolus calculated to load V_1, followed by the infusion; C, bolus calculated to load V_{ss}, followed by the infusion. The result of a compound infusion as defined in equation (7) is not illustrated, since the concentration rises to C^{ss} at t=0, and remains unchanged throughout (pethidine model)

only V_1 will result in a concentration which, although appropriate at the moment of injection, declines rapidly as a result of distribution to V_2, and only later climbs slowly to C^{ss}. This strategy, although avoiding excessive concentrations, may result in an appreciable period of unrelieved pain. A compromise approach, in which the bolus is based upon an intermediate volume, may reduce the degrees of 'overshoot' and 'dip', but one must always be traded off against the other.

To the theoretical pharmacokineticist, there is no real problem. To a bolus dose ($V_1 \times C^{ss}$) and a maintenance infusion ($C^{ss} \times k_{10}$) is added a second infusion, whose rate declines exponentially according to the rate at which drug is distributed from V_1 to V_2, and eventually diminishes to zero (Vaughan and Tucker, 1976). The compound infusion is calculated according to the following expression:

$$k'_{01} = C^{ss} \cdot V_1 \cdot k_{10} + X^0\,(\alpha - k_{21})\,(\beta - k_{21})^2 \cdot k_{21} \cdot e^{-k_{21}t} \tag{7}$$

However, the scheme presents several difficulties to the clinician. First, he must devise some means of administering the drug, since few infusion systems (except those under computer control) can follow such a complex programme.

Secondly, there is a low probability that the scheme would result in the desired plasma concentration profile. This is because the equations depend upon a high degree of system identification, and the considerable variation between subjects makes this difficult. In particular, the distributional parameters k_{12}, k_{21} have large coefficients of variation in most studies, and assumptions as to their values in an individual is likely to lead to large deviations from C^{ss} during the early phases of management. The problem is compounded by the fact that the pharmacokinetic profiles of many drugs are profoundly modified during and after surgery, and such changes for pethidine have been reported (Tamsen *et al.*, 1982a). Austin, Stapleton and Mather (1981) showed that prediction of pethidine clearance could be improved greatly by taking into account such simple variables as weight, standing and lying girth, and haemoglobin concentration. This is of great value in determining the maintenance infusion rate, but predictors of distribution volume are hard to find. Certainly, body weight is of very limited value (Mather *et al.*, 1975).

Lastly, and possibly most important, the clinician must select a value for the target concentration. Austin, Stapleton and Mather (1980) showed that for pethidine the minimal effective analgesic concentration (MEAC) in 9 patients varied between 240 and 760 ng/ml, with a coefficient of variation of 39%. Moreover, the coefficient of variation within subjects (i.e. the variation in each patient's pain : drug response over a 2-day period) was 31%. Tamsen *et al.* (1982b) found values in 20 patients ranging between 94 and 754 ng/ml, which also showed considerable within-patient variation. It is evident that the choice of C^{ss} lies between a low value which will satisfy few but harm none, a high value which will relieve pain in all cases but risk overdosage in a few sensitive individuals, or some compromise value between the two.

Clearly, the clinician needs more initial information than can be obtained from studies on patient groups, and must devise some means of tailoring the regimen to the changing needs of individual patients.

Clinical development of kinetic-based regimens

Church (1979) showed that a very simple bolus + infusion regime (using pethidine) could yield good results in approximately 80% of patients, if the clinician was prepared to adjust the infusion rate to suit the patient's needs in the first 48 h. In comparable groups of patients given i.m. and 'infusion' regimens, the incidences of unacceptable pain were 35% and 11% respectively. In the majority of cases, pain was least effectively relieved in the first few hours; this follows the prediction (*Figure 2.3*) that a 'bolus + infusion' regimen will suffer from low concentrations in the early infusional period.

Nayman (1979) devised a flexible regimen for morphine, in which a 3 mg bolus dose was followed by a 'nurse-adjusted' infusion. Here, even better results were obtained, with a nil incidence of unacceptable pain in the infused patients.

Stapleton, Austin and Mather (1979) developed a 3-segment infusion regimen based upon a previously derived pharmacokinetic model. Here, an initial infusion of 1 mg/min was given for 45 min, 0.53 mg/min for 28 min and then, finally, a maintenance rate of 0.4 mg/min. Despite greater sophistication, this regimen resulted in poor early analgesia in some 40% of patients. The authors concluded that their initial estimate of 200 ng/ml as the minimum effective concentration, based on the previous work of Shih, Robinson and Au (1976), was too low and that a target of 400 ng/ml would have yielded satisfactory results. It is also likely that such a 'model-dependent' approach would have yielded some non-conforming patients with unacceptably high or low concentrations. Their strategy could also be criticized on the choice of an initial infusion, in preference to a bolus. While it can be argued that the concentration profile following a short infusion is more predictable than that after a bolus, it must be conceded to be less satisfactory from the patient's point of view. An initial period of up to 30 min in unrelieved pain could hardly be considered the best start to an 'ideal' solution to postoperative pain!

At this point it might fairly be asked 'if intravenous regimens are so difficult to manage, what's so wrong with giving nice simple intramuscular injections?' The response is equally simple: putting drug into a 'depot' from which it is then absorbed does not simplify matters; it complicates them.

In compartmental model terms (*Figure 2.4*) we now have the same structure as before, but with the added complication of a drug depot and an uptake rate constant k_a. Now, the time course for plasma concentrations follows a three-term exponential equation:

$$C = A \cdot e^{-\alpha t} + B \cdot e^{-\beta t} + D \cdot e^{-k_a t} \quad (8)$$

where A, B and D are complex constants, derived from all the model parameters. Even this structure may be a gross oversimplification, since it assumes that uptake will be strictly first order (i.e. the rate of uptake is always proportional to the concentration gradient between depot and plasma). If the uptake constant were modified by the drug concentration, as might occur if the drug had an effect on muscle perfusion, then the assumption of first-order uptake might be considered unsafe. This caveat could well apply in the case of pethidine.

Figure 2.4 illustrates a second difficulty; not only is prediction of plasma concentration more hazardous, but there is a latent period between injection and the appearance of an effective plasma concentration. Rapid uptake will be associated with short latency and high peak values, while slow uptake will result in longer latency and lower (and delayed) peak concentrations.

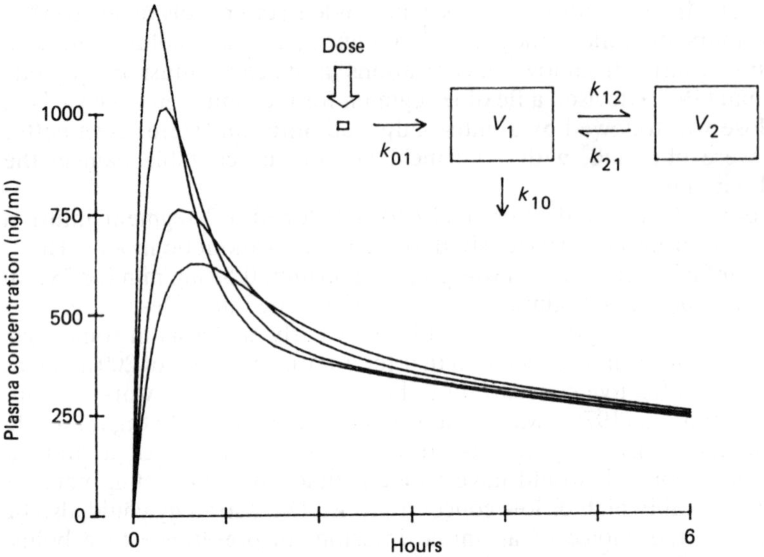

Figure 2.4. The two-compartment model developed to account for an elementally small i.m. injection depot. The simulated concentration curves predict the plasma concentrations following 150 mg i.m., with uptake half-times of 5, 10, 20 and 30 min (pethidine model)

The time taken for drug to diffuse to the site of action, the rate of association with receptors and uptake latency will summate to cause an inevitable delay between injection and the onset of effect. Clearly, this delay will be greatest in the case of a drug such as morphine, which, being poorly lipid soluble, would be expected to exhibit slow rates of both uptake and biophase diffusion. Studies in both dog and man have confirmed this expectation (Finck *et al.*, 1977; Rigg *et al.*, 1978; Stanski, Greenblatt and Lowenstein, 1978).

The general properties of i.m. regimens are illustrated by *Figure 2.5*. When given as a standard dose on a regular schedule (i.e. pethidine 100 mg 4-hourly), the initial dose is seen to have a short duration of useful effect because rapid distribution of drug to an 'empty' deep compartment causes the plasma concentration to fall quickly below the effective level.

Subsequent doses yield higher concentrations which persist longer at effective levels; thus, the patient is likely to suffer pain for much of the first inter-dose interval, but progressively less after successive doses. However, it is not difficult to see how the inexperienced nurse or clinician may conclude (on the basis of the first dose) that the drug is both ineffective and short-acting, and decide to increase the dose, with overdosage the likely outcome.

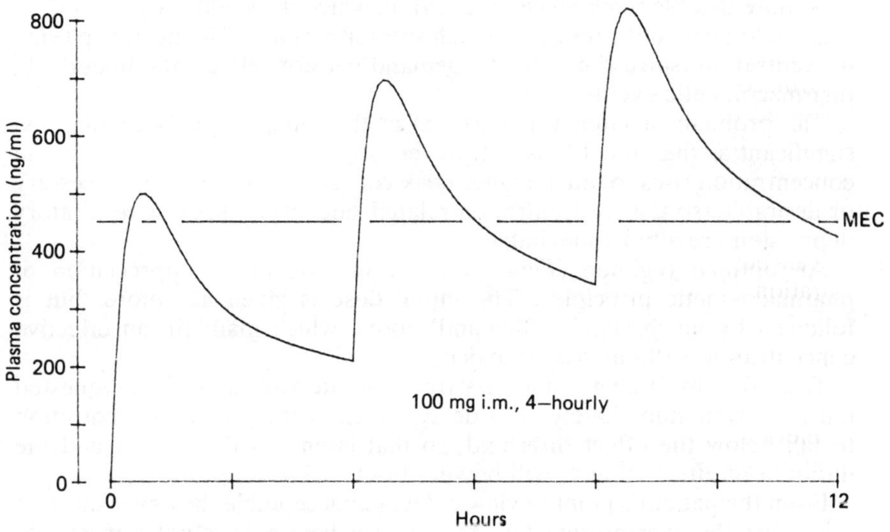

Figure 2.5. Predicted plasma concentrations following 100 mg i.m., 4-hourly (pethidine model)

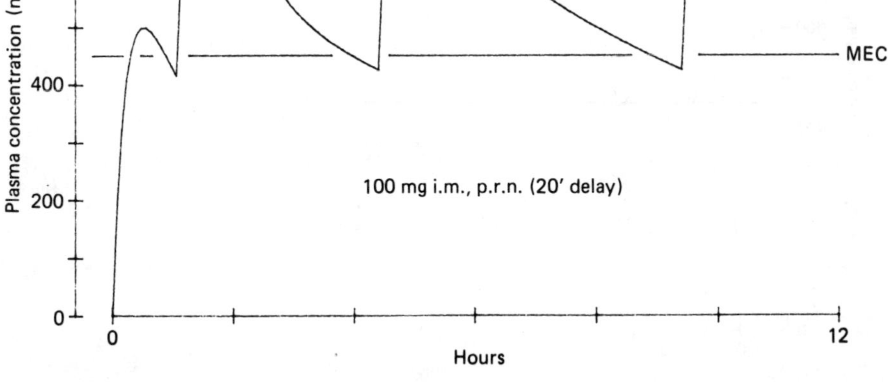

Figure 2.6. Predicted plasma concentrations following 100 mg i.m., given whenever the concentration falls below the effective level (pethidine model)

A more flexible regimen (*Figure 2.6*), in which the standard dose of drug is given 'on demand', results in much shorter periods of ineffective plasma concentration, since the patient's demand pattern reflects the underlying pharmacokinetic events.

The problem of latency is maximal at the initial dose, becoming less significant as the model 'fills'. However, after following doses the plasma concentration rises to much higher peak concentrations than are necessary or desirable, so that concentration-related side effects such as respiratory depression are almost inevitable.

An optimal regimen (*Figure 2.7*) makes use of an appreciation of pharmacokinetic principles. The initial dose is given as before, but is followed by much smaller 'demand' doses, which maintain an effective concentration without risk of toxicity.

True, they must be given at very frequent intervals, and when requested must be given immediately. Any delay will allow the plasma concentration to fall below the effect threshold, so that latency will reappear and the duration of effect (if any) will be very brief.

From the patient's point of view delay is unacceptable, however short. It reinforces the ever-present fear that his (or her) pain is not a matter of great concern to others and that the present discomfort will become intolerable agony before relief is given. If this fear is realized, then both confidence and rapport are likely to be destroyed and the postoperative period may become a nightmare for both patient and attendants alike. Of course, the converse is true; the patient whose pain is always relieved rapidly becomes progressively *less* anxious and *more* confident that pain is not a problem. It is tempting to speculate that psychological conditioning of the classical type may play an active role, with rapid pain relief and unrelieved pain acting as positive and negative conditioning factors.

If decreasing the interval between intramuscular doses is a logical step toward continuous, safe analgesia, then it is logical to propose that very

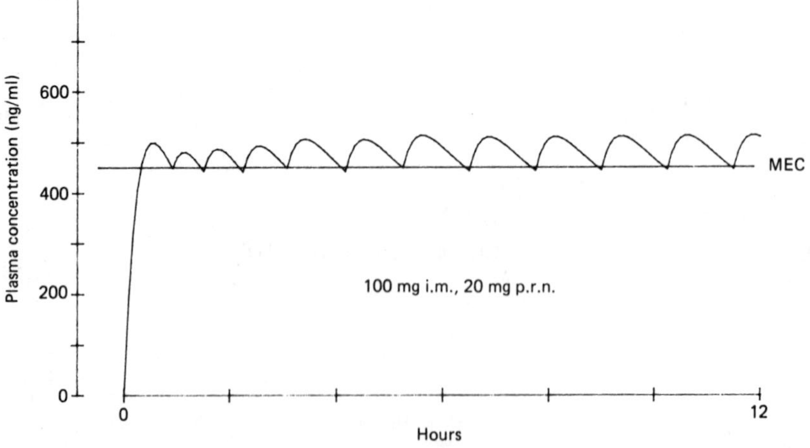

Figure 2.7. Predicted plasma concentrations following 100 mg i.m., followed by 20 mg i.m. given whenever the concentration falls below the effective level (pethidine model)

small doses given intravenously 'on demand' would be even better (*Figure 2.8*). In this case the principle of titration, by which the rate of drug administration is always appropriate to the patient's needs, becomes a practical proposition. Uptake latency is eliminated altogether and the patient need never be kept waiting for analgesia. Far from being a potential hazard, the 'spikes' in plasma concentration following each dose will ensure a transiently high plasma–biophase concentration gradient, thus promoting the rapid onset of analgesia.

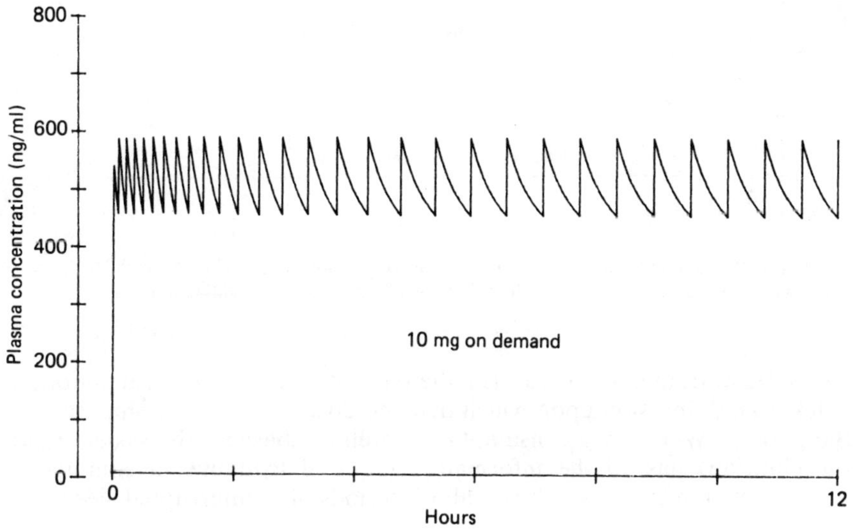

Figure 2.8. Predicted plasma concentrations following 10 mg i.v., given whenever the concentration falls below the effective level (pethidine model)

It can be argued that if the duration of each 'demand dose' is short, then each time the patient falls asleep he will awake in pain a few minutes later. In the case of a crude system, this objection holds true, but can be overcome by the simple expedient of giving an intramuscular dose to cover the sleep period.

A more sophisticated approach might be based upon the following principle: *Each patient needs an optimal plasma concentration, which will fluctuate with changing circumstances such as physiotherapy, movement, sleep, etc. The analgesia delivery system should take account of patient-opinion, then deliver the correct regimen.*

Figure 2.9 shows that, by adding a simultaneous infusion, the number of demands may be reduced, with a more gradual decline in plasma concentration after each bolus. Of course, an inappropriately rapid infusion will result in a steady-state concentration above the effective level, with cessation of demand dosing and risk of overdosage. In practice, the infusion should be based upon the patient's recent requirements. The Newcastle system (Hull, Sibbald and Johnson, 1979; Hull and Sibbald, 1981) *appears* to behave like a simple on-demand system, but in fact

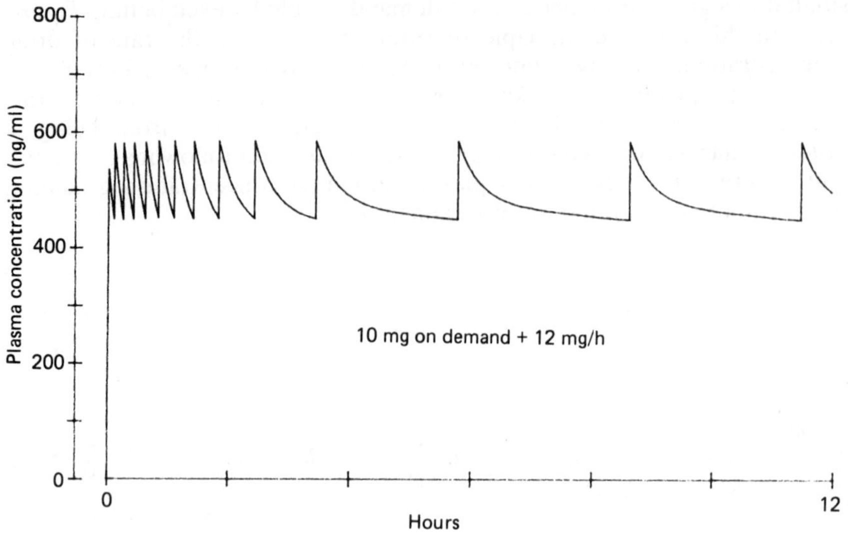

Figure 2.9. Predicted plasma concentrations following an infusion of 12 mg/h, with 10 mg i.v. given whenever the concentration falls below the effective level (pethidine model)

computes at frequent intervals (on the basis of recent drug consumption) a 'background' infusion upon which demand doses can be superimposed by the patient. When drug consumption is well established, the system (and the clinician) has all the information required to deliver a continuous programmed infusion which will allow periods of uninterrupted sleep.

The clinical experience

While patient-feedback devices may appear to have important theoretical advantages over 'open-loop' regimens, they have no clinical role to play until proven to be safe, effective and practical in the busy surgical environment.

Sechzer (1968, 1971) showed that a very simple device could achieve high grade analgesia, without any evidence that, given the opportunity, patients would dose themselves into oblivion. Indeed, Keeri-Szanto and Heaman (1972) recorded wide variation in patient demand rates, so that while some did consume more pethidine than those given an 'i.m.' regimen, some others needed significantly less. While only 5% of 'demand' patients complained of pain during the early postoperative period, 40% of patients given routine i.m. analgesia complained of incomplete pain control. These authors emphasized the importance of *appropriate* dosage, and showed that as much as 25% of i.m. administered drug is 'wasted' [*sic*] by producing greater peak concentrations than those actually required.

As has been reported by subsequent studies, 30% of 'demand' patients complained of increased discomfort when returned to an i.m. regimen at the end of the study period. These results contrast sharply with those of

Ellis *et al.* (1982), in which it was shown that when i.m. morphine is given in adequate dosage (68 mg in 48 h), the treatment groups can be difficult to separate. However, it is only fair to comment that Keeri-Szanto's 'IM regimen' patients were simply a sample of routinely managed cases receiving a variety of agents, with no stated criteria for dosage or timing, so that the two studies cannot be regarded as comparable.

While patients differ greatly, each individual tends to consume drug at a consistent rate (Sechzer, 1971; Hull and Sibbald, 1981; Tamsen *et al.*, 1982c), suggesting that several hours of patient-control may provide sufficient information to specify the required delivery rate during 'patient-asleep' periods.

In contrast to the conclusions of the Australian group (Austin, Stapleton and Mather, 1980), both Chakravarty *et al.* (1979) and Tamsen *et al.* (1982c) found that individual pethidine requirements could not be predicted from data such as the patient's age, sex or body weight. In a series of 56 cases, Tamsen *et al.* (1982c) found a high incidence (92%) of patient-acceptance, with no evidence of overt respiratory depression in most patients. The principal reported side effect was drowsiness, which occurred in 68% of patients. However, they did identify two patients who became hypercapnoeic, and one who was too confused to understand what was required of him. A similar case was reported by Hull and Sibbald (1981).

From measurements of plasma concentration during patient-controlled analgesia, Tamsen *et al.* (1982b) were able to estimate the minimum effective concentration for pethidine to be 455 ± 174 ng/ml, and confirmed their conclusion (from drug consumption alone) that age, sex and weight were of no predictive value.

A number of opioids have been evaluated for their suitability. Pethidine has been successfully used by a number of investigators (i.e. Sechzer, 1971; Keeri-Szanto and Heaman, 1972; Chakravarty *et al.*, 1979; Tamsen *et al.*, 1979, 1982c; Ellis *et al.*, 1982). It is of interest that patients consume pethidine at an average rate of approximately 25 mg/h, which is very close to the maintenance rate calculated by Stapleton, Austin and Mather (1979).

Fentanyl and alfentanil, having rapid onset and offset of effect, would seem to have ideal pharmacological profiles (Hull, Sibbald and Johnson, 1979; White, Pearce and Norman, 1979; Kay, 1981), but would be expected to give unsatisfactory results unless delivered by a sophisticated system capable of simultaneous 'background infusion'.

To the reviewer, morphine would not seem well suited to a rapid-response environment. However, in a recent paper with the modest title 'Patient-controlled analgesia. A new concept of postoperative pain relief', Bennett *et al.* (1982) showed that patient-controlled analgesia using this agent yielded superior analgesia to that following routine i.m. administration. Dahlstrom *et al.* (1982) also found morphine to be a satisfactory agent, with a mean consumption rate of 2.6 mg/h. These authors reported one patient who became hypercapnoeic when hypovolaemic, but did not require corrective measures.

Buprenorphine, having slow onset and a longer duration of action than morphine, would appear even less attractive. Although several studies have shown that good analgesia can be achieved, Gibbs, Johnson and Davis (1982) reported two cases of severe respiratory depression and warned of the possible hazard with this agent. From a purely theoretical standpoint, overdosage is likely to be a problem when analgesia does not rapidly follow each increment, and especially when (as a last resort) antagonists are not readily available.

The use of pentazocine (Harmer *et al.*, 1983) and meptazinol (Slattery *et al.*, 1981) have been reported. In view of the incidence of psychotomimetic side effects (Wood *et al.*, 1974), the former would seem best avoided. Meptazinol was found to be associated with a higher incidence of nausea, and one patient (out of 109) could not achieve satisfactory analgesia at a demand rate of 181 mg/h!

Conclusions

Patient-controlled analgesia is a powerful tool for the control of severe pain. Although it is highly effective in many cases, it must be accepted that some patients are not suitable and alternative strategies must be considered.

Throughout the literature runs an undercurrent of concern regarding patient safety, and this has been the principal reservation put forward by surgical colleagues whose patients have been studied by the reviewer. So far as a simple electromechanical device comprising motors, timers, switches, etc., is concerned, the safety factor will always be governed by the probability of failure of any one component, and the likelihood of this resulting in 'give drug' or 'stop' fail modes. Accordingly, the 'Cardiff' system (Evans *et al.*, 1976) was designed so that the dose of drug in the syringe *at any time* could be regarded as safe if given (in error) as a bolus. Of course, this does mean that syringe reloading becomes a logistic problem, and later devices have sought to achieve a true 'fail-safe' design philosophy, which would permit the drug reservoir to contain more than the 'safe-as-a-bolus' quantity.

Fail-safe operation can be achieved using micro-processor technology. In essence, the processor delivers drug by sending correctly timed and phased pulses directly to a stepping drive-motor, only sending the next pulse when the motor is observed to have responded appropriately to that before, and if all of a large number of 'device status' checks have been completed satisfactorily. Thus, there is no final common signal pathway by which a 'fail active' state could continue to deliver drug. This approach permits many checks and counter-checks against malfunction, and may be expected to yield devices which *never* fail in an active state.

Whether patient-controlled administration achieves wide popularity remains to be seen, but the recent availability of several sophisticated delivery systems designed according to the above philosophy has made large-scale evaluation possible. It is possible that the method will also find favour in other areas, such as the management of intractable or terminal pain, and those who have been concerned with technical development programmes and early clinical studies await the outcome with interest.

References

AUSTIN, K. L., STAPLETON, J. V. and MATHER, L. E. (1980). Relationship between blood meperidine concentrations and analgesic response. *Anesthesiology,* **53,** 460–466

AUSTIN, K. L., STAPLETON, J. V. and MATHER, L. E. (1981). Pethidine clearance during continuous intravenous infusions in postoperative patients. *British Journal of Clinical Pharmacology,* **1,** 25–30

BENNETT, R. L., BATENHORST, R. L., BIVINS, B. A., BELL, R. M., GRAVES, D. A., FOSTER, T. S., WRIGHT, B. D. and GRIFFEN, W. O. (1982). Patient-controlled analgesia. A new concept of postoperative pain relief. *Annals of Surgery,* **195,** 700–704

BOWER, S. and HULL, C. J. (1982). The comparative pharmacokinetics of fentanyl and alfentanil. *British Journal of Anaesthesia,* **54,** 871–877

BOYLE, P. and PARBROOK, G. D. (1977). The interrelation of personality and postoperative factors. *British Journal of Anaesthesia,* **49,** 259–263

CHAKRAVARTY, K., TUCKER, W., ROSEN, M. and VICKERS, M. D. (1979). Comparison of buprenorphine and pethidine given on-demand to relieve postoperative pain. *British Medical Journal,* **2,** 895–897

CHAN, K., KENDALL, M. J., MITCHARD, M., WELLS, W. D. E. and VICKERS, M. D. (1975). The effect of ageing on plasma pethidine concentration. *British Journal of Clinical Pharmacology,* **2,** 297–302

CHURCH, J. J. (1979). Continuous narcotic infusions for relief of postoperative pain. *British Medical Journal,* **1,** 977–979

CRONIN, M., REDFERN, P. A. and UTTING, J. E. (1973). Psychometry and postoperative complaints in surgical patients. *British Journal of Anaesthesia,* **45,** 879–886

DAHLSTROM, B., TAMSEN, A., PAALZOW, L. and HARTVIG, P. (1982). Patient-controlled analgesic therapy, part IV: Pharmacokinetics and plasma concentrations of morphine. *Clinical Pharmacokinetics,* **7,** 266–279

ELLIS, R., HAINES, D., SHAH, R., COTTON, R. and SMITH, G. (1982). Pain relief after abdominal surgery – a comparison of I.M. morphine, sublingual buprenorphine and self-administered I.V. pethidine. *British Journal of Anaesthesia,* **54,** 421–428

EVANS, E. F., PROCTOR, J. D., FRATKIN, M. J., VELANDIA, J. and WASSERMAN, A. J. (1975). Blood flow in muscle groups and drug absorption. *Clinical Pharmacology and Therapeutics,* **17,** 44–47

EVANS, J. M., ROSEN, M., MACCARTHY, J. and HOGG, M. I. J. (1976). Apparatus for patient-controlled administration of intravenous narcotics during labour. *Lancet,* **i,** 17–18

EYSENCK, S. G. B. and EYSENCK, H. J. (1969). Scores on three personality variables as a function of age, sex and social class. *British Journal of Social and Clinical Psychology,* **8,** 69–76

FINCK, A. D., BERKOWITZ, B. A., HEMPSTEAD, J. and NGAI, S. H. (1977). Effects of hypercarbia on serum and brain morphine concentrations in the dog. *Anesthesiology,* **47,** 407–410

GIBBS, J. M., JOHNSON, H. D. and DAVIS, F. M. (1982). Patient administration of i.v. buprenorphine for postoperative pain relief using the 'Cardiff' demand analgesia apparatus. *British Journal of Anaesthesia,* **54,** 279–284

GOURLAY, G. K., WILSON, P. R. and GLYNN, C. J. (1982). Pharmacodynamics and pharmacokinetics of methadone during the perioperative period. *Anesthesiology,* **57,** 458–467

HAMBROOK, J. M. and RANCE, M. J. (1976). The interaction of buprenorphine with the opiate receptor. In *Opiates and Endogenous Opioid Peptides* (Kosterlitz, H. W., Ed.), pp. 295–301. Amsterdam; Elsevier/North-Holland

HARMER, M., SLATTERY, P. J., ROSEN, M. and VICKERS, M. D. (1983). Comparison between buprenorphine and pentazocine given IV on demand in the control of postoperative pain. *British Journal of Anaesthesia,* **55,** 21–24

HULL, C. J. (1979). Pharmacokinetics and pharmacodynamics. *British Journal of Anaesthesia,* **51,** 579–594

HULL, C. J. and SIBBALD, A. (1981). Control of postoperative pain by interactive demand analgesia. *British Journal of Anaesthesia,* **53,** 385–391

HULL, C. J., SIBBALD, A. and JOHNSON, M. K. (1979). Control of postoperative pain by demand analgesia. *British Journal of Anaesthesia,* **51,** 570P

KAY, B. (1981). Postoperative pain relief. Use of an on-demand analgesia computer (ODAC) and a comparison of the rate of use of fentanyl and alfentanil. *Anaesthesia,* **36,** 949–951

KEERI-SZANTO, M. and HEAMAN, S. (1972). Postoperative demand analgesia. *Surgery, Gynecology and Obstetrics,* **134,** 647–651

KLOTZ, U., MCHORSE, T. S., WILKINSON, G. R. and SCHENKER, S. (1975). The effect of cirrhosis on the disposition and elimination of meperidine in man. *Clinical Pharmacology and Therapeutics,* **16,** 667–675

LASAGNA, L. and BEECHER, H. K. (1954). The optimal dose of morphine. *Journal of the American Medical Association,* **156,** 220

LOAN, W. B. and MORRISON, J. D. (1967). The incidence and severity of post-operative pain. *British Journal of Anaesthesia,* **39,** 695–698

MATHER, L. E., TUCKER, G. T., PFLUG, A. E., LINDOP, M. J. and WILKERSON, C. (1975). Meperidine kinetics in man. Intravenous injection in surgical patients and volunteers. *Clinical Pharmacology and Therapeutics,* **17,** 21–30

MCINNES, C. (1976). Cancer ward. *New Society,* **36,** 232

MITENKO, P. A. and OGILVIE, R. I. (1972). Rapidly achieved plasma concentration plateaus with observations on theophylline kinetics. *Clinical Pharmacology and Therapeutics,* **13,** 329–335

NAYMAN, J. (1979). Measurement and control of postoperative pain. *Annals of the Royal College of Surgeons of England,* **61,** 419–426

NILSSON, M. I., MERESAAR, U. and ANGGARD, E. (1982). Clinical pharmacokinetics of methadone. *Acta Anaesthesiologica Scandinavica,* suppl. 74, 66–69

RIGG, J. R. A., BROWNE, R. A., DAVIS, C., KHALDELWAL, J. K. and GOLDSMITH, C. H. (1978). Variation in the disposition of morphine after I.M. administration in surgical patients. *British Journal of Anaesthesia,* **50,** 1125–1130

SECHZER, P. H. (1968). Objective measurement of pain. *Anesthesiology,* **29,** 209–210

SECHZER, P. H. (1971). Studies in pain with the analgesic-demand system. *Anesthesia and Analgesia,* **50,** 1–10

SHIH, A. P. L., ROBINSON, K. and AU, W. Y. W. (1976). Determination of therapeutic serum concentrations of oral and parenteral meperidine by liquid chromatography. *European Journal of Clinical Pharmacology,* **9,** 451–456

SIMPSON, B. R. J. and PARKHOUSE, J. (1961). The problem of postoperative pain. *British Journal of Anaesthesia,* **33,** 336–344

SLATTERY, P. J., HARMER, M., ROSEN, M. and VICKERS, M. D. (1981). Comparison of meptazinol and pethidine given IV on demand in the management of postoperative pain. *British Journal of Anaesthesia,* **53,** 927–930

STANSKI, D. R., GREENBLATT, D. J. and LOWENSTEIN, E. (1978). Kinetics of intravenous and intramuscular morphine. *Clinical Pharmacology and Therapeutics,* **24,** 52–59

STAPLETON, J. V., AUSTIN, K. L. and MATHER, L. E. (1979). A pharmacokinetic approach to postoperative pain: continuous infusion of pethidine. *Anaesthesia and Intensive Care,* **7,** 25–32

TAMSEN, A., HARTVIG, P., DAHLSTROM, B., LINDSTROM, B. and HOLMDAHL, M. H. (1979). Patient-controlled analgesic therapy in the early postoperative period. *Acta Anaesthesiologica Scandinavica,* **23,** 462–470

TAMSEN, A., HARTVIG, P., FAGERLUND, C. and DAHLSTROM, B. (1982a). Patient-controlled analgesic therapy. Part I: Pharmacokinetics of pethidine in the per- and postoperative periods. *Clinical Pharmacokinetics,* **7,** 149–163

TAMSEN, A., HARTVIG, P., FAGERLUND, C. and DAHLSTROM, B. (1982b). Patient controlled analgesic therapy. Part II: Individual analgesic demand and analgesic plasma concentrations of pethidine in postoperative pain. *Clinical Pharmacokinetics,* **7,** 164–175

TAMSEN, A., HARTVIG, P., FAGERLUND, C., DAHLSTROM, B. and BONDESSON, U. (1982c). Patient controlled analgesic therapy: clinical experience. *Acta Anaesthesiologica Scandinavica,* suppl. 74, 157–160

VAUGHAN, D. P. and TUCKER, G. T. (1976). General derivation of the ideal intravenous drug input required to achieve and maintain a constant plasma drug concentration. Theoretical application to lignocaine therapy. *European Journal of Clinical Pharmacology,* **10,** 433–440

VON CUBE, B., TESCHEMACHER, HJ., HERZ, A. and HESS, R. (1970). Permeation of morphine-like acting substances to their sites of anti-nociceptive action in the brain after intravenous and intraventricular application and dependence upon lipid-solubility. *Naunyn-Schmiedebergs Arch. Pharmak.,* **265,** 455–473

WHITE, W. D., PEARCE, D. J. and NORMAN, J. (1979). Postoperative analgesia: a comparison of intravenous on-demand fentanyl with epidural bupivacaine. *British Medical Journal,* **2,** 166–167

WOOD, A. J. J., MOIR, D. C., CAMPBELL, C., DAVIDSON, J. F., GALLON, S. C., HENNEY, E. and MCALLION, S. (1974). Medicines evaluation and monitoring group: central nervous system effects of pentazocine. *British Medical Journal,* **1,** 305–307

Chapter 3

Newer analgesics in the control of postoperative pain

J. E. Charlton

Introduction

A review article on postoperative analgesia published in 1979 quoted no less than seven editorials and 12 articles citing the inadequacy of postoperative pain control. Several of the articles were personal descriptions of the pain encountered after surgery and a recurrent theme was one of shock and disbelief that the pain could be so severe and yet so inadequately relieved (Utting and Smith, 1979).

Postoperative pain is probably one of the most common forms of acute pain requiring alleviation. Figures from the USA and Finland suggest that about 1 in every 15 people will undergo surgery each year and thus are likely to have postoperative pain (Bunker, 1976; Tammisto and Tigerstedt, 1982). Narcotic analgesics are the commonest method of achieving pain relief, but the need for these agents depends upon numerous factors and may vary greatly. Racial, cultural, educational and environmental factors may all influence the report of pain and, furthermore, there are wide individual differences (Merskey, 1978).

As well as the above factors, the site of surgical incision, type of operation and anaesthetic technique will be the main determinants of postoperative pain. Thoracotomies, upper abdominal operations and nephrectomies are painful operations, while superficial operations are usually less painful. The maximum intensity of the pain tends to be immediately after the operation has been completed and diminishes with time. For adequate relief of postoperative pain, all these factors must be taken into account when analgesic regimens and agents are selected.

Figures quoted by Tammisto and Tigerstedt (1982) suggest that 48% of patients will have severe pain, and 50% moderate pain after upper abdominal surgery. After superficial surgery, 10% report severe pain and 50% moderate pain. However, not all of these will require narcotics, and there will be a very widespread individual variation among those who do. In many cases, pain relief is adequately achieved by the standard prescription of 'p.r.n.' narcotics, but for some patients this is totally inadequate. These patients may also face ingrained prejudice and ignorance about narcotics on the part of the nursing and medical professions. Two American studies illustrate this, and there is no reason to believe that matters are any different in any other part of the world. In a review of nursing practice in postoperative analgesia (Cohen, 1980), it was found that 75% of patients were in moderate or marked pain and that their pain was inadequately assessed; further, complete pain relief after surgery was not considered to be a major priority. Nurses were over-concerned with the possibility of addiction, choices of analgesics were irrational and knowledge of drugs was inadequate. Things were no better in a study by Marks and Sachar which revealed that many physicians underestimated the effective dose range, overestimated the duration of action and exaggerated the dangers of addiction for medical inpatients with acute pain treated with narcotics (Marks and Sachar, 1973).

When faced with failure of this magnitude, the response of the profession has frequently been to ignore the possibility that the pain-relieving agents we have are effective. Instead of finding the correct way to administer them, attention has been directed to the use of newer and, hopefully, more effective agents. The correct answer probably lies in a mixture of approaches. First, that the medical and nursing profession should be better educated as to the use of narcotic analgesics. Secondly, more effective methods of administration of existing agents should be sought such as 'on-demand' analgesia machines, sustained-release formulations, or delivery by another route such as intrathecally or epidurally. Finally, that new agents should be introduced which are suitable for postoperative pain relief and offer advantages over existing agents.

Newer analgesic agents

Since the discovery of the encephalins, increasingly complex endogenous opioid systems have been uncovered in the central nervous system (Hughes *et al.*, 1975). A review of the multiple opiate receptors and their actions will aid understanding of the actions of the newer analgesic agents – most of which have an effect at more than one receptor.

Opioid receptors

Martin and his colleagues were the first to ascribe differences in effects among the opiates to different receptor sites (Martin *et al.*, 1976). Three receptor types were suggested: mu (μ), kappa (κ) and sigma (σ). The μ-receptor, at which morphine was a typical agonist, mediated such effects as analgesia with dependence, bradycardia, miosis and hypothermia. Proposed μ-receptor agonists produced morphine-like tolerance and dependence and substituted for morphine in dependent animals. Ketocyclazocine and ethylketocyclazocine (ethyl ketazocine) were proposed as κ-agonists. These agents did not substitute for morphine in dependent animals and produced a physical dependence and withdrawal syndrome that was quite distinct from that produced by morphine and similar μ-agonists. The analgesic effects were produced without respiratory depression, but were accompanied by sedation. The proposed σ-receptor was associated with excitatory symptoms such as tachycardia, hypertonia, tachypnoea, mydriasis and mania. Subsequently, this receptor has been associated with the psychotomimetic actions of many opioid derivatives. A typical agonist at the σ-receptor was *N*-allyl norcyclazocine (SKF 10 047).

Since Martin's work at least two other receptors have been identified delta (δ) and epsilon (ε). It seems likely that the δ-receptor is responsible, at least in part, for respiratory depression and does not mediate analgesia. The ε-receptor is only found in the rat vas deferens and so far has proved of interest solely to rats and research scientists. Work by Pasternak has further subdivided the μ-receptor into those with high affinity (μ_1) and those with low affinity (μ_2). Under this classification, analgesia was associated with μ_1-receptors and not the low affinity μ_2- and δ-receptors (Pasternak, 1982).

Drugs acting at different receptors

By using highly selective agents working at the various receptors it is now possible to state more accurately the nature, distribution, function and clinical relevance of receptor subtypes. For the purposes of this chapter only the clinical application will be mentioned, but it should be emphasized that no definitive study has yet been published which has been designed to evaluate the receptor sensitivity of drugs in clinical use.

The μ-receptor

Drugs such as diamorphine, codeine and pethidine are clearly agonists at the μ-receptor by their pharmacology and their ability to substitute for morphine in dependent subjects. Fentanyl also shows μ selectivity. Of the mixed agonist–antagonist drugs currently available, only buprenorphine appears to have partial μ-agonist activity, as shown by its ability to partially suppress abstinence in the withdrawn morphine-dependent dog and to precipitate abstinence in non-withdrawn animals (Jasinski, Pevnick and Griffith, 1978; Heel *et al.*, 1979). There are human studies which support its role as a μ-partial agonist.

The κ-receptor

There are several κ-receptor agonists available – ethylketocyclazocine and bremazocine are examples – but few clinical data are available. However, many of the antagonist analgesics have κ-agonist properties. The antagonist analgesics can be divided into two subgroups: the partial agonists of the morphine type and the mixed agonist–antagonists which show agonist and antagonist action at different receptor subtypes. Nalorphine is the first example of this sort of drug and shows agonist activity at κ-receptors, together with antagonist action at μ sites. Agonist activity at κ-receptors appears to mediate analgesia associated with sedation and there is also a separate type of physical dependence which is not as severe as that associated with μ-agonists. κ-Agonists appear to be almost free of euphoric effect, which could be interpreted as an advantage or disadvantage depending upon clinical circumstances.

Examples of the mixed agonist–antagonist class are pentazocine, nalbuphine and butorphanol. They may show μ-antagonist properties and κ-agonist activity and all show analgesic activity (Houde, 1979).

Meptazinol is also an agonist–antagonist, but appears to have other modes of action that are as yet unclear. It is claimed that this class of analgesic shows a 'ceiling effect' with regard to the depression of respiration. These claims should be treated with suspicion until they can be investigated according to stricter protocols and with a less liberal interpretation of the results than has been the case so far. All these drugs produce far less in the way of psychotomimetic side effects than does nalorphine; this property is thought to be mediated through the σ-receptor and will be considered below. Finally, it is highly likely that the mixed agonist–antagonists will show a much lower potential for addiction than the pure μ-agonists.

The σ-receptor

It has been suggested that this receptor may mediate the psychotomimetic side effects seen with mixed agonist–antagonist drugs. It has even been postulated that there is a connection between the σ-receptor and a previously identified phencyclidine receptor (Quirion, Hammer and Herkenham, 1981).

Buprenorphine (Temgesic – Reckitt and Colman)

This drug is an oripavine derivative and has mixed agonist–antagonist activity. It is almost certainly unique in having partial agonist activity at the μ-receptor and in showing unusual receptor kinetics (Hambrook and Rance, 1976). The drug binds with the receptor most avidly and has a high bioavailability when administered intravenously, intramuscularly or sublingually (Brewster, Humphrey and McLeavy, 1981). This property has been ascribed to its high lipophilicity. Animal testing has shown buprenorphine to be a potent analgesic, with long duration and a low dependence liability.

Buprenorphine has been the subject of intensive clinical evaluation and initial studies confirmed its prolonged length of action (Kamel and Geddes, 1978; Kay, 1978). In a double-blind study comparing buprenorphine 0.3 mg and morphine 10 mg given intravenously, Kay found that those patients given buprenorphine had adequate postoperative pain relief for twice as long as those given morphine. Other studies (Downing, Leary and White, 1977; Kay, 1980) have shown this dosage of buprenorphine to be as effective as intramuscular morphine 10 mg and to last from 6 to 18 h. It has been claimed that even larger doses produce a dose-related increase in duration of analgesic action (Budd, 1981).

Other studies have investigated the use of sublingual buprenorphine. In a study of 20 patients, sublingual buprenorphine 0.4 mg was compared to intramuscular morphine 10 mg (Edge, Cooper and Morgan, 1979). Both drugs were effective, but buprenorphine had a slower onset and a longer duration of action. In other, largely anecdotal, studies sublingual buprenorphine 0.4 mg was shown to be as effective as intramuscular papaveretum 20 mg, to have a longer duration of action (Fry, 1979) and also, unsurprisingly, to be vastly superior to an inadequate dose of oral dihydrocodeine (Masson, 1981).

A series of studies from Oxford have tried to correlate the clinical effects and pharmacokinetics of buprenorphine (McQuay *et al.*, 1980; Bullingham *et al.*, 1981; Watson *et al.*, 1982). In the first of these studies, buprenorphine 0.3 mg was given intravenously during operation; 3 h postoperatively a further 0.3 mg was given intravenously or intramuscularly. Six hours after the first dose of buprenorphine, the patients were connected to an on-demand analgesia apparatus, enabling a continuous record to be made of analgesic requirements. There was no difference in the duration of analgesia for either intravenous or intramuscular group (median duration 480 min). They also found that there were smaller postoperative analgesic requirements when the second dose was given intramuscularly. Bullingham has suggested that the bioavailability of buprenorphine given by the intramuscular route is close to 100% (Bullingham *et al.*, 1980), and this finding alone would suggest no difference in effect between the intravenous and intramuscular routes of administration. Plasma concentration after a given period of time following the same dose given by these two routes shows no significant difference.

Very similar results were seen in another study where the second dose of buprenorphine was 0.4 mg sublingually (Bullingham *et al.*, 1981). Herewith lies one of the almost unique attributes of this drug, in that sublingual doses of potent analgesics avoid initial hepatic passage and are as convenient as the oral route for patients and nursing staff. In addition, the high first pass effect then acts as a safety factor should the drug be swallowed. A third study used the same protocol to measure the analgesic effect of a single intravenous dose of 0.3 mg or 0.6 mg of buprenorphine (Watson *et al.*, 1982). Their data suggest that analgesic duration was longer and that the requirement for further analgesia was less after the larger dose. However, the statistical methods used to arrive at their conclusions have been questioned (Hull, 1982).

Other studies using different designs have shown buprenorphine to be as effective as morphine when given intramuscularly (Cook *et al.*, 1982; Ouellette, 1982; Ellis *et al.*, 1982). In the latter study, the postoperative analgesia afforded by sublingual buprenorphine 0.4 mg given 6-hourly was compared with that of morphine 10 mg intramuscularly or pethidine intravenously via an on-demand patient-controlled machine – the Cardiff Palliator (Evans *et al.*, 1976). All afforded a similar degree of analgesia as measured with a visual analogue scale. This study also examined postoperative pulmonary function as an index of postoperative analgesia. It was found that the visual analogue pain scores exhibited the best correlation with peak expiratory flow rate and confirmed that the correlation with the forced expiratory volume in 1 second ($FEV_{1.0}$) was slightly better than that for the functional residual capacity (FRC) – expressed as a percentage of preoperative values.

This study showed the intramuscular and intravenous methods of delivery at their optimum and yet the authors felt that the analgesia provided by regular sublingual buprenorphine was just as good.

A further study of buprenorphine 0.4 mg given regularly every 8 h for postoperative pain has shown it to be efficacious (Bullingham *et al.*, 1984). Although the incidence of side effects was high, only 5 patients out of 74 were withdrawn from the trial for this reason. The authors even go so far as to suggest that since most side effects appeared in the early postoperative period, they are due to surgery and anaesthesia rather than the postoperative analgesic employed. A lot more work would need to be done to sustain this conclusion, but it must raise doubts about the value of single dose studies of any analgesic agent with regard to the incidence of side effects.

Patient-controlled on-demand analgesia has been advocated frequently as being the ideal way to provide postoperative analgesia. Harmer and colleagues have studied buprenorphine requirements for postoperative pain relief using an on-demand system (the Palliator) utilizing both intravenous (Harmer *et al.*, 1983a) and intramuscular routes (Harmer *et al.*, 1983b). In both studies buprenorphine provided adequate postoperative analgesia, and in the intramuscular study buprenorphine was felt to be significantly more effective than pethidine but not against the other drugs tested – morphine and meptazinol. In another study utilizing the Palliator (Gibbs, Johnson and Davis, 1982), the drug was delivered in 0.1 mg or 0.2 mg intravenous boluses and both dosage levels gave excellent postoperative analgesia in 47 out of 51 patients. However, 1 patient in each group had significant ventilatory depression which necessitated withdrawal from the trial and 4 elderly patients had difficulty in operating the demand apparatus.

The absence of a product licence for a particular method of delivery of any recently introduced agent seems to act as a positive incentive for its use. Accordingly, buprenorphine has been tried rectally, intrathecally and epidurally (Budd, 1983). In the case of buprenorphine this is not quite as dangerous as it may appear, as it has been suggested that the lipophilic opiates are less likely to cause respiratory depression and to have better tissue redistribution, thus resulting in smaller plasma and CNS levels. It is possible that buprenorphine may provide more reliable and rapid analgesia than a hydrophilic opiate like morphine because of better tissue penetration (Cahill *et al.*, 1983). The epidural administration of buprenorphine 0.6 mg in 10 ml of saline has been compared with morphine 2 mg in a similar volume of saline. Both gave good postoperative analgesia when used for up to 48 h. Side effects were minimal with both drugs and further studies are clearly indicated. At least one misuse of epidural buprenorphine has been reported (Christensen and Andersen, 1982).

Other possible effects of buprenorphine of more than passing interest are the report of reversal of the postoperative hyperglycaemia and associated hormonal changes in man by sublingual buprenorphine 0.4 mg. This is suggested to indicate that at least some aspects of the stress response are suppressed (Moore, McQuay and Bullingham, 1980). Another report suggests a possible antidepressant activity, possibly due to activation of central opiate receptors (Emrich *et al.*, 1982).

Effects upon the central nervous system are similar to those seen with other opiates. The most commonly observed effects are those of drowsiness and sedation. In some reports this has been reported in 75% (Kay, 1978; Ouellette, 1982) or more (Robertson and Laing, 1980) of the patients studied, while others have made no mention of it at all. The Oxford group noted less sedation with sublingual, as opposed to parenteral, buprenorphine but gave no figures (Bullingham *et al.*, 1981), while Ellis and colleagues noted greater sedation and nausea only in the buprenorphine group of patients in their study and wondered whether this was due to the regular administration of the buprenorphine, whereas the other drugs in their investigation were being given on patient request (Ellis *et al.*, 1982). They noted further that regular anti-emetics were not given to the buprenorphine group but were to the others. The incidence of nausea and vomiting is reported as varying from less than 5% (Kay, 1978; Ouellette, 1982) to 30% (Edge, Cooper and Morgan, 1979; Cook *et al.*, 1982) or greater (Gibbs, Johnson and Davis, 1982). Dizziness has also been reported as occurring in up to 12% of patients (Ouellette, 1982).

The effect of buprenorphine on the cardiovascular system is minimal, as studies in patients with cardiovascular pathology (Rosenfeldt *et al.*, 1978; Hayes, Fraser and Hampton, 1979) and normal patients (Harcus, Ward and Smith, 1979; Moore, McQuay and Bullingham, 1980) have shown.

Initial studies have suggested a respiratory depressant effect similar to that seen with morphine (Orwin *et al.*, 1976) and clinical usage would tend to confirm this (Ouellette, 1982). However, Budd has suggested that the respiratory depressant effect may begin to level off at between 0.3 and 0.6 mg intramuscularly (Budd, 1983). In addition, the same author has used extremely high intravenous doses without seeing any respiratory depression (Budd, 1981). Other studies and reports have shown severe respiratory depression (Cook *et al.*, 1982; Gibbs, Johnson and Davis, 1982; Papworth, 1983; Faroqui, Cole and Curran, 1983) which necessitated ventilation or reversal. Various drug interactions with other opiates and with benzodiazepines have been suggested and it seems most likely that the latter group of drugs may well act synergistically with buprenorphine and may cause a profound respiratory depression (Faroqui, Cole and Curran, 1983).

The respiratory depression caused by buprenorphine can only be partially reversed by high doses of naloxone. An infusion of doxapram (1.0 mg/kg) will reverse the respiratory depression caused by buprenorphine 0.3 mg (Orwin, 1977). In practice, it may require an initial infusion and then a continued infusion or injection of doxapram to sustain the reversal of respiratory depression.

Buprenorphine has a low potential for drug abuse and has even been used to treat drug addicts (R. A. Boas, personal communication). Buprenorphine has a high affinity for the receptor sites. It will displace 4 times more fentanyl from the receptor site than naloxone, and thus it will occupy the receptor so comprehensively that an addict will have no subjective signs if he injects another opiate. Boas has also suggested that buprenorphine (0.3 mg/kg) be used in a similar fashion for postoperative analgesia after high dose fentanyl anaesthesia (27.2 μg/kg).

The most commonly used dosage has been between 0.3 mg and 0.6 mg for parenteral use and 0.2–0.8 mg for the sublingual route. Although higher doses have been used (Budd, 1981) there is little evidence to date that much benefit ensues. Indeed, it is interesting to speculate that the use of reduced doses (0.1 mg) sublingually may yield the same analgesic benefits, but with a reduced incidence of side effects. For the control of postoperative pain, there is some pharmacokinetic evidence to suggest that an initial intravenous dose of 0.3 mg with intramuscular supplementation of a similar amount may yield the optimum analgesic response (McQuay *et al.*, 1980).

Butorphanol (Stadol – Bristol)

This is a completely synthetic morphinan derivative with mixed agonist–antagonist opioid properties. It is a strong κ-receptor agonist and probably has agonist actions at the σ-receptor. It also has weak antagonist actions at the μ-receptor. It is 5 times more potent that morphine (Tavakoli, Corssen and Caruso, 1976) and 30 times as potent as pethidine (Gilbert *et al.*, 1976). That butorphanol is an analgesic agent is undoubted, but there are confusing aspects to its clinical use. It is cited as being effective for 3–5 h for the control of postoperative pain (Tavakoli, Corssen and Caruso, 1976; Gilbert *et al.*, 1976), but there is some evidence from experimental work in animals that suggests that its analgesic activity is limited and that there is a 'ceiling effect' to even this limited activity (Murphy and Hug, 1982b). In addition, there is some human evidence to support this. In a study of high dose butorphanol for cardiac surgery, doses of 0.15 and 0.3 mg/kg (equivalent to 0.75 and 1.5 mg/kg of morphine) did not anaesthetize patients or even render them unconscious. Even after anaesthesia was induced, some patients reacted to surgery (Moldenhauer, Hug and Nagle, 1981). However, other studies have found butorphanol to be satisfactory as an adjuvant for routine general and cardiac surgery (Stehling and Zander, 1978; Aldrete *et al.*, 1983), but intraoperative hypertension, suggesting inadequate analgesia, was noted in both reports.

Further confusion arises from study of butorphanol's haemodynamic effects. Popio and colleagues (Popio *et al.*, 1978) demonstrated an increased cardiac index and mean pulmonary artery pressure after a single intravenous dose (a similar effect is seen with pentazocine). Other workers have failed to observe this and showed no significant change other than a mild reduction of left and right ventricular work indices concomitant with a reasonable reduction of myocardial oxygen demand (Lippman *et al.*, 1984).

Some opioids are known to cause spasm of the spincter of Oddi and cause biliary tract hypertension. Agonist–antagonist agents such as butorphanol and nalbuphine are not thought to exert this effect (Radnay *et al.*, 1982; McCammon, Stoelting and Madura, 1984) – or do they? (Martin and Joehl, 1983).

Adverse effects upon the central nervous system are those common to other strong opioids and a similar or slightly less frequent incidence of drowsiness, nausea and vomiting to that seen with morphine has been reported (Houde *et al.*, 1976). The same authors report that side effects were dose-related and that at doses of 4 mg or greater, psychotomimetic side effects such as dysphoria and hallucinations may occur. Butorphanol causes respiratory depression and any 'ceiling effect' which may occur is at the same dosage where other side effects may become a problem.

The normal adult dose is 2 mg (range 1–4 mg) for intramuscular and 1 mg (range 0.5–2.0 mg) for intravenous use, with a length of action of only 2–4 h. Oral tablets of 4 mg are available. Because of its agonist–antagonist nature, it has a low abuse potential and should be used with care where conventional opiates are being employed, as it is an excellent reversal agent. Butorphanol can be reversed with naloxone. Care should be exercised in its employment in patients with respiratory depression and, possibly, those with cardiovascular disease. It is no longer marketed in the UK, but is still available in the USA and elsewhere.

Nalbuphine (Nubain – DuPont)

This drug is structurally related to the pure μ-agonist oxymorphone and the pure μ-antagonist naloxone. It is likely that nalbuphine has actions at all three major receptors and is unique in probably being a partial agonist at the κ-receptor. It also has weak partial agonist activity at the σ-receptor and is a competitive antagonist at the μ-receptor.

There are relatively few well-controlled studies of the use of nalbuphine in postoperative pain. In a crossover study comparing nalbuphine and morphine, the results suggest that the drugs are approximately equipotent. However, the degree of analgesia obtained with nalbuphine was about 0.8 of that seen after the exhibition of morphine. Nalbuphine may have a slightly longer duration of action in doses that were equi-analgesic in terms of peak analgesic effect (Beaver and Feise, 1978). In a study of 6 normal subjects, analgesia to experimental (tourniquet) pain was similar when equivalent doses of nalbuphine (0.15 mg/kg) and morphine were used. The subjects also experienced similar amounts of respiratory depression. Increasing doses of morphine produced increasing analgesia; increasing doses of nalbuphine produced neither respiratory depression nor analgesia. Indeed, there was a marked variability of analgesic response (Gal, DiFazio and Moscicki, 1982).

There are two well-designed double-blind crossover studies in patients with postoperative pain that compare nalbuphine with pentazocine (Houde *et al.*, 1976; Tammisto and Tigerstedt, 1977). These suggest that nalbuphine is about 3 times as potent as pentazocine and when given intramuscularly has a lower peak effect but somewhat longer duration of action. There was a wide variation in analgesic effect of nalbuphine which made the determination of an equi-analgesic dose more difficult. There is only one published report comparing nalbuphine with pethidine (Waye and Braunfeld, 1982). This double-blind parallel group study compared the two drugs as analgesics during colonoscopy. Nalbuphine was not thought to be as effective as pethidine. Other, as yet unpublished, work has reported similar analgesic effects with nalbuphine and pethidine for a variety of procedures (Errick and Heel, 1983).

Nalbuphine does not seem to be a particularly powerful analgesic, as has been demonstrated in animal (Murphy and Hug, 1982b) and human anaesthetic studies (Lake *et al.*, 1982). In the animal study, nalbuphine 0.5 mg/kg reduced the enflurane MAC for dogs by 8%. Three to fortyfold increases in the nalbuphine dosage produced no further reduction. Butorphanol 0.1 mg/kg reduced enflurane MAC for dogs by 11% and similar three to fortyfold increases in dosage produced no further reduction. By contrast, morphine 0.5 mg/kg reduced enflurane MAC by 17%, progressively increasing to 63% at a dose of 5 mg/kg. A further fourfold increase in morphine dosage produced no further change. A similar effect is seen with fentanyl, with a maximum depression of 66% (Murphy and Hug, 1982a). In humans, nalbuphine 2–3 mg/kg intravenously provided insufficient analgesia for the proposed coronary artery or valvular surgery (Welch and Feldman, 1981; Lake *et al.*, 1982). Thus there is evidence of a 'ceiling effect' for analgesia – as has been shown, this is present for 'conventional' opiates, but at a much higher level.

Adverse effects are not dissimilar from those of morphine-like drugs. Drowsiness and sedation are quite prominent, although it could be argued that this represents an advantageous clinical effect as this is not usually associated with much respiratory depression. However, it has to be considered in conjunction with its limited effect as an analgesic. Much stress has been placed upon the 'ceiling effect' for respiratory depression that is alleged to occur at a dosage of 30 mg (Romagnoli and Keats, 1980). Up to that dosage, the respiratory depression is the same as morphine and as the clinical dosage range is 10–20 mg this 'advantage' appears illusory. The methods of measuring this 'ceiling effect' are open to question. In addition, psychotomimetic effects have been reported in this lower dose range (Houde *et al.*, 1976; Gal, DiFazio and Moscicki, 1982), although lower in incidence and severity than those seen with pentazocine (Houde *et al.*, 1976).

Nalbuphine does appear to have at least one advantage in that it has virtually no effect upon the cardiovascular system – an observation confirmed by several groups of researchers (Romagnoli and Keats, 1978; Lee *et al.*, 1981; Lake *et al.*, 1982; Fahmy, Sunder and Soter, 1984). There are equally confusing effects upon biliary tract dynamics, similar to those seen with butorphanol (Martin and Joehl, 1983; McCammon, Stoelting and Madura, 1984). However, until confirmation of the latter work, both nalbuphine and butorphanol would appear to offer at least theoretical advantages as analgesics for use where an increase in biliary tract pressure is undesirable.

Nalbuphine is thought likely to have the same abuse potential as pentazocine (Jasinski and Mansky, 1972). It can be reversed by naloxone and is itself an excellent reversal agent of agonist opiates (Julien, 1982; Murphy and Hug, 1983; Tabatabai, Collins and Kitihata, 1983).

The normal adult dose is considered to be 10 mg/70 kg (range 5–20 mg/70 kg) given intravenously or intramuscularly. Oral nalbuphine is not yet available in the UK, but its use has been reported and it appears to be about one-third as potent as the parenteral form.

Dezocine (Wy-16 225 – Wyeth)

This new drug is one of a series of novel bridged aminotetralins and is structurally related to pentazocine. It has shown analgesic activity in both animals and man. Its mode of action is unknown, but it has been suggested that it has an action at the μ-receptor, coupled with an action at a second receptor – possibly the σ-receptor. Thus it is not like other conventional agonist–antagonists. In a study in rats, cyclopropane MAC was reduced by 50%, more than twice that seen with other agonist–antagonists (pentazocine, butorphanol and nalbuphine). Of note was that dezocine and morphine together further reduced cyclopropane MAC, but by less than the sum of their individual values, suggesting an antagonistic effect (Rowlingson, Moscicki and DiFazio, 1983).

There are few worthwhile published studies of its use in postoperative pain. In a multiple dose study comparing dezocine 5, 10 and 15 mg against 10 mg of morphine, for the relief of postoperative pain following lower abdominal surgery, dezocine was found to be effective. Patients were allocated to one of two groups where pain was assessed as moderate or severe and the two larger doses were found to be superior to dezocine 5 mg in the moderate pain group. No significant differences were seen between the drugs or dosages tested in the group with severe pain. Side effects were reported as minimal (Downing *et al.*, 1981). Another study has compared dezocine intramuscularly at two dosage levels (10 mg and 15 mg against morphine 10 mg and placebo (Vinik *et al.*, 1982). Dezocine was faster in onset than morphine, but of shorter duration. Dezocine 15 mg is reported as producing better analgesia, but at the expense of a higher incidence of nausea and vomiting. In addition, a dose-related respiratory depression was seen.

An early review suggested that adverse reactions were minimal, and less than those observed with equi-analgesic doses of morphine (Petro, 1983). However, nausea and vomiting were prominent in one study (Vinik *et al.*, 1982) and in another volunteer study of ventilatory effects, dezocine demonstrated respiratory depressant properties at least as severe as those of morphine. Both analgesia and respiratory depression increased up to a dosage of 0.3 mg/kg intravenously, but further increase in dosage produced no further effect – thus a 'ceiling effect' seems likely (Gal and DiFazio, 1983).

It is likely that dezocine will have a low abuse potential, although it has been described as morphine-like (Jasinski, Pevnick and Griffith, 1976). It is naloxone reversible. Preliminary indications are that it is equipotent in terms of dosage and analgesic effect to morphine. Further studies are proceeding.

Bremazocine (AW-14 707 – Sandoz)

A benzomorphan analogue, bremazocine is reported in animal experiments as being a potent, long-acting κ-agonist, with analgesic potency twice that of morphine (Römer, Büscher and Hill, 1980). Only a brief report of animal work has so far been published in the anaesthetic literature (Freye, Hartung and Schenk, 1983). This suggests an action at other receptors, possibly σ, and thus raises the possibility of psychotomimetic side effects if this drug is used in humans.

Meptazinol (Meptid – Wyeth)

This drug belongs to a chemical series known as hexahydroazepines. It is known to act as a mixed agonist–antagonist at opiate receptors, but differs from all conventional drugs of this type by having an analgesic action which is independent of this. It is postulated, from animal studies, that this is attributable to an effect at central cholinergic synapses (Green, 1983).

The initial study of meptazinol tested four different doses of meptazinol (25, 50, 75, 100 mg) in a single blind study (Paymaster, 1976). The lowest dose had no analgesic effect and the others appeared to be effective in a dose-related manner. A second trial from the same source (Paymaster, 1977) compared meptazinol 100 mg intramuscularly with pentazocine 60 mg and pethidine 100 mg administered in a similar fashion. Results indicated little difference between these drugs in their efficacy at relieving postoperative pain. Claims were made for an earlier onset of analgesia with meptazinol, but these were offset by a more rapid decline in analgesia. In a double-blind crossover study, intramuscular meptazinol at three dose levels (60, 75 and 100 mg) was compared with pethidine 100 mg intramuscularly (Hedges, Turner and Wadsworth, 1980). Analysis of the results indicated no difference in postoperative analgesia between the two larger doses of meptazinol and pethidine, although pethidine was preferred by both patients and observers.

These studies indicated that meptazinol given intramuscularly had a similar potency to pethidine. However, when given intravenously via a patient-controlled analgesia machine, the consumption of meptazinol was 2.4 times greater than that of pethidine in a comparative study (Slattery *et al.*, 1981). This difference in potency may be accounted for by the fact that the intravenous study was carried out on patients with upper abdominal incisions, and hence more severe pain, than the early studies which were carried out on patients suffering from pain from lower abdominal and orthopaedic surgery. Effective postoperative analgesia was reported with both drugs. The same group of workers used a similar on-demand machine to compare pethidine, buprenorphine, morphine and meptazinol given intramuscularly (Harmer *et al.*, 1983b). They felt that meptazinol was relatively more effective when given intramuscularly as compared to their previous study.

Two other comparative studies have been made between meptazinol 100 mg and omnopon 20 mg (Moyes, Miller and Aldridge, 1979) and meptazinol 100 mg and morphine 15 mg (Major, Cohen and Continho, 1982). In both, meptazinol was claimed to be as effective as the other drug under study, but for a shorter period of time. Indeed, the short duration of action seems to be a feature of meptazinol and it seems unrealistic to expect any more than 4 h of effective analgesia and often much less on the basis of published work. Another disappointing feature is the unpredictable nature of the analgesia achieved (J. G. Jones, personal communication).

Side effects reported are sedation, which may be dose related (Paymaster, 1976; Harmer *et al.*, 1983b), and nausea and vomiting in a similar proportion to that seen with conventional agents (Paymaster, 1977; Harmer *et al.*, 1983a), or possibly slightly greater and accompanied by dizziness when meptazinol is given intravenously (Slattery *et al.*, 1981). No psychotomomimetic side effects have been reported. Cardiovascular effects that have been reported include a possible mild positive inotropic activity and antidysrhythmic activity in rats (Rashid and Waterfall, 1979) and this good news for rodents is mirrored in the lack of any report of haemodynamic upset in any human study (Budd, 1976; Paymaster, 1977; Moyes, Miller and Aldridge, 1979). No respiratory depression was seen in a comparative study of equi-analgesic intramuscular doses of meptazinol, morphine and pentazocine (Jordan *et al.*, 1979), although this side effect has been reported when intravenous meptazinol was compared to intravenous pethidine (Slattery *et al.*, 1983).

Meptazinol is thought to have a low abuse potential (Evans *et al.*, 1983) and is partially reversible with naloxone. The recommended adult dose is 75–100 mg intramuscularly, repeated 2–4 hourly. Intravenously, a dosage of 50–100 mg by slow injection is suggested. For infusion, a dosage of 0.45 mg/kg per hour is claimed to be effective. Oral meptazinol has recently been introduced, but would appear to have little place in the treatment of anything but the most minor postoperative pain.

Morphine

Another approach to the control of postoperative pain is to take existing drugs and to improve methods of delivery. Examples of this are patient-controlled on-demand analgesia machines, different routes of delivery such as intrathecal or epidural opiates or novel formulations which allow for a longer duration of action of the drug.

Morphine has been the subject of various attempts to improve its length of action.

Slow release tablets (MST Continus – Napp Laboratories)

These have been extensively used for the control of chronic pain from malignant and, to a lesser extent, non-malignant causes. Use in postoperative pain has been sporadic and there are few data to support its use. Two studies from Leicester indicate that further work is worth considering (Fell, Chmielewski and Smith, 1982; Derbyshire *et al.*, 1984). Both have shown that satisfactory analgesia can be achieved via the oral route and is comparable to that achieved by intramuscular morphine, sublingual buprenorphine and patient-controlled intravenous and intramuscular injections (Harmer *et al.*, 1983b). There are other anecdotal reports of the value of slow release morphine tablets following abdominal surgery, although no benefit was found in postoperative dental pain (Hanks *et al.*, 1981). This may have been due to the peculiarities of postoperative dental pain as in another study opiates have been shown to be ineffective (Seymour and Rawlins, 1981).

Sustained release hydrogen suppository

The Leicester group has submitted a pilot study showing that effective plasma levels of morphine can be achieved with a polyethylene oxide gel morphine suppository (Hanning *et al.*, 1983). It is presumed that clinical trials are proceeding.

Microcrystalline injections (Duromorph – Laboratories for Applied Biology)

There is a single anecdotal report of the use of these injections in postoperative pain (Johnson, 1983). Regular injections were said to give a twofold increase in duration of postoperative analgesia and lower incidence of side effects than that seen with ordinary parenteral morphine.

Intrathecal and epidural opiates

After the discovery of the endorphins and opiate receptors there came the initial report of analgesia mediated by the direct spinal action of opiates (Yaksh and Rudy, 1976). This was followed by reports of the clinical use of opiates in man by the intrathecal (Wang, Nauss and Thomas, 1979) and epidural (Behar *et al.*, 1979) routes. Since then, hundreds of reports of the use of intrathecal or epidural opiates have appeared and from these some general statements can be made. However, a full review of this topic is beyond the scope of this chapter.

Spinal and epidural opiates produce, at least initially, segmental, dose-related analgesia especially effective for visceral-type pain, but not effective for severe acute or somatic pain. In other words, one cannot use this technique for an operation itself. Compounds with strong receptor binding and, in the case of morphine, low lipid solubility, give intense long-lasting analgesia. The more lipid-soluble drugs give intense analgesia of far shorter duration. Spinal opiates do not produce sympathetic or motor blockade and may have advantages over local anaesthetics in certain clinical situations.

Side effects of intrathecal or epidural opiates include pruritis, nausea, vomiting, drowsiness, dizziness, urinary retention and respiratory depression. Morphine in particular produces significant and consistent respiratory depression in relatively large doses and this is thought to be due to its high water solubility and poor lipid solubility. Lipid-soluble opiates appear to have relatively little respiratory depressant effect (Shnider, 1983). With conventional opiates, all side effects are naloxone reversible, but this may not be the case with mixed agonist–antagonist drugs.

Although intrathecal and epidural analgesics can provide excellent analgesia of long duration, much work remains to be done to establish dose requirements and methods of reducing side effects. The safe limits of dosage and volume have yet to be defined and their use should be restricted to patients who can be closely and constantly monitored for many hours. It should be remembered that these drugs are being introduced close to their site of action, and great care should be exercised especially when this technique is employed in conjunction with oral or parenteral opiates.

References

ALDRETE, J. A., DECAMPO, T., USUBIAGA, J., RENCK, R., SUZUKI, D. and WITT, W. D. (1983). Comparison of butorphanol and morphine as analgesics for coronary bypass surgery. A double blind randomized study. *Anesthesia and Analgesia,* **62,** 78–83

BEAVER, W. T. and FEISE, G. A. (1978). A comparison of the analgesic effect of intramuscular nalbuphine and morphine in patients with postoperative pain. *Journal of Pharmacology and Experimental Therapeutics,* **204,** 487–496

BEHAR, M., OLSHWANG, D., MAGORA, F. and DAVIDSON, J. T. (1979). Epidural morphine in the treatment of pain. *Lancet,* **i,** 527–528

BREWSTER, D., HUMPHREY, M. J. and MCLEAVY, M. A. (1981). The systemic bioavailability of buprenorphine by various routes of administration. *Journal of Pharmacy and Pharmacology,* **33,** 500–506

BUDD, K. (1976). Meptazinol, a new analgesic. Effects on haemodynamic stability. *Acta Anaesthesiologica Belgica,* **27,** 151–154

BUDD, K. (1981). High dose buprenorphine for postoperative analgesia. *Anaesthesia,* **36,** 900–903

BUDD, K. (1983). Buprenorphine. In *Clinics in Anaesthesiology* (Bullingham, R. E. S., Ed.), vol. 1, no. 1. London, Philadelphia, Toronto; Saunders, pp. 147–152

BULLINGHAM, R. E. S., MCQUAY, H. J., DWYER, D., ALLEN, M. C. and MOORE, R. A. (1981). Sublingual buprenorphine used postoperatively: clinical observations and preliminary pharmacokinetics. *British Journal of Clinical Pharmacology,* **12,** 117–122

BULLINGHAM, R. E. S., MCQUAY, H. J., MOORE, R. A. and BENNET, M. R. D. (1980). Buprenorphine kinetics. *Clinical Pharmacology and Therapeutics,* **28,** 667–672

BULLINGHAM, R. E. S., O'SULLIVAN, G., MCQUAY, H. J., POPPLETON, P., ROLFE, M., WEIR, L. and MOORE, R. A. (1984). Mandatory sublingual buprenorphine for postoperative pain. *Anaesthesia,* **39,** 329–334

BUNKER, J. P. (1976). Manpower problems in anesthesiology. In *Manpower and Examinations in Anesthesia* (Djokovic, J., Ed.). *International Anesthesiology Clinics,* vol. 14. Boston; Little, Brown, pp. 1–13

CAHILL, J., MURPHY, D., O'BRIEN, D., MULHALL, J. and FITZPATRICK, G. (1983). Epidural buprenorphine for pain relief after major abdominal surgery – a controlled comparison with epidural morphine. *Anaesthesia,* **38,** 760–764

CHRISTENSEN, F. R. and ANDERSEN, L. W. (1982). Adverse reaction to extradural buprenorphine. *British Journal of Anaesthesia,* **54,** 476

COHEN, F. L. (1980). Postsurgical pain relief: patients' status and nurses' medication choices. *Pain,* **9,** 265–274

COOK, P. J., JAMES, I. M., HOBBS, K. E. F. and BROWNE, D. R. G. (1982). Controlled comparison of IM morphine and buprenorphine for analgesia after abdominal surgery. *British Journal of Anaesthesia,* **54,** 285–290

DERBYSHIRE, D. R., VATER, M., MAILE, C. I. D., LARSSON, I. M., AITKENHEAD, A. R. and SMITH, G. (1984). Non-parenteral postoperative analgesia. A comparison of sublingual buprenorphine and morphine (slow release) tablets. *Anaesthesia,* **39,** 324–328

DOWNING, J. W., BROCK-UTNE, J. G., BARCLAY, A. and SCHWEGMANN, I. L. (1981). Wy 16 225 (Dezocine): a new synthetic opiate agonist–antagonist and potent analgesic: comparison with morphine for relief of pain after lower abdominal surgery. *British Journal of Anaesthesia,* **53,** 59–64

DOWNING, J. W., LEARY, W. P. and WHITE, E. S. (1977). Buprenorphine: a new potent long acting synthetic analgesic. Comparison with morphine. *British Journal of Anaesthesia,* **49,** 251–255

EDGE, W. G., COOPER, G. M. and MORGAN, M. (1979). Analgesic effects of sublingual buprenorphine. *Anaesthesia,* **34,** 463–467

ELLIS, R., HAINES, O., SHAH, R., COTTON, B. R. and SMITH, G. (1982). Pain relief after abdominal surgery. A comparison of IM morphine, sublingual buprenorphine and self administered IV pethidine. *British Journal of Anaesthesia,* **54,** 421–427

EMRICH, H. M., VOGT, P., HERZ, A. and KISSLING, W. (1982). Antidepressant effects of buprenorphine. *Lancet,* **ii,** 709

ERRICK, J. K. and HEEL, R. C. (1983). Nalbuphine. A preliminary review of its pharmacological properties and therapeutic efficacy. *Drugs,* **26,** 191–211

EVANS, J. M., ROSEN, M., MCCARTHY, J. and HOGG, M. I. S. (1976). Apparatus for patient controlled administration of intravenous narcotics during labour. *Lancet,* **i,** 17–18

EVANS, M., ROBSON, P. J., CHADD, M. A., EVANS, C. M. and FRY, D. M. (1983). Administration of meptazinol to opiate-dependent patients. *Postgraduate Medical Journal,* **59,** Supplement 1, 78–84

FAHMY, N. R., SUNDER, N. and SOTER, N. A. (1984). A comparison of histamine-releasing properties and hemodynamic effects of morphine and nalbuphine in humans (Abstract). *Anesthesia and Analgesia,* **63,** 210

FAROQUI, M. H., COLE, M. and CURRAN, J. (1983). Buprenorphine, benzodiazepines and respiratory depression. *Anaesthesia,* **38,** 1002–1003

FELL, D., CHMIELEWSKI, A. and SMITH, G. (1982). Postoperative analgesia with controlled release morphine sulphate: comparison with intramuscular morphine. *British Medical Journal,* **ii,** 92–94

FREYE, E., HARTUNG, E. and SCHENK, G. K. (1983). Bremazocine: an opiate that induces sedation and analgesia without respiratory depression. *Anesthesia and Analgesia,* **62,** 483–488

FRY, E. N. S. (1979). Relief of pain after surgery: a comparison of sublingual buprenorphine and intramuscular papaveretum. *Anaesthesia,* **34,** 549–551

GAL, T. J. and DIFAZIO, C. A. (1983). Ventilatory and analgesic effects of dezocine. *Anesthesiology,* **59,** A526

GAL, T. J., DIFAZIO, C. A. and MOSCICKI, J. (1982). Analgesic and respiratory depressant activity of nalbuphine: a comparison with morphine. *Anesthesiology,* **57,** 367–374

GIBBS, J. M., JOHNSON, H. D. and DAVIS, F. M. (1982). Patient administration of IV buprenorphine for postoperative pain relief using the Cardiff demand analgesia apparatus. *British Journal of Anaesthesia,* **54,** 279–284

GILBERT, M. S., HANOVER, R. M., MOYLAN, D. S. and CARUSO, F. S. (1976). Intramuscular butorphanol and meperidine in postoperative pain. *Clinical Pharmacology and Therapeutics,* **20,** 359–364

GREEN, D. (1983). Current concepts concerning the mode of action of meptazinol as an analgesic. *Postgraduate Medical Journal,* **59,** Supplement 1, 9–12

HAMBROOK, J. M. and RANCE, M. J. (1976). The interaction of buprenorphine and the opiate receptor: lipophilicity as a determining factor in drug receptor kinetics. In *Opiates and Endogenous Opioid Peptides* (Kosterlitz, H. W., Ed.). Amsterdam; Elsevier/North-Holland Biomedical Press, pp. 295–301

HANKS, G. W., ROSE, N. M., AHERNE, G. W., PIALL, E. M., FAIRFIELD, S. and TRUEMAN, T. (1981). Controlled release morphine tablets: a double blind trial in dental surgery patients. *British Journal of Anaesthesia,* **53,** 1259–1264

HANNING, C. D., SMITH, G., MCNEILL, M. and GRAHAM, N. B. (1983). Rectal administration of morphine from a sustained release hydrogel suppository. *British Journal of Anaesthesia,* **55,** 236P–237P

HARCUS, A. W., WARD, A. E. and SMITH, D. W. (1979). Methodology of monitored release of a new preparation: buprenorphine. *British Medical Journal,* **ii,** 163–165

HARMER, M., SLATTERY, P. J., ROSEN, M. and VICKERS, M. D. (1983a). Comparison between buprenorphine and pentazocine given IV on demand in the control of postoperative pain. *British Journal of Anaesthesia,* **55,** 21–25

HARMER, M., SLATTERY, P. J., ROSEN, M. and VICKERS, M. D. (1983b). Intramuscular on demand analgesia: double blind controlled trial of pethidine, buprenorphine, morphine and meptazinol. *British Medical Journal,* **i,** 680–682

HAYES, M. J., FRAZER, A. R. and HAMPTON, J. R. (1979). Randomized trial comparing buprenorphine and diamorphine for chest pain in suspected myocardial infarction. *British Medical Journal,* **ii,** 300–302

HEDGES, A., TURNER, P. and WADSWORTH, J. (1980). A double-blind comparison of meptazinol with pethidine in postoperative pain. *British Journal of Anaesthesia,* **52,** 295–298

HEEL, R. C., BROGDEN, R. N., SPEIGHT, T. M. and AVERY, G. S. (1979). Buprenorphine: a review of its pharmacological properties and therapeutic efficacy. *Drugs,* **17,** 81–110

HOUDE, R. W. (1979). The analgesic effectiveness of the narcotic agonist antagonists. *British Journal of Clinical Pharmacology,* **7,** Supplement 3, 297S–308S

HOUDE, R. W., WALLENSTEIN, S. L., ROGERS, A. and KAIKO, R. F. (1976). Annual Report of the Analgesic Studies Section of the Memorial Sloan–Kettering Cancer Center. *Problems of Drug Dependence Committee Proceedings,* pp. 149–168

HUGHES, J., SMITH, T. W., KOSTERLITZ, H. W., FOTHERGILL, L. A., MORGAN, B. A. and MORRIS, H. R. (1975). Isolation of two related penta peptides from brain with potent opiate activity. *Nature,* **258,** 577–579

HULL, C. J. (1982). Postoperative buprenorphine. *British Journal of Anaesthesia,* **54,** 1144

JASINSKI, D. R. and MANSKY, P. A. (1972). Evaluation of nalbuphine for abuse potential. *Clinical Pharmacology and Therapeutics,* **13,** 78–90

JASINSKI, D. R., PEVNICK, J. S. and GRIFFITH, J. D. (1976). Assessment of WY-16 225 for morphine-like subjective effects and miosis. Progress report on studies from the Clinical Pharmacology Section of the Addiction Research Center. In *Proceedings of the 38th Annual Scientific Meeting Committee on Problems of Drug Dependence,* pp. 122–128, Richmond, Virginia

JASINSKI, D. R., PEVNICK, J. S. and GRIFFITH, J. D. (1978). Human pharmacology and abuse potential of buprenorphine. *Archives of General Psychiatry,* **35,** 501–516

JOHNSON, C. D. (1983). Methods for relief of postoperative pain. *Annals of the Royal College of Surgeons of England,* **65,** 137

JORDAN, C., LEHANE, J. R., ROBSON, P. J. and JONES, J. G. (1979). A comparison of the respiratory effects of meptazinol, pentazocine and morphine. *British Journal of Anaesthesia,* **51,** 497–502

JULIEN, R. M. (1982). Effects of nalbuphine on normal and oxymorphone-depressed ventilatory responses to CO_2 challenge. *Anesthesiology,* **57,** A320

KAMEL, M. M. and GEDDES, I. C. (1978). A comparison of buprenorphine and pethidine for immediate postoperative pain relief by the intravenous route. *British Journal of Anaesthesia,* **50,** 599–603

KAY, B. (1978). A double-blind comparison of morphine and buprenorphine in the prevention of pain after operation. *British Journal of Anaesthesia,* **50,** 605–609

KAY, B. (1980). A double blind comparison between fentanyl and buprenorphine in analgesic supplemented anaesthesia. *British Journal of Anaesthesia,* **52,** 453–457

LAKE, C. L., DUCKWORTH, E. N., DIFAZIO, C. A., DURBIN, C. G. and MAGRUDER, M. R. (1982). Cardiovascular effects of nalbuphine in patients with coronary or valvular heart disease. *Anesthesiology,* **57,** 498–503

LEE, G., LOW, R. I., AMSTERDAM, E. A., DEMARIA, A. N., HUBER, P. W. and MASON, D. T. (1981). Hemodynamic effects of morphine and nalbuphine in acute myocardial infarction. *Clinical Pharmacology and Therapeutics,* **29,** 576–581

LIPPMAN, M., MOK, M. S., STEEN, S. N., HARLEY, D. and APPEL, P. (1984). Butorphanol as an intravenous adjunct in balanced anaesthesia for cardiac surgery (Abstract). *Anesthesia and Analgesia,* **63,** 243

MAJOR, E., COHEN, D. G. and CONTINHO, P. E. (1982). A comparison between meptazinol and morphine for relief of postoperative orthopaedic pain. *Proceedings of the Sixth European Congress of Anesthesiology,* Session 81, Paper 353. London and New York; Grune and Stratton

MARKS, R. M. and SACHAR, E. J. (1973). Undertreatment of medical inpatients with narcotic analgesics. *Annals of Internal Medicine,* **78,** 173–181

MARTIN, D. E. and JOEHL, R. J. (1983). Butorphanol and nalbuphine cause human bile duct obstruction. *Anesthesiology,* **59,** A324

MARTIN, W. R., EADES, C. G., THOMPSON, J. A., HUPPLER, R. E. and GILBERT, P. E. (1976). The effect of morphine- and nalorphine-like drugs in the non-dependent and morphine-dependent chronic spinal dog. *Journal of Pharmacology and Experimental Therapeutics,* **197,** 517–532

MASSON, A. H. B. (1981). Sublingual buprenorphine versus oral dihydrocodeine in postoperative pain. *Journal of International Medical Research,* **9,** 506–510

MCCAMMON, R. L., STOELTING, R. K. and MADURA, J. A. (1984). Effects of butorphanol, nalbuphine and fentanyl on intrabiliary tract dynamics. *Anesthesia and Analgesia,* **63,** 139–142

MCQUAY, H. J., BULLINGHAM, R. E. S., PATTERSON, G. M. C. and MOORE, R. A. (1980). Clinical effects of buprenorphine during and after operation. *British Journal of Anaesthesia,* **52,** 1013–1019

MERSKEY, H. (1978). Pain and personality. In *The Psychology of Pain* (Sternback, R. A., Ed.). New York; Raven Press, pp. 111–127

MOLDENHAUER, C. C., HUG, C. C. JR. and NAGLE, D. M. (1981). High dose butorphanol (Stadol) in anesthesia for aortocoronary bypass surgery (Abstract). *3rd Annual Meeting of the Society of Cardiovascular Anesthetists,* San Francisco, 10–13 May, pp. 59–60

MOORE, R. A., MCQUAY, H. J. and BULLINGHAM, R. E. S. (1980). Reversal of postoperative hyperglycaemia by buprenorphine. *Lancet,* **ii,** 597–598

MOYES, D. G., MILLER, M. T. and ALDRIDGE, N. J. (1979). A comparison between meptazinol and omnopon in the relief of postoperative pain. *South African Medical Journal,* **59,** 908–911

MURPHY, M. R. and HUG, C. C. JR. (1982a). The anaesthetic potency of fentanyl in terms of its reduction of enflurane MAC. *Anesthesiology,* **57,** 485–488

MURPHY, M. R. and HUG, C. C. JR. (1982b). The enflurane sparing effect of morphine, butorphanol and nalbuphine. *Anesthesiology,* **57,** 489–492

MURPHY, M. R. and HUG, C. C. JR. (1983). Efficacy of fentanyl in reducing isoflurane MAC: antagonism by naloxone and nalbuphine. *Anesthesiology,* **59,** A334

ORWIN, J. M. (1977). The effect of doxapram on buprenorphine induced respiratory depression. *Acta Anaesthesiologica Belgica,* **28,** 93–106

ORWIN, J. M., ROBSON, P. J., ORWIN, J. and PRICE, M. (1976). The effects of buprenorphine and morphine on respiration following administration by the intramuscular route in man. *Sixth World Congress of Anesthesiology,* Mexico City, SEC. 5/5, p. 157. Belgium; Societé d'Anesthesie de Charleroi

OUELLETTE, R. D. (1982). Buprenorphine and morphine efficacy in postoperative pain: a double-blind multiple-dose study. *Journal of Clinical Pharmacology,* **22,** 165–172

PAPWORTH, D. P. (1983). High dose buprenorphine for postoperative analgesia. *Anaesthesia,* **38,** 163

PASTERNAK, G. W. (1982). High and low affinity opioid binding sites: relationship to mu and delta sites. *Life Sciences,* **31,** 1303–1305

PAYMASTER, N. J. (1976). Clinical evaluation of meptazinol, a new analgesic, in postoperative pain. *British Journal of Anaesthesia,* **48,** 599–606

PAYMASTER, N. J. (1977). Analgesia after operation. A controlled trial of meptazinol, pentazocine and pethidine. *British Journal of Anaesthesia,* **49,** 1139–1146

PETRO, D. J. (1983). Dezocine. In *Clinics in Anaesthesiology* (Bullingham, R. E. S., Ed.), vol. 1, no. 1. London, Philadelphia, Toronto; Saunders, pp. 159–163

POPIO, K. A., JACKSON, D. N., ROSS, A. M., SCHREINER, B. P. and YU, P. N. (1978). Hemodynamic and respiratory effects of morphine and butorphanol. *Clinical Pharmacology and Therapeutics,* **23,** 281–287

QUIRION, R., HAMMER, R. P. and HERKENHAM, M. (1981). Phencyclidine (angel dust)/σ-opiate receptor: visualization by tritium sensitive film. *Proceedings of the American National Academy of Sciences,* **78,** 5881–5885

RADNAY, P. A., DUNCALF, D., NOVAKOVIC, M. and BENOIT, J. (1982). Effect of fentanyl, morphine, meperidine, butorphanol and naloxone on common bile duct pressure. *Anesthesiology,* **57,** A351

RASHID, S. and WATERFALL, J. F. (1979). Cardiovascular actions of meptazinol in comparison with pentazocine and morphine. *General Pharmacology,* **10,** 459–469

ROBERTSON, D. H. and LAING, A. W. (1980). Intravenous buprenorphine (Temgesic): use following fentanyl analgesic anaesthesia. *Clinical Trials Journal,* **17,** 51–55

ROMAGNOLI, A. and KEATS, A. S. (1978). Comparative hemodynamic effects of morphine and nalbuphine in patients with coronary artery disease. *Bulletin of the Texas Heart Institute,* **5,** 19–24

ROMAGNOLI, A. and KEATS, A. S. (1980). Ceiling effect for respiratory depression by nalbuphine. *Clinical Pharmacology and Therapeutics,* **27,** 478–485

RÖMER, D., BÜSCHER, H. and HILL, R. C. (1980). Bremazocine: a potent, long-acting opiate kappa agonist. *Life Sciences,* **27,** 971–978

ROSENFELDT, F. L., HOUSTON, B., THOMPSON, D., NAQUI, N., MALCOLM, A. D., WILLIAMS, B. T. and COLTART, D. J. (1978). Haemodynamic effects of buprenorphine after heart surgery. *British Medical Journal,* **ii,** 1602–1603

ROWLINGSON, J. C., MOSCICKI, J. C. and DIFAZIO, C. A. (1983). Anesthetic potency of dezocine and its interaction with morphine in rats. *Anesthesia and Analgesia,* **62,** 899–902

SEYMOUR, R. A. and RAWLINS, M. D. (1981). Paracetamol (Acetominophen), aspirin, dihydrocodeine tartrate and postoperative dental pain. Third World Congress of the International Association for the Study of Pain, Edinburgh, 4–11 September, 1981. *Pain,* Supplement, **1,** S248

SHNIDER, S. M. (1983). Extradural and intrathecal narcotics. *American Society of Anesthesiologists Annual Refresher Course Lectures,* p. 503

SLATTERY, P. J., HARMER, M., ROSEN, M. and VICKERS, M. D. (1981). Comparison of meptazinol and pethidine given i.v. on demand in the management of postoperative pain. *British Journal of Anaesthesia,* **53,** 927–931

SLATTERY, P. J., HARMER, M., ROSEN, M. and VICKERS, M. D. (1983). Comparison of the respiratory depressant effect of IV meptazinol and pethidine. *British Journal of Anaesthesia,* **55,** 245P

STEHLING, L. C. and ZANDER, H. L. (1978). Double blind comparison of butorphanol tartrate and meperidine HCl in balanced anesthesia. *Journal of International Medical Research,* **6,** 384–387

TABATABAI, M., COLLINS, J. G. and KITIHATA, L. M. (1983). Disruption of the activity of inspiratory neurons by high-dose fentanyl and reversal with nalbuphine. *Anesthesiology,* **59,** A485

TAMMISTO, T. and TIGERSTEDT, I. (1977). Comparison of the analgesic effects of intravenous nalbuphine and pentazocine in patients with postoperative pain. *Acta Anaesthesiologica Scandinavica,* **21,** 390–394

TAMMISTO, T. and TIGERSTEDT, I. (1982). Narcotic analgesics in postoperative pain relief in adults. *Acta Anaesthesiologica Scandinavica,* Supplement 74, 161–164

TAVAKOLI, M., CORSSEN, G. and CARUSO, F. (1976). Butorphanol and morphine: a double blind trial of their parenteral analgesic activity. *Anesthesia and Analgesia,* **55,** 394–401

UTTING, J. E. and SMITH, J. M. (1979). Postoperative analgesia. *Anaesthesia,* **34,** 320–332

VINIK, H. R., MCFARLAND, L., WRIGHT, D. and BAKER, W. (1982). Double-blind postoperative study comparing multiple doses of dezocine (WY 16 225) with morphine and placebo. *Anesthesiology,* **57,** A189

WANG, J. K., NAUSS, L. A. and THOMAS, J. E. (1979). Pain relief can be controlled by intrathecally applied morphine in man. *Anesthesiology,* **50,** 149–151

WATSON, P. J. Q., MCQUAY, H. J., BULLINGHAM, R. E. S., ALLEN, M. C. and MOORE, R. A. (1982). Single dose comparison of buprenorphine 0.3 mg and 0.6 mg IV given after operation: clinical effects and plasma concentrations. *British Journal of Anaesthesia,* **54,** 37–44

WAYE, J. D. and BRAUNFELD, S. F. (1982). A randomized double-blind study of nalbuphine as an analgesic for colonoscopy. *Gastrointestinal Endoscopy,* **28,** 86–87

WELCH, G. W. and FELDMAN, H. S. (1981). Intravenous nalbuphine. *Anesthesia and Analgesia,* **60,** 168

YAKSH, T. L. and RUDY, T. A. (1976). Analgesia mediated by a direct spinal action of narcotics. *Science,* **192,** 1357–1358

Chapter 4

Effects of anaesthesia and surgery on drug kinetics and action

N. D. S. Bax and H. F. Woods

Introduction

The physiological changes caused by anaesthesia and surgery might so influence the absorption, distribution and elimination of a drug that its therapeutic effect becomes altered. These changes include alterations of the gastric emptying rate, cardiac output and regional blood flow. Of particular importance are disturbances of the hepatic blood flow and variable effects on the activity of hepatic drug metabolizing enzymes. In addition, drug kinetics and pharmacological effect may be altered by changes in drug–protein binding, the body temperature, acid–base status and by the hormonal response to stress.

In this chapter these factors are discussed and the clinical relevance of changes in drug disposition brought about by anaesthesia and surgery are evaluated.

Changes in gastric emptying

Following oral administration of a drug, its rate of absorption is largely dependent upon the gastric emptying rate. A delay in gastric emptying would increase the lag-time between dosing and the drug appearing in the blood and also delay the time at which peak blood concentrations occurred. In healthy volunteers, the peak plasma concentration of lignocaine occurs between ½ and 1 h after oral dosing, whereas in patients undergoing laparoscopy the peak concentration is seen at 3 h (Adjepon-Yamoah, Scott and Prescott, 1973). However, this change may be quite unrelated to the effect of anaesthesia or surgery since in this study atropine, which would have slowed gastric emptying, was used as premedication. Although the patients did not all receive an identical anaesthetic regimen, with only half being administered halothane, its omission was shown to have no influence on lignocaine absorption.

It is well recognized that gastric and intestinal motility may be decreased for a few days after abdominal surgery (Devine, 1946; Kock, 1963) and may also be decreased after trauma not directly involving the gut (Howard, 1955). In addition, both premedication and postoperative analgesia regimens usually contain opiates which will decrease gastrointestinal motility irrespective of their route of administration. It has been suggested that 1 d after elective cholecystectomy, postoperative opioid analgesia is a more important factor in delaying gastric emptying than the operation itself (Ingram and Sheiner, 1981).

Nimmo *et al.* (1978) investigated the effects on gastric emptying of a number of analgesic regimens following hysterectomy. They studied 21 patients. Fourteen received extradural analgesia with bupivacaine; 8 of these patients received intramuscular diamorphine in addition. A further group of 7 patients received intramuscular diamorphine alone. All had a decreased gastric emptying rate 1 d postoperatively when compared with the 7th postoperative day. The decrease was greatest in those patients who received diamorphine alone.

These authors conclude that patients receiving extradural analgesia as opposed to diamorphine alone may, because of a lesser disturbance of gastric function, experience less nausea and vomiting and commence oral food and drug intake sooner. They provided no data to support this view and thus the clinical significance of their findings is unclear. Indeed, the literature appears to contain no data showing an alteration in the pharmacological effect of an orally dosed drug when administered together with an opiate.

Changes in blood flow

Most general anaesthetics are cardiac depressants and thus may lower the cardiac output and both hepatic and renal blood flow. Anaesthetic-induced changes in hepatic blood flow are of pharmacokinetic importance for many drugs. Hepatic blood flow during an operation may be lowered in man by up to 50% by halothane (Epstein *et al.,* 1968), cyclopropane (Levy *et al.,* 1961; Price *et al.,* 1965) and methoxyflurane (Libonati *et al.,* 1973). For certain co-administered drugs whose removal from the circulation is related to the magnitude of hepatic blood flow, this might result in an increase in their blood concentration with a risk of resultant toxicity. Although most anaesthetics alter hepatic perfusion indirectly by an effect on the heart, nitrous oxide anaesthesia in dogs causes a dose-dependent decrease in hepatic arterial blood flow without causing any significant change in cardiac output (Thomson *et al.,* 1982). A similar haemodynamic response has been seen in man with high spinal anaesthesia with lignocaine (Kennedy *et al.,* 1970).

In sheep, high spinal anaesthesia with amethocaine with fluid preloading, as opposed to general anaesthesia with thiopentone and halothane (1.5%), has recently been found to cause no significant changes in cardiac output, hepatic and renal blood flows or in the elimination of a number of marker compounds (Mather, Runciman and Ilsley, 1982). However, spinal anaesthesia without fluid preloading may be accompanied by decreases in both hepatic and renal blood flow (Bonica, 1978). Any intraoperative decrease in hepatic blood flow may be further accentuated by artificial ventilation (Prys-Roberts *et al.,* 1967; Cooperman, Warden and Price, 1968), but the extent of this change may be lessened if there is an accompanying fall in the $PaCO_2$, which causes a fall in the splanchnic vascular resistance.

The nature of the operation, however, may be of greater influence on blood flow than the anaesthetic agent used. Using the same halothane regimen in two groups of patients, hepatic blood flow was decreased to a far greater extent by abdominal surgery than by non-abdominal surgery (Gelman, 1976). Although hepatic perfusion may fall during an operation with a general anaesthetic, postoperatively it may increase (Wicklund, 1975; Austin, Stapleton and Mather, 1981). This rise may in part be related to the increase in plasma adrenaline concentration seen in the immediate postoperative period (Halter, Pflug and Porte, 1977; Nistrup Madsen *et al.*, 1978). It may be significant that none of the patients in the study of Wicklund (1975) received halothane, since this agent has been shown to lower adrenaline secretion both *in vitro* and *in vivo* (Roizen *et al.*, 1974; Halter, Pflug and Porte, 1977).

The factors influencing changes in hepatic and renal blood flow during an operation are numerous, with the degree and even direction of change being somewhat unpredictable, as may be the extent of any accompanying alterations in drug metabolism or effect.

Changes in drug distribution

Perioperative changes in the perfusion of some vascular beds, together with any fluid volume changes, might alter the distribution of drugs within the body.

Following normovolaemic haemodilution with dextran 40, Schuh (1981) found the neuromuscular blocking drugs suxamethonium, pancuronium and tubocurarine to have greater potency. This shift of the dose–response curve to the left might be explained by a decrease in blood viscosity with an improvement in blood flow to skeletal muscle or a decrease in serum protein concentration, resulting in increase in the free concentration of drug.

The total body water volume may be estimated from measurement of the volume of distribution of antipyrine and the plasma (and blood) volume measured by determining the volume of distribution of indocyanine green. Provided that there is no significant blood loss during an operation, there is little evidence that either of these physiological volumes are altered by anaesthesia or surgery (*Table 4.1*). The clinical significance of these findings is that modification of the loading doses of many drugs administered in the perioperative period is probably unnecessary.

Table 4.1. Body fluid volumes – the effect of a surgical operation

Physiological compartment	*N*	*Volume* (l) ± *s.d.* Preoperative	Postoperative
Total body water (antipyrine volume of distribution*)	11	38.7 ± 14.3	37.9 ± 5.5
Blood volume (from indocyanine green volume of distribution)†	8	3.5 ± 0.4	3.5 ± 0.6

* Elfström (1978) (Antipyrine dose 10 mg/kg; weight of subjects not given and for calculation of $V_{d\,extrap}$ was assumed to be 70 kg).

† Austin, Stapleton and Mather (1981).

Changes in hepatic drug metabolism

As a preliminary to describing the effect of anaesthesia and operation on drug metabolism, a brief description of factors influencing drug metabolism is necessary.

The main organ involved in drug metabolism is the liver. The capacity of the liver to clear drugs from the circulation depends upon (a) the intrinsic activity of the drug metabolizing enzymes, (b) the hepatic blood flow, and (c) the extent of drug binding to blood constituents.

One pharmacokinetic measurement that reflects the ability of an organ to remove a drug from the systemic circulation is the blood (or plasma) clearance of that drug. This is the volume of blood (or plasma) from which the drug is removed irreversibly in unit time. In concept, it is no different from the assessment of renal function by the measurement of creatinine clearance.

Drugs that are eliminated by the liver may be divided into two groups depending upon the fraction of drug that is removed during a single passage of blood through this organ. This fraction is termed the extraction ratio and is high (>0.7) for drugs whose clearance is primarily dependent upon hepatic blood flow (flow limited) and low (<0.3) for drugs whose hepatic clearance is mostly dependent upon hepatic enzyme function (function limited). Examples of these two classes of drug are shown in *Table 4.2*.

Table 4.2. Examples of drugs with high or low extraction ratios

High extraction ratio ($E_H \geq 0.7$)* 'Flow limited' drugs	*Low extraction ratio* ($E_H \leq 0.3$) 'Function limited' drugs
Pethidine	Phenytoin
Morphine	Benzodiazepines
Althesin	Thiopentone
Lignocaine	Warfarin
Propranolol	

* E_H = hepatic extraction ratio.

The extent of drug–protein binding further influences the hepatic clearance of function-limited drugs. Following parenteral administration, the clearance of these compounds is related to the unbound (free) drug blood concentration, whereas the clearance of flow-limited drugs is related to the total (free plus bound) concentration. The plasma proteins to which drugs bind mainly are albumin and α_1 acid glycoprotein. The concentration of both of these proteins may be changed by surgery, with associated changes in the fraction of the drug which is unbound.

In addition to lowering hepatic blood flow, general anaesthetics may also decrease the activity of enzymes responsible for the metabolism of a wide range of substrates (Pessayre *et al.*, 1978; Stacey, Priestly and Hall, 1978; Sear and McGivan, 1979; Da Rocha-Reis and Hipolito-Reis, 1982). A prediction of the change in the kinetics and thus possibly the dynamics of a hepatically eliminated drug may thus be made from the known effects of anaesthesia and surgery upon the physiological variables of hepatic blood flow, hepatic function and drug–protein binding (*Table 4.3*).

Table 4.3. Factors affecting hepatic total drug clearance

Physiological changes	*Changes in clearance* Low E_H drugs	High E_H drugs
↓ Hepatic blood flow	⟷	↓
↓ Hepatic 'function'	↓	↓
↓ Drug–protein binding	↑	⟷
↑ Drug–protein binding	↓	⟷

The effect of surgery on the plasma clearance of antipyrine ($E_H = 0.03$) has been studied by Pessayre *et al.* (1978). Antipyrine was administered on three occasions: before surgery and both 3 and 6 d after surgery. A summary of the findings of this study is shown in *Figure 4.1*. However, one difficulty of interpreting these findings is due to the heterogeneity of the patients studied, as is demonstrated by the clinical details shown in *Table 4.4*.

Pessayre *et al.* (1978) found that the longer the operation, the greater the inhibitory effect on hepatic function. This had also been demonstrated by Geller and Tagnon (1950). In this earlier study, bromosulphthalein retention tests were performed pre- and postoperatively in 20 patients undergoing major abdominal surgery. Five patients had operations lasting 2 h or less and in these the mean percentage bromsulphthalein retention

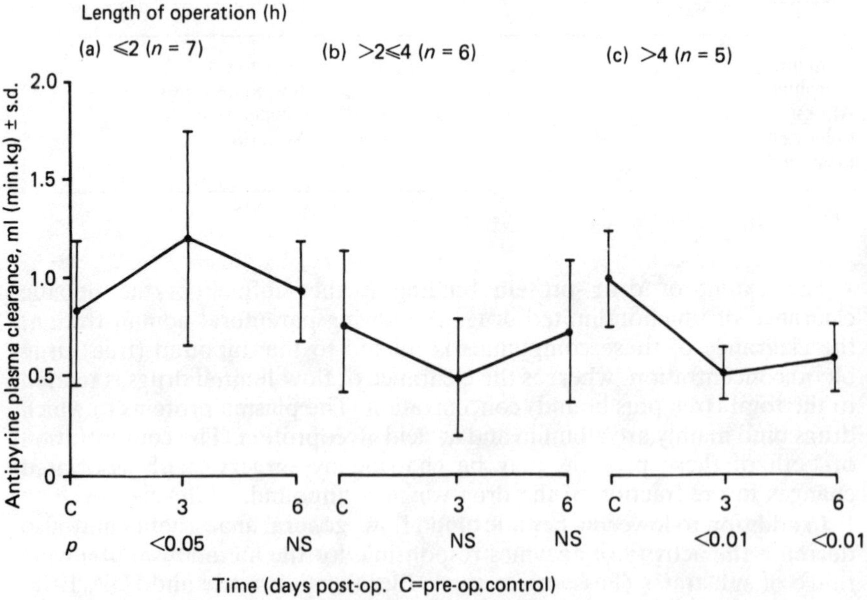

Figure 4.1. Changes in antipyrine clearance caused by surgery under general anaesthesia (After Pessayre *et al.*, 1978)

Table 4.4. Clinical details of the patients studied by Pessayre *et al.* (1978)

Clinical details	*No. of patients*
Abdominal operation	17
Arthrodesis of ankle fracture	1
Identical procedure performed (cholecystectomy)	4
Identical anaesthetic regimen	2
Intravenous infusion	15
Duration of i.v. infusion:	
6 d	8
2 d	1
1 d	6

increased from 5 to 15, whereas in 5 patients whose operations lasted 4 h or more the mean percentage retention increased from 6 to 29. As in the study of Pessayre *et al.* (1978) there was great diversity in both the types of operation and the anaesthetic regimens. Tagnon, Robbins and Nichols (1948) also showed that the longer an operation, the greater the likelihood of an abnormal bromosulphthalein retention test. Pessayre *et al.* (1978) have suggested that their results might be explained by short operations having little depressant effect on drug metabolism, thus permitting the inducing effect of drugs administered perioperatively to be detected. Long operations, by means not understood, but possibly related to the length of exposure to general anaesthetic drugs, might more than counteract the induction of hepatic drug-metabolizing enzymes and have an inhibitory effect. Other workers have also shown that antipyrine clearance may be increased after operations that were probably of mostly short duration and their findings are compared with those of Pessayre *et al.* (1978) in *Table 4.5*.

Postoperatively patients, particularly those on an intensive care unit, may receive a large number of drugs many of which could alter hepatic drug-metabolizing ability. This possibility was examined by Reitbrock *et al.* (1981), who measured hexobarbitone plasma clearance at various times after admission of patients to an intensive care unit after surgery. Hexobarbitone was used as a model drug in this instance because, like antipyrine, it has a low hepatic extraction ratio, is extensively metabolized by the liver and is an indicator of hepatic oxidative drug metabolizing activity. Three different groups of patients were given hexobarbitone intravenously. The resulting plasma hexobarbitone clearance data are shown in *Figure 4.2* and compared with a control group who were otherwise healthy, not operated upon and not receiving other drugs. Although Reitbrock *et al.* (1981) have shown that there were statistically significant differences between hexobarbital clearances for the groups studied, the variability in the data is such that the clinical relevance of these findings is questionable. Furthermore, the nature of the control group makes comparisons between it and the treatment groups somewhat difficult. One explanation offered for the increased hexobarbitone clearance in the longer stay patients was that these groups had received multiple drug treatments that may have induced hepatic drug-metabolizing

Table 4.5. Changes in antipyrine clearance postoperatively

Authors	*Anaesthetic agents*	*Length of operation* (h)	*N*	*Mean antipyrine clearance** (ml/min/kg ± s.e.m.) Preoperatively	Postoperatively	*Mean* Δ% *clearance*	*Postoperative day of 2nd antipyrine clearance estimation*
Pessayre *et al*. (1978)	Various†	⩽2	7	0.83 ± 0.36‡	1.21 ± 0.53‡	+48	3
		>4	5	0.98 ± 0.22‡	0.52 ± 0.12‡	−47	
Duvaldestin *et al*. (1981)	Halothane	Not stated	25	0.85 ± 0.05	1.02 ± 0.07	+20	4–8
	NLA§	Not stated	29	0.67 ± 0.05	0.78 ± 0.05	+16	
Nimmo, Thompson and Prescott (1981)	Halothane	<2	5	0.51 ± 0.06	0.73 ± 0.13	+43	7

* All differences between pre- and postoperative antipyrine clearance were significant at $p < 0.05$.
† The drugs used for anaesthesia with numbers of patients receiving them were: alfadolone, 3; droperidol, 7; fentanyl, 9; gallamine, 1; halothane, 4; nitrous oxide, 2; pancuronium, 9; phenobarbitone, 3; succinylcholine, 9; thiopentone, 9.
‡ Standard deviation.
§ NLA = neuroleptanaesthesia.

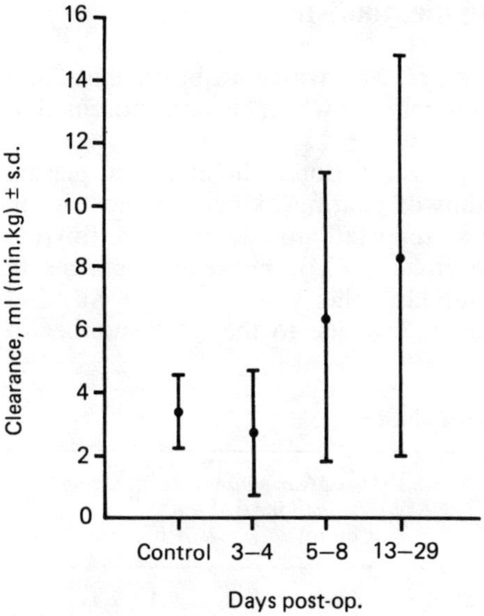

Figure 4.2. Hexobarbitone clearance in postoperative patients on an intensive care unit (After Reitbrock *et al.*, 1981)

enzymes. However, fever is also recognized as increasing the clearance of some drugs (Ballard, 1974; Elin, Vessell and Wolff, 1975; Trenholme *et al.*, 1976), and increased hexobarbitone clearance in the study of Reitbrock *et al.* (1981) was always associated with the presence of septicaemia. Postoperative changes in arterial oxygen tension may also alter drug metabolism, and Cumming (1976) has suggested that antipyrine half-life increases when the arterial oxygen tension falls below 50 mm Hg (6.8 kPa).

There are many animal studies which examine the effect of anaesthetics on drug metabolism, but most however are of uncertain relevance as regard to man. In the intact rat, a progressive increase in the aminopyrine elimination half-life was found when these animals were exposed to increasing concentrations of halothane (Wood and Wood, 1982) and a decrease in hepatic microsomal aminopyrine demethylase activity has also been found after rats were exposed to enflurane (Da Rocha-Reis and Hipolito-Reis, 1982). The mechanisms of these effects are unknown, but might be related to decreases in hepatic microsomal cytochrome concentration, as was found in rats exposed to halothane (Ross and Cardell, 1978). A more recent animal study which may be of clinical relevance is that of Mather, Runciman and Ilsley (1982). Using intact sheep, they demonstrated that general anaesthesia with thiopentone and halothane not only decreased the cardiac output and blood flow to the liver and kidney, but also decreased the metabolic capabilities of the vital organs as shown by lower extraction ratios of a number of marker drugs. Spinal anaesthesia with amethocaine after fluid preloading was without effect on either blood flow or extraction ratios. The minimal effect of spinal as compared with general anaesthesia on hepatic function in humans was recognized some time ago (Schmidt, Unruh and Chesky, 1942).

Effect of surgical stress on drug metabolism

The stress response to surgery consists of cardiovascular, biochemical and hormonal changes (Savege, 1978), a number of which have the potential to alter hepatic drug metabolism.

One hormonal component of the stress reaction is the increased plasma concentrations of cortisol. It was thus of pharmacokinetic interest when hydrocortisone administration was reported to decrease antipyrine elimination half-life (Breckenridge *et al.*, 1973). However, changes in antipyrine kinetics have not been found by other workers (*Table 4.6*), but the statistical power of these studies is low due to the small number of subjects.

Table 4.6. Effects of hydrocortisone on antipyrine kinetics

Authors	*N*	*Mean antipyrine elimination half-life* (h ± s.d.)	
		Control	+ hydrocortisone
Breckenridge *et al.* (1973)	5	16.0 ± 3.1	9.3 ± 2.4
		Antipyrine plasma clearance (ml/min) ± s.d.	
Flanagan and Richens (1974)*	4	52.0 ± 15.1	59.5 ± 9.4
Shiveley *et al.* (1978)	4	50.2 ± 13.9	48.5 ± 14.2
Elfström and Lindgren (1978):*			
3 d pre-dosing with hydrocortisone	9	44.1 ± 10.9	46.6 ± 10.2
Immediate effect of hydrocortisone	5	45.3 ± 10.6	43.9 ± 8.9

* Clearance values derived from the quoted volume of distribution and elimination half-life measurements. In the case of Elfström and Lindgren (1978), body weight for each subject was assumed to be 70 kg.

The elimination half-life of a drug as measured by Breckenridge *et al.* (1973) is a dependent kinetic variable, its value being influenced by both the clearance and the volume of distribution of the drug. The blood or plasma clearance of a drug rather than the elimination half-life is now recognized as being the pharmacokinetic measurement that reflects the drug-removing capacity of the eliminating organ. In addition to the data in adults showing a lack of effect of hydrocortisone on antipyrine clearance (*Table 4.6*), neither dexamethasone nor ACTH, when given for up to 4 d, altered the clearance, half-life or apparent volume of distribution of antipyrine in children (Saenger, Rifkind and Pareira, 1978).

Changes in drug–protein binding

The changes in the concentration of albumin and α_1 acid glycoprotein that occur postoperatively may temporarily alter the free concentration of drugs, with potential alterations of their pharmacological effect (*Table 4.7*).

In patients undergoing thyroidectomy, propranolol protein binding increased by 5% postoperatively and the free fraction fell by 30% (Feely *et al.*, 1980). However, the total (free plus bound) plasma concentration of propranolol rose by over 200% and despite the free *fraction* falling, the free plasma *concentration* of propranolol also rose significantly. These disproportionate changes in total and free plasma propranolol concentrations suggest that the effect of anaesthesia and surgery on the hepatic elimination of this drug are greater than changes in protein binding.

None of the studies describing the protein binding changes shown in *Table 4.7* reported whether or not there were altered pharmacodynamic effects of therapy and therefore, although the findings are of scientific interest, their clinical importance is unknown.

Table 4.7. Drug–protein binding perioperatively

Drug	*Binding protein*	*N*	*Mean percentage of drug–protein bound* Preoperatively	Postoperatively (24–96 h)
Phenytoin*	Albumin	9	87.5	86.2
Quinidine*	α_1 acid glycoprotein	9	78.5	87.5
Propranolol†	α_1 acid glycoprotein	30	85.2	89.6

* Fremstad *et al.* (1976).
† Feely *et al.* (1980).

Free fatty acid plasma concentrations may rise after trauma (Birke, Carlson and Liljedahl, 1965) and it has been suggested that in patients with pre-existing hypoalbuminaemia the rise may be sufficient to cause displacement of phenytoin from its albumin binding sites (Elfström, 1977). As with propranolol, these findings are of unknown clinical relevance, however, since no pharmacodynamic data were given.

Changes in other factors affecting drug metabolism

A variety of other factors may alter the pharmacokinetics of drugs in the perioperative period, but as with much of the data already discussed the clinical implications of these changes are largely unknown.

Temperature

The hepatic blood flow, hepatic enzyme activity, renal blood flow and glomerular filtration rate all decrease during hypothermia and, together with changes in the physicochemical properties of drugs induced by variations in temperature, may cause altered drug kinetics and action. The effect of temperature changes on pharmacokinetics has been reviewed by Ballard (1974).

Drug metabolism by the liver may be decreased during both hypothermia and pyrexia (Elin, Vessell and Wolff, 1975; Trenholme *et al.*, 1976; Kadar, Tang and Conn, 1982). A temperature rise of just under 2°C, such as might be seen in a patient with a postoperative infection, lowered antipyrine clearance by 16% and prolonged the elimination half-life by

29% (Elin, Vessell and Wolff, 1975). However, this degree of change in the activity of hepatic drug-metabolizing enzymes is unlikely to require changes in the dosages of most drugs.

Much of the work concerning the effect of hypothermia on the kinetics and pharmacodynamics of drugs has been performed in animals, and caution is needed in the extrapolation of such animal data to man. Low core temperatures decreased the clearance of tubocurarine in cats (Ham *et al.*, 1978), but no such changes were found in hypothermic humans (Ham *et al.*, 1981). Although, in the cat, hypothermia decreased the sensitivity of the neuromuscular junction to tubocurarine, this was not seen in man, where the only pharmacodynamic change was a delay in the onset of paralysis (Ham *et al.*, 1978, 1981), possibly due to a decreased blood flow and thus rate of drug delivery to the muscles.

Alterations in acid–base status

For drugs whose pK_a is close to physiological pH, slight changes in acid–base balance might alter their degree of ionization and thus their distribution and clinical effect.

The uptake of the weak base fentanyl into the brain was slower but more extensive after injection into hypocapnic dogs as compared with those that were normo- or hypercapnic (Ainslie, Eisele and Corkill, 1979). This might be because the lowered arterial carbon dioxide tension caused a decrease in cerebral perfusion, but at the same time increased the un-ionized fraction of the drug in the blood. Thus, more drug was potentially available to cross the blood–brain barrier, but it was delivered there more slowly.

The elimination half-lives from brain of both fentanyl and another weak base, morphine, were prolonged in hypercapnic dogs as compared with those dogs with normal blood gas tensions (Finck *et al.*, 1977; Ainslie, Eisele and Corkill, 1979). In both instances this may have been due to the phenomenon of ion trapping. In a more acidic environment, such as might exist intracellularly in the hypercapnic dogs, both of these drugs will be more extensively ionized with resultant lowering of their lipid solubility, thus rendering them less able to leave the brain cells.

Respiratory depression is a well-recognized adverse effect of many strong analgesics, most of which are basic drugs with pK_a values close to physiological pH. Drugs such as fentanyl and morphine have a depressant effect on the respiratory centre and thus indirectly prolong their elimination from brain. These factors might also account for the clinical observation that patients with chronic lung disease are more sensitive to morphine than those with normal lung function.

Conclusions

There is much evidence showing that the three main physiological determinants of a drug's kinetics, namely blood flow, drug-metabolizing enzyme activity and plasma drug–protein binding, are altered by anaesthesia and surgery during and for some time after an operation.

There is a paucity of information as to whether these kinetic changes are clinically relevant. This stems in part from research being directed mainly towards measuring drug concentrations, rather than first identifying a clinical problem concerning the use of a drug and then trying to solve it in the laboratory.

Controlled studies, however, are very difficult to perform and it is not easy to determine whether clinical deterioration is due to the adverse effects or lack of effect of a drug or to the underlying disease. The animal work of Mather, Runciman and Ilsley (1982) is interesting in that it shows the great difference in both the metabolic and cardiovascular effects between a spinal and general anaesthetic, and their findings might well have clinical implications for patients, especially those with diseases of the heart, liver or kidneys.

Postoperatively, analgesics probably are administered more frequently than other groups of drugs, yet they are rarely cited as the cause of death in surveys of deaths associated with anaesthesia (Harrison, 1978; Hovi-Viander, 1980). This does not imply that opiate analgesics are not a cause of morbidity. Recording postoperative adverse drug reactions might reveal a pattern that could give a clinical basis for any subsequent scientific investigation.

The few investigations reported in the literature of an altered drug effect caused by anaesthesia or surgery may indeed be a true reflection of the situation. It is possible that there is no significant clinical problem. Indeed, Hovi-Viander (1980) reported that 72% of all deaths associated with anaesthesia were due to the primary disease. Furthermore, the normally cautious drug manufacturers make scant mention of adverse effects resulting from altered drug metabolism caused by general anaesthetics (ABPI, 1984).

For many drugs, the degree of change of a pharmacokinetic parameter would have to be at least 50% before one might see an altered drug effect. A summary of the percentage changes in the postoperative plasma clearances of a number of marker drugs is shown in *Table 4.8*. All the drugs listed are metabolized by the liver. The lack of change in morphine clearance is of interest, as unlike the other drugs which are oxidatively metabolized (phase 1 metabolism) it undergoes mainly conjugation (phase 2 metabolism). Perhaps anaesthesia and surgery, like liver disease and old age, spare this latter pathway.

One possible reason that the changes in drug kinetics, both intra- and postoperatively, are only infrequently held responsible for adverse clinical effects or lack of efficacy is that such changes are transient. The longer the operation or period on an intensive care unit, the longer lasting is the disturbance of drug elimination (Pessayre *et al.*, 1978; Reitbrock *et al.*, 1981), but in these patients it is not known whether such kinetic disturbances were clinically relevant.

Recommendations that one might make for clinical practice are:

(1) Modify drug dosage and the frequency of dosing according to the underlying disease, rather than anticipated and possibly short-lived changes in drug disposition caused by anaesthesia and surgery.

Table 4.8. Postoperative changes in total drug plasma clearance

Drug	*Hepatic extraction ratio* (high or low)	*Mean Δ% plasma clearance**	*Time of postoperative study*	*General anaesthetic*	
Antipyrine	Low	↑ 48 and ↓ 47	3 and 6 d postoperatively	Various	Pessayre *et al.* (1978)
Antipyrine	Low	↑ 44	7 d postoperatively	Halothane	Nimmo, Thompson and Prescott (1981)
Antipyrine	Low	↑ 16–20	4–8 d postoperatively	Halothane or neuroleptanaesthesia	Duvaldestin *et al.* (1981)
Thiopentone	Low	No change	During operation†	Enflurane	Ghoneim and Van Hamme (1978)
Hexobarbitone	Low	↑ 143	13–29 d† postoperatively	Not stated	Reitbrock *et al.* (1981)
Morphine	Low	No change	3 or 7 d postoperatively	Neuroleptanaesthesia	Dahlstrom *et al.* (1982)
Morphine	Low	No change	§	Fentanyl	Rigg *et al.* (1978)
Indocyanine green	High	↑ 30	8 h postoperatively	Various	Austin, Stapleton and Mather (1981)
Propranolol	High	↓ ‡	1–14 d postoperatively	Fentanyl or halothane	Feely *et al.* (1980)

* Compared with preoperative value.
† Comparisons of clearance made with normal volunteer subjects.
‡ Deduced from the change in steady-state plasma concentrations or propranolol.
§ Precise details not given.

(2) Consider the use of regional anaesthesia in patients who might be at a high risk of complications because of changes in haemodynamics or drug elimination that might be caused by a general anaesthetic.
(3) If a drug is either ineffective or toxic, keep a record of the event and suspect that it might be due to the anaesthetic or surgery.
(4) When conducting studies of the kinetics of a drug, if at all possible, relate these measurements to its therapeutic effect.

References

ABPI (1984). *Data Sheet Compendium.* London; Datapharm Publications

ADJEPON-YAMOAH, K. K., SCOTT, D. B. and PRESCOTT, L. F. (1973). Impaired absorption and metabolism of oral lignocaine in patients undergoing laparoscopy. *British Journal of Anaesthesia,* **45,** 143–147

AINSLIE, S. G., EISELE, J. H. and CORKILL, G. (1979). Fentanyl concentrations in brain and serum during respiratory acid–base changes in the dog. *Anesthesiology,* **51,** 293–297

AUSTIN, K. L., STAPLETON, J. V. and MATHER, L. E. (1981). Pethidine clearance during continuous intravenous infusions in postoperative patients. *British Journal of Clinical Pharmacology,* **11,** 25–30

BALLARD, B. E. (1974). Pharmacokinetics and temperature. *Journal of Pharmaceutical Sciences,* **63,** 1345–1358

BIRKE, G., CARLSON, L. A. and LILJEDAHL, S.-O. (1965). Lipid metabolism and trauma. III. Plasma lipids and lipoproteins in burns. *Acta Medica Scandinavica,* **178,** 337–350

BONICA, J. J. (1978). Hemodynamic changes of local and regional anesthesia. In *Haemodynamic Changes in Anaesthesia,* Proceedings of the Vth European Congress of Anaesthesiology, (3), Paris, pp. 1137–1187

BRECKENRIDGE, A., BURKE, C. W., DAVIES, D. S. and ORME, M. L'E. (1973). Immediate decrease by hydrocortisone of the plasma half-life of antipyrine. *British Journal of Pharmacology,* **47,** 434–436

COOPERMAN, L. H., WARDEN, J. C. and PRICE, H. L. (1968). Splanchnic circulation during nitrous oxide anesthesia and hypocarbia in normal man. *Anesthesiology,* **29,** 254–258

CUMMING, J. F. (1976). The effect of arterial oxygen tension on antipyrine half-time in plasma. *Clinical Pharmacology and Therapeutics,* **19,** 468–471

DAHLSTROM, B., TAMSEN, A., PAALZOW, L. and HARTVIG, P. (1982). Multiple and single-dose kinetics of morphine in patients with post-operative pain. *Acta Anaesthesiologica Scandinavica,* Supplement 74, 44–46

DA ROCHA-REIS, M. G. F. and HIPOLITO-REIS, C. (1982). Effects of the inhalation of enflurane on hepatic microsomal enzymatic activities in the rat. *British Journal of Anaesthesia,* **54,** 97–101

DEVINE, J. (1946). A concept of paralytic ileus: a clinical study. *British Journal of Surgery,* **34,** 159–179

DUVALDESTIN, P., MAZZE, R. I., NIVOCHE, Y. and DESMONTS, J.-M. (1981). Enzyme induction following surgery with halothane and neurolept anaesthesia. *Anesthesia and Analgesia,* **60,** 319–323

ELFSTRÖM, J. (1977). Plasma protein binding of phenytoin after cholecystectomy and neurosurgical operations. *Acta Neurologica Scandinavica,* **55,** 455–464

ELFSTRÖM, J. (1978). Effects of surgery on the pharmacokinetics of phenazone and phenytoin. Linkoping University Medical Dissertations, No.53

ELFSTRÖM, J. and LINDGREN, S. (1978). Metabolism of phenazone in man after hydrocortisone administration. *European Journal of Clinical Pharmacology,* **13,** 69–72

ELIN, R. J., VESSELL, E. S. and WOLFF, S. M. (1975). Effects of etiocholanone-induced fever on plasma antipyrine half-lives and metabolic clearance. *Clinical Pharmacology and Therapeutics,* **17,** 447–457

EPSTEIN, R. M., DEUTSCH, S., COOPERMAN, L. H., CLEMENT, A. J. and PRICE, H. L. (1968). Splanchnic circulation during halothane anaesthesia and hypercapnia in normal man. *Anesthesiology,* **27,** 654–661

FEELY, J., FORREST, A., GUNN, A., HAMILTON, W., STEVENSON, I. and CROOKS, J. (1980). Influence of surgery on plasma propranolol levels and protein binding. *Clinical Pharmacology and Therapeutics,* **28,** 759–764

FINCK, A. D., BERKOWITZ, B. A., HEMPSTEAD, B. S. and NGAI, S. H. (1977). Pharmacokinetics of morphine: effects of hypercarbia on serum and brain morphine concentrations in the dog. *Anaesthesiology,* **47,** 407–410

FLANAGAN, R. J. and RICHENS, A. (1974). The influence of elevated plasma hydrocortisone concentrations on antipyrine metabolism in man. *British Journal of Clinical Pharmacology,* **1,** 409–412

FREMSTAD, D., BERGERUD, K., HAFFNER, J. F. W. and LUNDE, P. K. M. (1976). Increased plasma binding of quinidine after surgery: a preliminary report. *European Journal of Clinical Pharmacology,* **10,** 441–444

GELLER, W. and TAGNON, H. J. (1950). Liver dysfunction following abdominal operations. *Archives of Internal Medicine,* **86,** 908–916

GELMAN, S. I. (1976). Disturbances in hepatic blood flow during anaesthesia and surgery. *Archives of Surgery,* **111,** 881–883

GHONEIM, M. M. and VAN HAMME, M. J. (1978). Pharmacokinetics of thiopentone: effects of enflurane and nitrous oxide anaesthesia and surgery. *British Journal of Anaesthesia,* **50,** 1237–1242

HALTER, J. B., PFLUG, A. E. and PORTE, D. (1977). Mechanism of plasma catecholamine increases during surgical stress in man. *Journal of Clinical Endocrinology and Metabolism,* **45,** 936–944

HAM, J., MILLER, R. D., BENET, L. Z., MATTEO, R. S. and RODERICK, L. L. (1978). Pharmacokinetics and pharmacodynamics of d-tubocurarine during hypothermia in the cat. *Anesthesiology,* **49,** 324–329

HAM, J., STANSKI, D. R., NEWFIELD, P. and MILLER, R. D. (1981). Pharmacokinetics and dynamics of d-tubocurarine during hypothermia in humans. *Anesthesiology,* **55,** 631–635

HARRISON, G. G. (1978). Death attributable to anaesthesia. A 10-year survey (1967–1976). *British Journal of Anaesthesia,* **50,** 1041–1046

HOVI-VIANDER, M. (1980). Death associated with anaesthesia in Finland. *British Journal of Anaesthesia,* **52,** 483–489

HOWARD, J. M. (1955). Studies of the absorption and equilibration of water (deuterium oxide) from the gastrointestinal tract following injury. *Surgery, Gynecology and Obstetrics,* **100,** 69–77

INGRAM, D. M. and SHEINER, H. J. (1981). Postoperative gastric emptying. *British Journal of Surgery,* **68,** 572–576

KADAR, D., TANG, B. K. and CONN, A. W. (1982). The fate of phenobarbitone in children in hypothermia and at normal body temperature. *Canadian Anaesthetists' Society Journal,* **29,** 16–23

KENNEDY, W. F., EVERETT, G. B., COBB, L. A. and ALLEN, G. D. (1970). Simultaneous systemic and hepatic haemodynamic measurements during high spinal anaesthesia in normal man. *Anesthesia and Analgesia,* **49,** 1016–1024

KOCK, N. G. (1963). Studies on intestinal motility during the first few days after partial gastrectomy. I. Response to jejunal feeding. *Acta Chirurgica Scandinavica,* **125,** 241–247

LEVY, M. L., PALAZZI, H. M., NARDI, G. L. and BUNKER, J. P. (1961). Hepatic blood flow variations during surgical anesthesia in man measured by radioactive colloid. *Surgery, Gynecology and Obstetrics,* **112,** 289–294

LIBONATI, M., MALASCH, E., PRICE, H. L., COOPERMAN, L. H., BAUM, S. and HARP, J. R. (1973). Splanchnic circulation in man during methoxyflurane anesthesia. *Anesthesiology,* **38,** 466–472

MATHER, L. E., RUNCIMAN, W. B. and ILSLEY, A. H. (1982). Anesthesia-induced changes in regional blood flow: implications for drug disposition. *Regional Anesthesia,* **7,** S24–S33

NIMMO, W. S., LITTLEWOOD, D. G., SCOTT, D. B. and PRESCOTT, L. F. (1978). Gastric emptying following hysterectomy with extradural analgesia. *British Journal of Anaesthesia,* **50,** 559–561

NIMMO, W. S., THOMPSON, P. G. and PRESCOTT, L. F. (1981). Microsomal enzyme induction after halothane anaesthesia. *British Journal of Clinical Pharmacology,* **12,** 433–434

NISTRUP MADSEN, S., FOG-MOLLER, F., CHRISTIANSEN, C., VESTER-ANDERSEN, T. and ENGQUIST, A. (1978). Cyclic AMP, adrenaline and noradrenaline in plasma during surgery. *British Journal of Surgery,* **65,** 191–193

PESSAYRE, D., ALLEMAND, H., BENOIST, C., AFIFI, F., FRANCOIS, M. and BENHARMON, J.-P. (1978). Effect of surgery under general anaesthesia on antipyrine clearance. *British Journal of Clinical Pharmacology,* **6,** 505–513

PRICE, H. L., DEUTSCH, S., COOPERMAN, L. H., CLEMENT, A. J. and EPSTEIN, R. M. (1965). Splanchnic circulation during cyclopropane anaesthesia in normal man. *Anesthesiology,* **26,** 312–319

PRYS-ROBERTS, C., KELMAN, G. R., GREENBAUM, R. and ROBINSON, R. H. (1967). Circulatory influences of artificial ventilation during nitrous oxide anaesthesia in man. II: Results: the relative influence of mean intrathoracic pressure and arterial carbon dioxide tension. *British Journal of Anaesthesia,* **39,** 533–548

REITBROCK, I., LAZARUS, G., RICHTER, E. and BREIMER, D. D. (1981). Hexobarbitone disposition at different stages of intensive care treatment. *British Journal of Anaesthesia,* **53,** 283–293

RIGG, J. R. A., BROWNE, R. A., DAVIS, C., KHANDELWAL, J. K. and GOLDSMITH, C. H. (1978). Variation in the disposition of morphine after i.m. administration in surgical patients. *British Journal of Anaesthesia,* **50,** 1125–1130

ROIZEN, M. F., MOSS, J., HENRY, D. P. and KOPIN, I. J. (1974). Effects of halothane on plasma catecholamines. *Anesthesiology,* **41,** 432–439

ROSS, W. T. and CARDELL, R. R. (1978). Proliferation of smooth endoplasmic reticulum and induction of microsomal drug-metabolizing enzymes after ether or halothane. *Anesthesiology,* **48,** 325–331

SAENGER, P., RIFKIND, A. B. and PAREIRA, J. (1978). Effect of glucocorticoids and ACTH on antipyrine clearance in children. *Clinical Pharmacology and Therapeutics,* **23,** 692–696

SAVEGE, T. (1978). Reduction or obliteration of reflex responses to surgery. In *Stress Free Anaesthesia* (Wood, C., Ed.), p. 11. London; Royal Society of Medicine

SCHMIDT, C. R., UNRUH, R. T. and CHESKY, V. E. (1942). Clinical studies of liver function. I. The effect of anaesthesia and certain surgical procedures. *American Journal of Surgery,* **57,** 43–50

SCHUH, F. T. (1981). Influence of haemodilution on the potency of neuromuscular blocking drugs. *British Journal of Anaesthesia,* **53,** 263–264

SEAR, J. W. and MCGIVAN, J. D. (1979). Cytotoxicity of i.v. anaesthetic agents on the isolated rat hepatocyte. *British Journal of Anaesthesia,* **51,** 733–739

SHIVELY, C. A., GAGLIARDI, C. L., HARTSHORN, R. D. and VESSELL, E. S. (1978). Failure of hydrocortisone to alter acutely antipyrine disposition. *Clinical Pharmacology and Therapeutics,* **23,** 408–413

STACEY, N. H., PRIESTLY, B. G. and HALL, R. C. (1978). Toxicity of halogenated volatile anesthetics in isolated rat hepatocytes. *Anesthesiology,* **48,** 17–22

TAGNON, H. J., ROBBINS, G. F. and NICHOLS, M. P. (1948). The effect of surgical operations on the bromsulfalein-retention test. *New England Journal of Medicine,* **238,** 556–559

THOMSON, I. A., HUGHES, R. L., FITCH, W. and CAMPBELL, D. (1982). Effects of nitrous oxide on liver haemodynamics and oxygen consumption in the greyhound. *Anaesthesia,* **37,** 548–553

TRENHOLME, G. M., WILLIAMS, R. L., RIECKMANN, K. H., FIRSCHER, H. and CARSON, P. E. (1976). Quinine disposition during malaria and during induced fever. *Clinical Pharmacology and Therapeutics,* **19,** 459–467

WICKLUND, L. (1975). Postoperative hepatic blood flow and its relation to systemic circulation and blood gases during splanchnic blockade and fentanyl anaesthesia. *Acta Anaesthesiologica Scandinavica,* **19,** Supplement 58, 5–28

WOOD, M. and WOOD, A. J. J. (1982). Contrasting effects of inhalation anesthetics on *in vivo* drug metabolism. *Anesthesiology,* **57,** A245

Part II

Fluid requirements

Chapter 5

Fluid and electrolytes

R. G. Clark

Introduction

The maintenance of fluid and electrolyte metabolism is an important aspect of the management of many surgical patients and represents a substantial element of the care and support of body function during acute illness which has contributed greatly to developments in surgical practice over the past 50 years. The beneficial impact of routine intravenous fluid and electrolyte therapy can be seen most readily in the management of acute disease and injury where there may be periods of time when the patient is unable to maintain hydration orally and where there may also be abnormalities in the distribution of fluid within the body. Many important body functions are threatened in the presence of such fluid shifts and inadequate hydration, in particular the circulating volume and renal function.

Prior to the institution of routine intravenous (i.v.) fluid and electrolyte therapy, shock and renal failure were not uncommon in the list of complications which led to fatal outcome in the surgical patient. However, intravenous infusions are not without hazard and their use demands care and supervision in conjunction with a knowledge of the factors which regulate water and electrolyte metabolism. In normal circumstances, the body exercises its control through a series of homeostatic mechanisms which influence intake by their effect on thirst and possibly taste together with regulation of the renal output of water and sodium. The prescription of i.v. fluid bypasses the central control of intake and i.v. fluid therapy must therefore be employed with an understanding of the renal factors involved.

Ultimate survival from any serious disease or injury depends on optimal function of the body cell mass and it is the objective of homeostasis to provide an appropriate environment within the extracellular space to support cell function. A wide range of tolerance is allowed by the influence of homeostatic mechanisms on the renal output of water and electrolytes within which the normal function of the extracellular fluid (ECF) is maintained. The daily renal excretion of water can vary from 600 ml to 10 l or more, while sodium output can range between 1–2 mmol and 400 mmol in the presence of a functionally acceptable ECF volume. This permits a great deal of latitude in intake, especially of water and sodium, which may be one of the reasons why there can be such divergent views on the ideal or proper method of management for many aspects of fluid and electrolyte management. In general terms, the maintenance of fluid and electrolyte metabolism is straightforward in the unstressed patient provided that the infusion regimen delivers fluid of a quantity and quality to enable the homeostatic responses to influence renal function in the normal manner to maintain a functional normal ECF. The difficulties which are encountered in fluid and electrolyte management in clinical practice tend to occur when there is incompatibility between the prescribed intake and the ability of the homeostatic mechanisms to respond normally to physiological stimuli.

Control of extracellular fluid

Between 50% and 60% of the body weight is accounted for by water which is partly dependent on sex (M>F) and age, whereby the body water diminishes with advancing years. The average adult contains between 35 l and 45 l of water which is apportioned between the ECF, compromising fluid in the circulating volume (3 l) with the interstitial fluid (12 l) and the intracellular fluid (ICF) which is a variable body compartment related to heredity, nutritional status and disease, but which is approximately 25 l in normal circumstances (Moore *et al.*, 1963). The composition of the fluids in the extracellular and intracellular spaces differs significantly in many respects – a factor of some importance which determines the distribution of fluid between the various compartments of the body.

The ICF is rich in potassium (150 mmol/l) and poor in sodium (10–12 mmol/l), contains substantial quantities of phosphate, sulphate and protein as anions and is the compartment in which the active processes of metabolism take place. The ECF equilibrates across the capillary membrane between the circulating volume and the interstitial fluid and is rich in sodium (140 mmol/l) and poor in potassium (4–4.5 mmol/l), with chloride as the predominant anion and a smaller component of organic and inorganic anions and protein.

The interstitial fluid performs a supportive function, both physical and physiological, in a medium which is composed of fluid within a mucopolysaccharide ground substance traversed by collagen fibres and applied to the skeleton and tendons. It has a sponge-like character in which the fluid content can vary considerably without large changes in pressure (Auckland and Nicolaysen, 1981).

The ECF is responsible for transport of nutrients and oxygen to the cells and for the movement of metabolites and carbon dioxide with cell products in the reverse direction. It is usually this aspect of ECF function which is most vulnerable in acute disease. It also provides the optimum physicochemical environment for function of the cells by maintaining a constant osmolality, pH and temperature. The volume of the ECF is related directly to the quantity of osmotically active particles within it and, as the sodium cation with its accompanying anions provide about 95% of the osmotic activity of the ECF, the two components of importance in the general care of fluid and electrolyte metabolism are water and sodium.

The means by which homeostatic responses combine to control water and sodium metabolism are complex and ill-understood and there is considerable overlap in the nature of many responses which may represent a fail-safe capability in homeostasis in view of the importance of the ECF to body economy. The afferent side of the homeostatic responses which control the ECF is dependent on a number of sensors which are located within the circulating volume, e.g. osmoreceptors, baroreceptors and volume sensors. The afferent side comprises both neural and humoral elements which function by their control of renal output. The distribution of fluid between the compartments of the body is maintained by physicochemical forces across the capillary and cell membranes. Volume and pressure of the fluid within the interstitial space is controlled by the hydrostatic and colloid osmotic pressures which operate across the capillary membrane and the ICF volume is dependent on the osmotic forces across the cell membrane.

Although hormones such as prolactin, growth hormone and oestrogen have obvious physiological influences by promoting water and sodium retention (Lockett and Roberts, 1963; Murlow and Boyd, 1972) and prostaglandin E_2 can induce antidiuresis (Zusman, 1981), it is likely that they perform merely a background controlling function and are not directly involved in the maintenance of water and sodium homeostasis. There is also experimental evidence of a natriuretic hormone which can induce a natriuresis in animals when the ECF is expanded, although its role in the human is not known (De Wardener and Clarkson, 1982). Adrenergic activity may have a more direct role, there being a rich sympathetic nerve supply to the kidney which can affect directly the glomerular filtration rate by its effect on renal haemodynamics, and it has also been established that α-adrenergic stimulation can depress antidiuretic function by inhibiting AVP release, whereas β-adrenergic stimulation has an antidiuretic effect (Shrier *et al.,* 1977). In addition, there are intrarenal mechanisms independent of neurohumoral control which may influence water and sodium balance to a greater degree than has been appreciated in the past. Glomerular filtration rate is directly dependent on arterial pressure, so that alterations in circulating volume which affect pressure will influence urine volume in conjunction with changes in peritubular capillary pressure.

Two hormones – antidiuretic hormone and aldosterone – have a major physiological role in water and sodium metabolism, although our understanding of their importance in the pathogenesis of abnormalities in clinical practice is less clear in the case of aldosterone. In the mammal, antidiuretic activity is provided by arginine vasopressin (AVP). This is synthesized in the supraoptic nuclei and released from the posterior lobe of the pituitary gland on stimulation of the osmoreceptors by hypertonicity of the plasma (Robertson, Athar and Shelton, 1977). Other stimuli, such as hypovolaemia, hypotension, acute pain, tissue trauma, especially tissue traction, and drugs such as opiates and barbiturates, can also induce an increase in AVP levels independent of plasma osmolality. Arginine vasopressin increases the permeability of the distal convoluted tubule of the kidney to water which decreases urine volume. Below a threshold plasma osmolality of 280 mosmol/l the level of plasma AVP remains low (<0.5 pg/m), enabling the kidney to produce a dilute urine. Above that level the AVP level increases linearly with osmolality, and maximal AVP activity with a high urine concentration can be identified after a 36–48 h fast. A much more immediate and intense AVP response is produced by a sudden decrease in circulating volume of 10–15% or by intense pain (Dunn *et al.*, 1973).

Aldosterone which promotes renal tubular sodium reabsorption and also potassium excretion is secreted by the zona glomerulosa in the adrenal cortex (Fraser *et al.*, 1979). It is sensitive to changes in the concentration of sodium in the plasma, but only to substantial differences of the order of 20 mmol/l. More important is the renin–angiotensin system which is activated by a decrease in circulating volume by releasing renin from the juxtaglomerular apparatus in the kidney, thus initiating the response which stimulates aldosterone synthesis and reduces urinary sodium excretion. By its action on the tubular reabsorption of sodium, aldosterone also affects indirectly water metabolism. Arginine vasopressin and aldosterone are activated by different stimuli, namely changes in plasma osmolality and sodium concentration, but both have greater and more dramatic responses to changes in volume and it is likely that they act in unison. The control of water and sodium equilibrium is not achieved by only one or two of the homeostatic responses, but is the resultant interaction of a large number of factors, principally the intrarenal regulatory mechanisms, catecholamines, AVP and aldosterone.

The state of the body fluids is normally determined by the balance between the intake of fluid and electrolytes and the rate at which they are lost from the body. The average daily intake of 3.0 l water and 100–150 mmol sodium maintains the distribution of fluids and electrolytes within the body at an optimal level and this is compensated by a daily urine loss of 1.5–2.0 l and 95 mmol sodium. The loss of water and sodium by extrarenal routes (1.0 l and 5 mmol Na), principally by evaporation from the skin and to a lesser extent from the lungs, are not under any direct control, but these losses are accommodated for by the influence of the homeostatic mechanisms on the kidney. Any variation in ECF volume or osmolality created by an abnormal intake is corrected by a change in urine volume and sodium excretion, there being a wide range of daily output from 500 ml to 6.0 l and in sodium from 1 mmol to 300–400 ml. Most abnormalities in fluid and electrolyte metabolism arise in clinical practice when intravenous fluid therapy is combined with excessive extrarenal losses in situations such as extensive burns, intestinal fistulae, vomiting and diarrhoea.

Metabolic response to injury

The postoperative state has been described as one of water and sodium retention and it has been a topic of clinical concern for almost 50 years. During the 1930s, a number of groups interested in the technique of i.v. fluid infusion demonstrated that water and sodium equilibrium could be maintained by infusion over many days in the unstressed patient with a wide range of water and sodium intake (Coller, Dick and Maddock, 1936). However, similar regimens infused in the immediate postoperative period were associated with oedema, dilution of plasma and hypoalbuminaemia, constituting a syndrome which became known as 'postoperative nutritional oedema' (Coller *et al.,* 1944). Despite intensive investigation at the time, no adequate reason could be found to explain the altered postoperative circumstances and therefore a policy of water and sodium restriction was advised for the postoperative patient.

Some time later, the studies of Dr F. D. Moore (Moore and Ball, 1952) and many other groups were able to characterize the nature of the response as water and sodium retention in the presence of a hypo-osmolar hyponatraemia with expansion of the ECF and features which suggested increased activity of antidiuretic hormone and aldosterone. These findings provided further support for the concept that the response was an obligatory feature of the postoperative patient and there was good reason to restrict fluids. This view was eventually challenged in the 1960s by evidence which suggested that the altered water and sodium metabolism of the postoperative patient was a physiological response to a deficit which developed in the ECF by translocation of fluid in traumatic oedema and by movement of water and sodium into the cells (Shires and Jackson, 1962). The deficit was estimated to be as high as 30% and it was recommended that large volumes of 'balanced salt' solution should be given during and after operation to compensate. The size of the deficit had been grossly overestimated because the technique employed for measurement was not applicable to the postoperative state (Roth, Lax and Maloney, 1969), and the result of the large volumes of infusate which were employed was that pulmonary and peripheral oedema were again encountered in the postoperative period, particularly in young injured men who were otherwise healthy.

The controversy which surrounded this radical change in approach served to remind us that deficits do occur, although they are much smaller than had originally been suggested. Apart from blood loss, there is translocation of ECF in traumatic oedema which is partly represented in a decrease in plasma volume which may be as much as 10–15% in major abdominal surgery (Williams *et al.,* 1962), insensible water loss by vaporization from exposed viscera and accumulation of intestinal fluid in the gut lumen (Kragelund, 1970). It is unlikely that the total of these deficits amounts to more than 700–1000 ml, which is readily accommodated by the infusion of 1 l of a salt solution intraoperatively in addition to the normal requirements.

Nevertheless, the liberation of the clinician from the constraints of severe restriction of fluids in the postoperative period demonstrated that there were at least two components in the genesis of the original description of the fluid and electrolyte response to injury. The first was an obligatory response associated with an alteration in endocrine status and renal function. This was potentiated by a 'physiological' response related to changes in the distribution of the body fluids which created a small deficit in the functional part of the ECF. Correction of the deficit by intraoperative replacement diminished the intensity of postoperative water and sodium retention and exposed the true nature of its obligatory element, which was much smaller than originally described. The 'art' of postoperative fluid and electrolyte management is therefore to steer a middle course between under-provision, when the risk of postoperative shock and pre-renal uraemia due to impairment of ECF function increases after major surgery, and over-provision, when the antidiuresis and antinatriuresis promotes retention of water and sodium and increases the risk of oedema formation.

Injury and operation are associated with a change in the endocrine environment which may persist for some days after the operation and may be potentiated or prolonged by complications such as ileus, sepsis or excessive extrarenal losses. The circulating levels of AVP (Sinnamtamby *et al.*, 1974; Thomas and Morgan, 1979), aldosterone (Yoshitake *et al.*, 1974) and catecholamines (Christensen *et al.*, 1984) are increased and the stimuli for these changes are to be found in the events associated with operation and trauma. In addition to preoperative dehydration, the effects of injury produce tissue trauma, pain and anxiety, haemorrhagic and evaporative fluid loss and transudation of ECF into areas of traumatic oedema which act as additional stimuli and to which must be added the central effects of therapy such as postoperative analgesia. As a conseqence of the neurohumoral responses to these stimuli, the urinary sodium output and volume are diminished but not in a fixed manner, and increasing intakes of water and sodium will be associated with increases in urine volume and sodium output although not sufficient to avoid an accumulation of water and sodium in the ECF (Tindall and Clark, 1981). Obviously, the method of management before, during and after operation can influence the metabolic response independent of the surgical trauma by its effect on the stimuli which promote water and sodium retention, so that meticulous care in preparation and management in conjunction with a high degree of technical operative skill will reduce the metabolic effects. However, the presence of the traumatic stimulus of surgery will always determine that there will be some reduction in the ability to excrete completely any administered load of water and sodium.

Should the postoperative patient be unable to hydrate orally and be deprived also of i.v. fluids, the ECF will decrease because of the shift in body fluids which have already been described and of continuing insensible losses from the body surface. The renal response to the injury is immediate and dramatic, with a rapid reduction in daily urine volume to 500–800 ml and almost no urinary sodium loss, a response which is much faster than could be created by total fasting without injury. When fluids are given during and after operation, the obligatory aspects of the response persist but are of lesser severity and there remains therefore a phase of antidiuresis and antinatriuresis, although the urine volume and sodium output are higher because of the i.v. fluids. The ultimate effect is the retention of some of the administered fluid and sodium with expansion of the ECF. Approximately 50%infused sodium is retained in the first 2 or 3 days after operation (Cochrane, 1978), and should the metabolic stimuli to promote increased tubular sodium reabsorption be maintained by postoperative complications the total exchangeable sodium may increase by one-third or more. The obligatory antidiuretic phase is of relatively short duration, 24–48 h, but should sodium retention persist there will be a secondary antidiuretic phase to expand the ECF in response to the increase in extracellular sodium to avoid hyperosmolality (Thomas and Morgan, 1979).

Hyponatraemia

All routine infusion regimens of fluid and electrolyte are iso-osmolar on administration, but those which contain 5% dextrose become hypo-osmolar when the dextrose is metabolized and the potential to dilute the ECF is normally corrected by the insensible losses which have a low sodium content and by the effect of the homeostatic mechanisms on the kidney. The limitation placed on renal function by the postoperative state impedes homeostasis, so that hypotonic expansion of the ECF becomes evident with the development of a dilutional hyponatraemia, of a degree dependent upon the quantity of dextrose infused and the renal response to surgery. The usual finding after operation is a modest decrease of serum sodium by 4–6 mmol/l during a 4-day infusion, but if the infusion is prolonged because of a postoperative complication the stage is set for severe dilution and eventual water intoxication in the absence of adequate care and attention.

Hyponatraemia is the most common abnormality found in the serum electrolyte pattern in clinical practice and its incidence has been reported at between 30% and 50% of all abnormalities (Flear and Singh, 1973), about two-thirds emanating from cases in the surgical wards, the majority in postoperative patients. In most surgical cases the hyponatraemia is dilutional in type, where the depressed plasma sodium occurs in association with a decrease in plasma osmolality, an increase in the ECF volume and in exchangeable sodium. The genesis of the dilution is partly iatrogenic, being the result of an intravenous fluid infusion which is iso-osmolar on infusion but becomes hypo-osmolar on metabolism of the dextrose at a time when there is an inhibition of the compensation normally provided by homeostatic mechanisms on renal water and sodium output.

One of the mechanisms which inhibit homeostasis is associated with an alteration in the sensitivity of the osmoregulatory cells in the hypothalamus which are unable to suppress AVP output in the presence of a decrease in plasma osmolality so that the circulating levels of AVP remain inappropriately high for the plasma osmolality and the kidney cannot produce a dilute enough urine to correct the hypo-osmolar state (Shirani *et al.*, 1983). In a patient who has a normal uncomplicated postoperative course, the return to a normal metabolic status occurs within a few days, and the extracellular dilution is of a modest degree and normality is restored on resumption of oral intake by a gradual diuresis and natriuresis. Where the postoperative course is prolonged by a complication which delays restoration of oral intake, the stimuli to maintain elevated levels of AVP persist and the trend to dilution continues with the development of serious hyponatraemia if supervision is inadequate. Osmoregulation, however, is not totally insensitive to changes in osmolality and remains capable of correcting hyperosmolar states by further increasing antidiuretic activity which produces a concentrated urine in response to a high sodium intake (Cochrane, 1978).

A much less common form of hyponatraemia is related to the underlying pathology, especially chronic debilitating diseases such as cardiac failure, infection and liver disease, and is not necessarily associated with intravenous fluid therapy. It is characterized by a decrease in the plasma sodium concentration without a concomitant fall in plasma osmolality (Flear and Singh, 1973). It has been postulated that although the total exchangeable sodium in the body may be unchanged the distribution of sodium between the extracellular and intracellular fluid is altered due to a change in cell membrane potential. The sodium content of the extracellular space decreases as sodium passes into the cell and, as there is no osmotic gradient across the cell membrane, osmotically active components move into the ECF from the cells. This form of hyponatraemia, sometimes known as the sick cell syndrome, is not responsive to manipulation of the water and sodium intake and resolution is possible only after successful treatment of the underlying pathology.

References

AUCKLAND, K. and NICOLAYSEN, G. (1981). Interstitial fluid volume: local regulatory factors. *Physiological Reviews,* **61,** 556–643

CHRISTENSEN, N. J., HILSTED, J., HEGEDUS, L. and MADSBAD, S. (1984). Effects of surgical stress and insulin on cardiovascular function and norepinephrine kinetics. *American Journal of Physiology,* **57,** E29–E34

COCHRANE, J. P. S. (1978). The aldosterone response to surgery and the relationship of this response to postoperative sodium retention. *British Journal of Surgery,* **65,** 744–747

COLLER, F. A., CAMPBELL, K. N., VAUGHAN, H. H. and MOYER, C. (1944). Post operative salt intolerance. *Annals of Surgery,* **119,** 533–542

COLLER, F. A., DICK, V. S. and MADDOCK, W. G. (1936). Maintenance of normal water exchange with intravenous fluid. *Journal of the American Medical Association,* **107,** 1522–1527

DE WARDENER, H. E. and CLARKSON, E. M. (1982). Natriuretic hormone: recent developments. *Clinical Science,* **63,** 415–470

DUNN, F. L., BRENNAN, T. J., NELSON, A. E. and ROBERTSON, G. L. (1973). The role of blood osmolality and volume in regulating vasopressin secretion in the rat. *Journal of Clinical Investigation,* **52,** 3212–3219

FLEAR, C. T. G. and SINGH, C. M. (1973). Hyponatraemia and sick cells. *British Journal of Anaesthesia,* **45,** 976–985

FRASER, R., BROWN, J. J., LEVER, A. F., MASON, P. A. and ROBERTSON, J. I. (1979). Control of aldosterone secretion. *Clinical Science,* **56,** 389–399

KRAGELUND, E. (1970). Changes in apparent ^{3}HOH, ^{82}Br, ^{125}I human albumin and ^{51}Cr red blood cell dilution volumes, before, during and after operation in human subjects. *Annals of Surgery,* **172,** 116–124

LOCKETT, M. F. and ROBERTS, C. M. (1963). Hormonal factors affecting sodium excretion in the rat. *Journal of Physiology,* **167,** 581–590

MOORE, F. D. and BALL, M. R. (1952). *The Metabolic Response to Surgery.* Illinois; Thomas

MOORE, F. D., OLESEN, K. H., MCMURRARY, J. D., PARKER, H. V., BALL, M. R. and BOYDEN, C. M. (1963). *The Body Cell Mass and Its Supporting Environment.* Philadelphia; Saunders

MURLOW, P. J. and BOYD, J. E. (1972). Hormonal effects on water and electrolyte metabolism. In *Clinical Disorders of Fluid and Electrolyte Metabolism* (Maxwell, M. H. and Kleeman, C. R., Eds). New York; McGraw-Hill

ROBERTSON, G. L., ATHAR, R. S. and SHELTON, R. L. (1977). Osmotic control of vasopressin function. In *Disturbance in Body Fluid Osmolality,* pp. 125–148 (Andreoli, T. E., Grantham, J. J. and Rector, E. C., Eds). Maryland; American Physiology Society

ROTH, E., LAX, L. C. and MALONEY, J. V. (1969). Ringer's lactate solution and extracellular fluid volume in the surgical patient. *Annals of Surgery,* **169,** 149–164

SHIRANI, K. Z., VAUGHAN, G. M., ROBERTSON, G. L., PRUITT, B. A., MCMANUS, W. F., STALLINGS, R. S. and MASON, A. D. (1983). Inappropriate vasopressin secretion (SIADH) in burned patients. *Journal of Trauma,* **23,** 217–224

SHIRES, G. T. and JACKSON, D. E. (1962). Post operative salt tolerance. *Annals of Surgery,* **176,** 288–295

SHRIER, R. W., BERL, T., ANDERSON, R. J. and MCDONALD, K. M. (1977). Nonosmolar control of renal water excretion. In *Disturbance in Body Fluid Osmolality,* pp. 149–178 (Andreoli, T. E., Grantham, J. J. and Rector, F. C., Eds). Maryland; American Physiology Society

SINNAMTAMBY, C., EDWARDS, C. R. W., KITAU, M. and IRVING, M. H. (1974). Antidiuretic response to high and conservative fluid regimens in patients undergoing operation. *Surgery, Gynecology and Obstetrics,* **139,** 715–719

THOMAS, T. H. and MORGAN, D. B. (1979). Post surgical hyponatraemia: the role of intravenous fluids and vasopressin. *British Journal of Surgery,* **66,** 540–542

TINDALL, S. F. and CLARK, R. G. (1981). The influence of high and low sodium intake on post operative antidiuresis. *British Journal of Surgery,* **68,** 639–644

WILLIAMS, J. A., GRABLE, E., FRANK, H. A. and FINE, J. (1962). Blood losses and plasma volume shifts during and following major surgical operation. *Annals of Surgery,* **156,** 648–654

YOSHITAKE, T., MIZUNO, A., SAIGUSA, M. and KATO, T. (1974). Relationship of plasma aldosterone concentration to electrolytes and acid-base balance in blood after open cardiac surgery. *Annals of Surgery,* **180,** 203–208

ZUSMAN, R. M. (1981). Prostaglandins and water excretion. *Annual Review of Medicine,* **41,** 359–374

Chapter 6

Fluid requirements in shock

J. A. R. Smith and J. A. Thornton

Introduction

As recently as 1979, 'shock' was defined as 'an abnormal state of the circulation in which cardiac output is reduced enough, that the tissues of the body are damaged for lack of adequate tissue blood flow' (Guyton, 1979). This definition is suitable for the classical low output shock syndrome, readily recognized clinically by the presence of tachycardia, hypotension, skin pallor and clamminess, but overlooks the equally important high output shock, seen in anaphylaxis and the early stages of sepsis. In such patients, the skin is warm, the pulse pressure increased and the degree of systolic hypotension less. Indeed, only the associated features of tachypnoea, pyrexia and toxicity indicate that the patient is gravely ill.

Thus, it is more suitable to define shock as 'a common and ill-defined state in which a reduction in tissue blood flow causes tissue hypoxia and widespread derangement of function' (Tinkler, 1979).

As a result of vasodilatation, shunting and increased capillary permeability, in both septic and anaphylactoid shock, there may be a degree of functional hypovolaemia, so that whatever the primary cause of the shock state, intravenous fluid therapy has an integral role in management. Indeed, only in cardiogenic shock could it be argued that intravenous fluids were contra-indicated, but even here a fluid challenge may be necessary before the aetiology becomes clear.

It must be emphasized that fluid therapy alone is seldom sufficient and must be considered only as part of the overall treatment regimen which will include the specific treatment of the underlying cause, together with pharmacological or mechanical support of the respiratory, renal and cardiovascular systems.

Septic shock

In view of the fact that septic shock is so different from other varieties of the shock syndrome, a brief consideration of the pathophysiology may be helpful. A number of components contribute to the shock state.

Functional hypovolaemia

In the early stages, there is peripheral vasodilatation, increased capillary permeability and the development of arteriovenous shunts. Thus, additional fluid must be infused to maintain the effective circulating blood volume.

Impaired oxygenation

As a result of pulmonary arteriovenous shunting, formation of microthrombi, the action of superoxide radicals, and alveolar collapse secondary to changes in surfactant production, there is ventilation–perfusion imbalance. The net result is impaired oxygenation of pulmonary arterial blood.

These effects are compounded by a shift of the oxyhaemoglobin dissociation curve to the left, because of reduced red cell 2,3-diphosphoglycerate concentrations. The result is an increase in the affinity of haemoglobin for oxygen and reduced delivery of oxygen in the microcirculation.

Toxins and impaired function of the reticulo-endothelial system

Probably the most important of all are the products released by bacteria or freed by bacterial cell death. These toxins have a number of actions, but best understood is the endotoxin released by the death of Gram-negative bacteria and consisting of the polysaccharide moiety of the cell wall. Endotoxin, when free in the systemic circulation, activates complement by the alternate pathway and thus produces activation of the coagulation system, increased capillary permeability (Wardle, 1979) and probably stimulation of sympathetic activity on the peripheral vessels (Fine and Minton, 1966). All these tend to compound the effects noted above.

Endotoxin is released in small amounts into the portal circulation in normal health, but is bound by the α_1 antitrypsin and α_2 macroglobulin. The macroglobule which results is consumed by the reticulo-endothelial system. In all shock states, but especially in septic shock, increased amounts of endotoxin are released, sufficient to overcome the available natural inhibitors. The function of the hypoxic reticulo-endothelial system is impaired, resupply of inhibitors is reduced and free endotoxin is then released into the systemic circulation with distressing results.

Other toxins, such as myocardial depressant factor (Brand and Lefer, 1966) or reticulo-endothelial depressant factor (Blattberg and Levy, 1962) have been investigated but their clinical relevance is far from clear.

Are intravenous fluids necessary?

The stimulus for such a rhetorical question comes from the claim that the major cause of refractoriness to conventional treatment of shock is the elaboration of a myocardial depressant factor. This substance has been shown to be present in the circulation of experimental animals after 3 h, but not after 1 h of haemorrhagic hypotension (Fisher *et al.*, 1973). The experimental protocol used failed to ensure cardiac filling, however, the importance of which has been emphasized (Rothe and Selkurt, 1964). On the other hand, a specific myocardial depressant factor has been purified and shown to depress the function of feline ventricular papillary muscle *in vitro* (Glenn and Lefer, 1970). The substance is believed to arise from the ischaemic pancreas in severe shock (Brand and Lefer, 1966).

Certainly, cardiogenic shock has a mortality second only to that reported for septic shock, so that a common myocardial deficit would be theoretically acceptable and would have significant implications for shock resuscitation.

It seems likely, however, that the lowered cardiac output encountered in some varieties of the shock syndrome reflects a poor venous return (Dudley, 1963) and that adequate cardiac filling is indeed essential (Rothe and Selkurt, 1964). As early as 1941, it was recognized that, in shock, the fluid requirements might be in volumes of up to three or four times the estimated blood volume (Grant and Reeves, 1941; Harkins, 1941) and more recent reports have confirmed this (Hunt, 1972).

In an experimental study of haemorrhagic hypotension in dogs, the myocardium remained tolerant of infused fluids even beyond the point of experimental irreversibility. In the same study, the importance of functional normovolaemia was re-emphasized (Smith and Norman, 1979).

Thus it is clear that, in shock, infusion of fluid often in surprisingly large volumes is an essential *part* of resuscitation. Controversy persists about the volume required and the nature of the fluids to be used.

How may overload be avoided?

It should be axiomatic that fluid overload should be prevented, but in the critically ill patients whose renal function may be impaired and in whom capillary permeability may be increased, the practice is often more difficult than the theory. Furthermore, inappropriate selection of the type of fluid used may induce electrolyte disturbances which compound the fluid problem yet further, e.g. hyponatraemia induced by excessive infusion of isotonic dextrose may affect cell function severely.

Once the clinical signs of fluid overload are present – ankle and sacral oedema, elevation of jugular venous pulse pressure, basal pulmonary crepitations on auscultation and, more rarely, a tender enlarged liver – the situation is already out of hand. The remedy usually proves more difficult in the postoperative period or in the shocked patient because of the altered responses to diuretic therapy, to the infusion of plasma proteins and in both renal and hepatic function in general.

A falling pulse rate in the presence of a blood pressure rising towards normal levels are encouraging signs, but as long ago as 1917 it was concluded 'we have focussed our attention too much on blood pressure' and noted that while the heart and arterial tree might function adequately, the peripheral circulation was deficient (Archibald and McLean, 1917). Recognizing that effective peripheral perfusion is the first priority in management, a number of parameters have been recommended to monitor adequacy without overload.

Urine volume

The renal circulation is relatively protected from the generalized vasoconstriction in shock, at least in the short term (Vatner, 1974). However, reduced output of urine is a frequent finding in shock and acute cortical failure – a serious complication. Before renal cortical necrosis supervenes, the measurement of urine output either hourly or half-hourly provides a simple and effective monitor of peripheral perfusion.

It is customary to aim for an hourly volume of over 40 ml or, more accurately, 1 ml/kg body weight. It must be remembered that where renal dysfunction results in loss of concentration, high volumes of dilute urine may be excreted and unwarranted optimism result.

Central venous pressure

Monitoring of the central venous pressure has become well established in general surgical practice and particularly in the postoperative care of the critically ill patient. It must be remembered that as an absolute measurement it is of no real value and must be considered only in the assessment of response to fluid infusion.

Furthermore, when the patient is supported by positive pressure ventilation, the central venous pressure should be maintained at a higher positive level than in the individual, breathing spontaneously. In sepsis, too, higher levels of central venous pressure are required (e.g. 10–15 cm H_2O) to take account of the vasodilatation and the increased capillary permeability.

Criticisms of central venous pressure monitoring have increased as alternative monitors such as pulmonary wedge pressure have become safer and more widely understood. The major criticism is that central venous pressure monitors right heart function only, and while in surgical practice it is unusual for the left and right ventricles to fail independently, more and more cases are reported in which a normal central venous pressure is associated with inadequate left ventricular function (D. E. Edbrooke, 1984, personal communication).

In younger patients, venospasm may produce significantly high central venous pressure readings which fall in response to infusion, only to rise again when adequate volume replacement is achieved.

Despite the above criticisms, central venous pressure monitoring is adequate for most patients after major surgery, and pulmonary wedge pressure can be reserved for the critically ill and for patients at particular risk of inadequate or excessive infusion, such as after emergency resection of aortic aneurysm.

Pulmonary wedge pressure

Monitoring pulmonary wedge pressure carries the significant advantage of monitoring left ventricular function, but has the additional benefit of allowing measurement of cardiac output by the method of thermodilution, provided the appropriate catheter is used. In the early stages of experience, difficulties may be encountered in passing the flow catheter into the pulmonary bed, but success increases with practice. Furthermore, there is a tendency for the balloon to dislodge and for readings to be less reliable after 48 h or so, but for critically ill patients in the early postoperative period, wedge pressure can prove invaluable.

How much fluid should be infused?

In both septic shock and in shock due to a combination of haemorrhage and trauma, it is now well recognized that it is frequently necessary to infuse fluid, in addition to any requirements for blood transfusion, in volumes up to three times the estimated blood volume (Harkins, 1941; Hunt, 1972). In the postoperative period, however, sufficient volume should be infused to ensure adequate hourly urine output – over 40 ml/h or 1 ml/kg/h – with restoration of normal pulse and blood pressure. A positive central venous pressure of 5 cm H_2O is usually adequate, although in patients on ventilatory support, 10–15 cm H_2O is more realistic. In patients at risk, a pulmonary wedge pressure of 15 mm Hg should be the aim.

Clearly, the above parameters and the clinical state of the patient must be considered together, as no one parameter provides effective monitoring.

What fluid should be infused?

The well-known claim of Shires and his colleagues regarding functional loss of extracellular fluid compartment in severe shock has encouraged the use of crystalloid solutions alone (Shires *et al.*, 1960; Shires *et al.*, 1964). Other workers have failed to reproduce the experimental work described by Shires (Roth, Lax and Maloney, 1969; Shizgal, Lopez and Gutelius, 1972) and have suggested the difference of reported results to be due to inappropriate understanding of the model used.

Greater volumes of Ringer lactate alone are required to maintain a low positive central venous pressure after transfusion, compared with a colloidal solution (Poole *et al.*, 1982), and in a canine shock model, crystalloid alone was associated with higher requirements for volume and a significantly higher incidence of pulmonary overload (Smith and Norman, 1982). Some others have argued that colloids are superior to crystalloid solutions because greater plasma volumes and higher oncotic pressures are achieved, with better pulmonary function as reflected by arterial blood gases, alveolar–arterial oxygen tension gradients and venous admixture (Esrig and Fulton, 1975; Transbaugh, Lewis and Christensen, 1980; Poole *et al.*, 1982). There is a lower mortality, primarily due to better cardiac haemodynamics. These experiments show that smaller volumes of colloid solutions will increase plasma volume more than larger volumes of crystalloids (Esrig and Fulton, 1975; Transbaugh, Lewis and Christensen, 1980; Kohler *et al.*, 1981; Poole *et al.*, 1982).

Smith and Norman (1982) used the canine haemorrhagic shock model to compare the efficacy of various solutions in maintaining a low positive central venous pressure after the reinfusion of shed blood. Each of the colloidal solutions (Dextran 70, Haemaccel or hydroxyethyl starch) produced restoration of oxygen balance more effectively than Ringer lactate alone, but a standard crystalloid–colloid mixture was more effective than either crystalloid or colloid alone. It was concluded that the effects on oxygen debt and oxygen consumption must suggest that the infusion of perfusate is the more effective method of restoring nutritive flow.

However, it does seem likely that the controversy that has persisted about whether crystalloid or colloid is the preferable solution to use in shock resuscitation is very largely artificial and that a combination of crystalloid and colloid will be required to produce not only effective restoration of blood volume but also improvement in regional flow.

In clinical practice, the risk of pulmonary oedema has been confirmed together with an increased incidence of the adult respiratory distress syndrome (Gruber, Sturm and Messmer, 1976).

The use of colloidal solutions – and indeed of albumin – in the resuscitation of shocked patients has been criticized on the basis of cost (although this must be a minor component of intensive care expenditure!) and of the risk of colloid escaping into the interstitial spaces through leaky capillaries and increasing interstitial oedema. There seems little doubt that such a phenomenon may occur, but it is not a common problem in clinical practice. The specific complications of colloidal solutions will be considered later.

Of course, both crystalloid and colloid solutions serve only to restore volume with no improvement in oxygen-carrying capacity. Indeed, in excessive haemodilution, by which is meant to below a haematocrit of 30 (i.e. haemoglobin concentration of 10 g/dl), the cardiac compensation which occurs above haematocrit 30 is insufficient to maintain the delivery of oxygen at tissue level (Bassenge *et al.*, 1972). Furthermore, where the heart is already diseased, the compensation may prove inadequate with less major degrees of dilution (Buckberg and Brazier, 1975).

For these reasons, experimentation into solutions capable of carrying and delivering oxygen without serious side effects in clinical use has been followed with great interest. Recent developments have included fluorocarbons and stroma-free haemoglobin solutions.

The use of blood transfusion should be reserved for the replacement of blood loss of sufficient severity to produce acute cardiovascular decompensation or a haemoglobin of less than 10 g/dl. For the reasons given below, as fresh blood as available should be transfused. Where there are deficiencies of specific blood fractions, these should be replaced individually.

Plasma – most commonly used as HPPF – is used for the resuscitation of severe burns and, less commonly, where shock is due to acute pancreatitis. It has been recommended for hypoalbuminaemia secondary to sepsis, but it is most unlikely that normal levels of albumin can be maintained unless the sepsis, which causes both increases in protein breakdown and reduction in albumin synthesis (Traynor and Hall, 1981), has been drained surgically.

Which colloid should be used?

Using the same canine model described above, no difference could be identified between Dextran 70, the gelatin solution Haemaccel or hydroxyethyl starch (HES), in terms of oxygen availability, consumption or the cardiovascular parameters studied. No comparative clinical studies are available, but experience with the individual colloidal solutions allows a theoretical comparison to be made.

The best known colloidal solutions are the Dextrans, initially developed from research for fluids to treat impaired capillary flow (Gelin and Ingleman, 1961). The solutions of different mean molecular weights had different properties, but the only two now in use are Dextran 70 and Dextran 40. Dextran 40 reduces platelet adhesiveness and improves blood flow (Guest and Bond, 1972), but as its molecular weight is considerably less than albumin's 68 000, its retention in the circulation is limited. On the other hand, Dextran 70 has been recommended for use in shock resuscitation (Gruber and Messmer, 1977) and in controlled haemodilution (Matheson, 1969; Messmer *et al.,* 1969; Carey, 1972). In addition to its effect as a plasma expander, Dextran 70 alters the morphology of fibrin to render it more readily lysed by the fibrinolytic system. An increased risk of haemorrhage has been reported (Hunt, 1972; Solanke, 1968) but more dangerous has been the serious anaphylactoid reactions recorded by a number of authors (Hunt, 1972; Schoning and Koch, 1975). Furthermore, the shelf life of Dextran 70 is limited and thus alternative solutions have been developed.

Hydroxyethyl starch (HES) has had a chequered clinical career, but is reported to have a longer shelf life, a lower incidence of anaphylaxis and to be as effective as Dextran 70 (Thompson *et al.,* 1970). The latter conclusion was shared in our own study (Smith and Norman, 1982), but concern has been expressed at the toxicity of HES (Gruber, 1969; Lindblad, 1970), and the fact that the higher molecular weight fractions of the solution are retained for long periods in the reticulo-endothelial tissues, especially the liver (Takaori, Safar and Galla, 1970). At least 25% of any infused volume will be retained for up to 72 h (Metcalf *et al.,* 1970). Blocking the reticulo-endothelial system, using carbon fragments, reduces the tolerance to experimental shock (Fine, Rutenberg and Schweinburg, 1959) and concern about the toxicity of such solutions has been expressed (Lindblad, 1970).

The relative viscosity of Dextran, HES and infused gelatin is similar (Gruber and Messmer, 1977). Haemaccel has been shown to achieve a similar degree of plasma expansion to Dextran or HES, despite its relatively short half-life of 4–5 h (Boon, 1973; Smith and Norman, 1982). No gelatin molecules are retained longer than 12 d and over 80% is excreted within 2 d (Zekorn, 1969). It is effective in treating hypovolaemia without impairment of hepatic or renal function (Boon, 1973). Haemaccel has no specific antithrombotic effect (Ehrly, 1969) and haemorrhagic complications have not been reported.

The ideal plasma expander has yet to be developed (Goodman and Gilman, 1970), but of those solutions in current use, the gelatin solution Haemaccel comes closest to that perfection (Froeschlin, 1962).

Dangers of blood transfusion

The problems associated with blood transfusion ought to be well recognized, but are not. In addition to the risk of overload shared with any fluid infusion, a number of specific complications exist. Such problems as transmission of disease and major incompatibility are seldom encountered in the western world because of improved screening, but minor incompatibility reactions are not uncommon especially in patients subjected to repeated transfusions. Particulate matter should be filtered, but pyrogens or leucocyte antibodies may still produce a febrile reaction.

The remaining complications relate to the dangers of blood storage. Old red cells haemolyse and release potassium, so that where large volumes are transfused, jaundice of haemolytic type or, more serious, hyperkalaemia may result. Potassium levels greater than 7 mmol/l are toxic to the heart. Alternatively, the use of acid citrate dextrose may produce hypocalcaemia, but it is rare for cardiac or coagulation problems to result, as the levels usually encountered cause tetany as the first symptom.

Storage results in consumption of platelets and the clotting factors, so that if fresh blood is not available, the risks of haemorrhage are increased.

The red cell concentration of 2,3-diphosphoglycerate falls on storage, with a consequent shift of the oxyhaemoglobin dissociation curve to the left. The resulting increase in affinity for oxygen reduces delivery at tissue level.

Thus, it is vitally important that careful consideration and reconsideration be made of the indications for any blood transfusion and that the patient concerned is monitored for the development of any untoward reaction.

Conclusions

Infusion of fluid to maintain a functionally normal blood volume is an essential part of the management of shock, whatever the primary cause may be. However, it should be seen as part only of the overall treatment regimen. Careful and intensive monitoring is essential to avoid fluid overload, but it is equally essential that sufficient volume is administered to ensure adequate tissue perfusion.

There is little point in pursuing the argument of crystalloid versus colloid, as both compounds will be required for most patients. Of the available colloidal solutions, the gelatin Haemaccel is as effective as any other and has a lower incidence of reported side effects. However, the hope for the future is the development of a safer solution capable of transporting and delivering oxygen at tissue level.

References

ARCHIBALD, E. W. and MCLEAN, W. S. (1917). Observations upon shock with particular reference to the condition as seen in war surgery. *Annals of Surgery,* **66,** 280–286

BASSENGE, E., SCHMID-SCHONBEIN, H., VON-RESTORFF, W. and VOLGER, E. (1972). Effects of haemodilution on coronary haemodynamics in conscious dogs. In *Haemodilution. Theoretical Basis and Clinical Application.* Basel; Karger, pp. 174–183

BLATTBERG, B. and LEVY, M. N. (1962). Mechanism of depression of reticulo-endothelial system in shock. *American Journal of Physiology,* **203,** 867–869

BOON, P. E. (1973). Gelatin solutions. In Proceedings of the Australian Society of Blood Transfusion Seminar, pp. 45–52

BRAND, E. D. and LEFER, A. M. (1966). Myocardial depressant factor in plasma from cats in irreversible post-oligaemic shock. *Proceedings of the Society of Experimental Biological Medicine,* **122,** 200–203

BUCKBERG, G. and BRAZIER, J. (1975). Coronary blood flow and cardiac function during haemodilution. In *Intentional Haemodilution. Bibl. Haemat.*, **41,** 173–189. Basel; Karger

CAREY, J. S. (1972). Colloids and crystalloids for volume replacement during and after surgery. In *Haemodilution. Theoretical Basis and Clinical Application.* Basel; Karger, pp. 229–246

DUDLEY, H. A. F.. (1963). Surgical shock and electrolyte balance. In *Recent Advances in the Surgery of Trauma* (Matthews, D. N., Ed.). London; Churchill, pp. 36–45

EHRLY, A. M. (1969). The effect of plasma substitutes on erythrocyte aggregates and blood viscosity. In *Modified Gelatins as Plasma Substitutes. Bibl. Haemat.*, **33,** 302–310. Basel; Karger

ESRIG, B. C. and FULTON, R. L. (1975). Sepsis, resuscitated haemorrhagic shock and 'shock lung' – an experimental correlation. *Surgery, Gynecology and Obstetrics,* **182,** 218

FINE, J. and MINTON, R. (1966). Mechanism of action of bacterial endotoxin. *Nature,* **210,** 97–98

FINE, J., RUTENBURG, S. and SCHWEINBURG, F. B. (1959). The role of the reticulo-endothelial system in haemorrhagic shock. *Journal of Experimental Medicine,* **110,** 547–569

FISHER, W. D., HEIMBACH, D. W., MCARDLE, C. S., MADDERN, M., HUTCHESON, M. M. and LEDINGHAM, I. MCA. (1973). A circulating depressant effect following canine haemorrhagic shock. *British Journal of Surgery,* **60,** 392–394

FROESCHLIN, W. (1962). The treatment of shock with haemaccel – a new plasma volume expander. *Deutsche Medizinische Wochenschrift,* **87,** 811–819

GELIN, L. E. and INGLEMAN, B. (1961). Rheomacrodex – a new dextran solution for rheological treatment of impaired capillary flow. *Acta Chirurgica Scandinavica,* **122,** 294–302

GLENN, T. M. and LEFER, A. M. (1970). Protective effect of thoracic lymph diversion in haemorrhagic shock. *American Journal of Physiology,* **219,** 1305–1310

GOODMAN, L. S. and GILMAN, A. (1970). *The Pharmacological Basis of Therapeutics* (Goodman, L. S. and Gilman, A., Eds). New York; McMillan, p. 629

GRANT, R. T. and REEVES, E. B. (1941). Clinical observations on air raid casualties. *British Medical Journal,* **2,** 293–297; 329–332

GRUBER, U. F. (1969). *Blood Replacement.* Berlin; Springer

GRUBER, U. F. and MESSMER, K. (1977). Colloids for blood volume support. *Proceedings of Surgery,* **15,** 49–76

GRUBER, U. F., STURM, V. and MESSMER, K. (1976). Fluid replacement in shock. In *Shock* (Ledingham, I. McA., Ed.). Amsterdam; Excerpta Medica, pp. 231–256

GUEST, M. M. and BOND, T. P. (1972). Effect of haemodilution on haemostatis and coagulation. In *Haemodilution. Theoretical Basis and Clinical Application.* Basel; Karger, pp. 298–308

GUYTON, A. C. (1979). *Physiology of the Human Body*, 5th edn. Philadelphia; Saunders

HARKINS, H. H. (1941). Recent advances in the study and management of traumatic shock. *Surgery,* **9,** 231–294; 447–482; 607–655

HUNT, A. C. (1972). *Pathology of Injury: Current Knowledge and Future Development* (Hunt, A. C., Ed.). The report of a working party of the Royal College of Pathologists. London; Harvey, Miller and Metcalf Ltd, pp. 53–64

KOHLER, J. P., RICE, C. L., ZARINS, C. K., GAMMACK, B. F. and MOSS, G. S. (1981). Does reduced colloid oncotic pressure increase pulmonary dysfunction in sepsis? *Critical Care Medicine,* **9,** 90

LINDBLAD, G. (1970). The toxicity of hydroxyethyl starch: investigations in mice, rabbits and dogs. *Excerpta Medica Congress*, Series 198, pp. 128–144

MATHESON, N. A. (1969). The micro circulation in shock. *Post-Graduate Medical Journal,* **45,** 530–533

MESSMER, K., BRENDEL, W., SUNDER-PLASSMANN, L. and HOLPER, K. (1969). The use of colloidal solutions for extreme haemodilution. In *Modified Gelatins as Plasma Substitutes. Bibl. Haemat.,* **33,** 261–269. Basel; Karger

METCALF, W., PAPADOPOULOS, A., TUFARO, R. and BARTH, A. (1970). A clinical phsyiological study of hydroxyethyl starch. *Surgery, Gynecology and Obstetrics,* **131,** 255–267

POOLE, G. V., MEREDITH, J. W., PENNELL, T. and MILLS, S. A. (1982). Comparison of colloids and crystalloids in resuscitation from haemorrhagic shock. *Surgery, Gynecology and Obstetrics,* **154,** 577

ROTH, E., LAX, L. C. and MALONEY, J. V. (1969). Ringer lactate solution and extracellular fluid volume in the surgical patient: a critical analysis. *Annals of Surgery,* **169,** 149–164

ROTHE, C. F. and SELKURT, E. E. (1964). Cardiac and peripheral failure in haemorrhagic shock in the dog. *American Journal of Physiology,* **207,** 203–214

SCHONING, B. and KOCH, H. (1975). Pathergiequote vershiedener plasmasubstitute an haut under respirationstrakt orthopadischer patienten. *Anaesthetist,* **24,** 507–516

SHIRES, T., BROWN, F. T., CABIZARO, P. C. and SOMERVILLE, N. (1960). Distributional changes in extracellular fluid during acute haemorrhagic shock. *Surgical Forum,* **11,** 115–117

SHIRES, T., COLN, D., CARRICO, J. and LIGHTFOOT, S. (1964). Fluid therapy in haemorrhagic shock. *Archives of Surgery,* **88,** 688–693

SHIZGAL, H. M., LOPEZ, G. A. and GUTELIUS, J. R. (1972). Effects of experimental haemorrhagic shock on extracellular water volume. *Annals of Surgery,* **176** (6), 736–741

SMITH, J. A. R. and NORMAN, J. N. (1979). Volume infusion in experimental refractory shock. *British Journal of Surgery,* **66,** 80–83

SMITH, J. A. R. and NORMAN, J. N. (1982). The fluid of choice for resuscitation of severe shock. *British Journal of Surgery,* **69,** 702–705

SOLANKE, T. F. (1968). Clinical trial of 6% hydroxyethyl starch (a new plasma expander). *British Medical Journal,* **31,** 783–785

TAKAORI, M., SAFAR, P. and GALLA, S. J. (1970). Changes in body fluid compartments during haemodilution with hydroxyethyl starch and Dextran 40. *Archives of Surgery,* **100,** 263–268

THOMPSON, W. L., FUKUSHIMA, T., RUTHERFORD, R. B. and WALTON, R. P. (1970). Intravascular persistence, tissue storage and excretion of hydroxyethyl starch. *Surgery, Gynecology and Obstetrics,* **131,** 965–972

TINKLER, J. (1979). A pharmacological approach to the treatment of shock. *British Journal of Hospital Medicine,* **21** (3), 261–268

TRANSBAUGH, R. F., LEWIS, F. R., CHRISTENSEN, J. M. and ELINGS, V. B. (1980). Lung water changes after thermal injury: the effect of crystalloid resuscitation and sepsis. *Annals of Surgery,* **192,** 479–490

TRAYNOR, C. and HALL, G. M. (1981). Endocrine and metabolic changes during surgery: anaesthetic implications. *British Journal of Anaesthesia,* **53,** 153

VATNER, S. F. (1974). Effects of haemorrhage on regional blood flow distribution in dogs and primates. *Journal of Clinical Investigation,* **54,** 225–235

WARDLE, N. (1979). Bacteraemia and endotoxic shock. *British Journal of Hospital Medicine,* **21** (3), 223–231

ZEKORN, D. (1969). Intravenous retention, dispersal, excretion and break-down of gelatin solutions. In *Modified Gelatins as Plasma Substitutes. Bibl. Haemat.,* **33,** 131–140. Basel; Karger

Chapter 7

The place of albumin, and nutritional therapy

A. The place of albumin

A. Fleck

Introduction

In recent years the chemistry, biology, metabolism and clinical aspects of albumin have been subject to extensive reviews (Davison, 1976; Rosenoer, Oratz and Rothschild, 1977; Peters and Sjöholm, 1978; Lundsgaard-Hansen, Pappora and Frei, 1981; Schwartzkopff *et al.,* 1981). Albumin is widely used in therapy and more than 10 000 kg were administered in the year 1978 in the USA (Peters and Reed, 1978), and an estimate from a blood products laboratory is that at least 10 000 kg of albumin were infused in 1983 in England and Wales alone. Several preparations suitable for intravenous administration are available (*Table 7.1*) and from the data given it can be calculated that the cost of albumin in these preparations ranges from about £1.45 to £2.00 per gram. It follows that the monetary value of the albumin administered to patients in England and Wales during 1983 was about £17 million.

The concentration of albumin in serum can now be determined simply, quickly and relatively cheaply (Peters, 1979) and perhaps, in consequence, it is frequently measured. Its amino acid composition and sequence are known and much also is known about its structure and chemical properties, although its three-dimensional configuration in space is not yet known. In this section only a few aspects of albumin can be selected for discussion: function or physiological aspects; diagnostic (including prognostic) aspects; and therapeutic aspects.

Physiological aspects

In normal adults albumin is the most abundant plasma protein (*see Figure 7.1* and *Table 7.2*), accounting for more than half the total circulating proteins. Usually, the concentration of albumin in the plasma of a normal adult is about 40 g/l. In contrast, the concentration of the next most abundant protein, IgG, is about 12 g/l and the concentration of fibrinogen is about 3 g/l (Blombäck and Hanson, 1976 – *Table 7.2*).

Table 7.1. Some preparations of albumin for therapeutic use

Product name	*Producer*	*Concentration of albumin* (g/l)	*Concentration of: Sodium* (mmol/l)	*Potassium* (mmol/l)	*Volume of pack* (ml)	*Approximate cost* (£)
Albuminkabi	Kabi Vitrum	200	<120	< 1	100	36
Albuminor	Armour Therapeutic Blood Products	250	130–160	< 1	20, 50, 100	10, –, 50
		200	<130	< 1	50, 100	14, 29
Buminate	Travenol	200	<130	<10	50, 100	18, 34
		50	130–160	< 2	250, 400, 500	21, 32, 40
Human Albumin 20%	Immino	200	<130	< 1	10, 50, 100	4, 19, 37
Plasma Protein Fraction (PPF–4.3%)		43	120–160	< 1	400	32
Salt Poor Albumin	NHS blood products laboratories	200	<140	<10	100	35*
Plasma Protein Fraction (PPF)		45	140–160	< 2	400	35*

* Supplied without charge to NHS; indicated cost is to private hospitals.

Table 7.2. Comparison of the concentration of some proteins in normal human plasma* (after Blombäck and Hanson, 1976)

	Mass concentration (g/l)	*Molar concentration* (μmol/l)
Pre-albumin		
(thyroxine-binding pre-alb.; 54 980)	0.25	4.0
Albumin	40	603
(66 400)	(53% of total)	
α_1-Globulins		
α_1-antitrypsin (54 000)	2.6	48
α_1-acid glycoprotein (41 000)	0.9	21
α_2-Globulins		
ceruloplasmin (151 000)	0.35	2.3
α_2-macroglobulin (752 000)	2.4	3.3
β-Globulins		
transferrin (76 500)	3.0	39
C3 (180 000)	0.82	4.4
γ-Globulins		
IgG (150 000)	12.5	83
IgA (160 000)	2.1	13
IgM (971 000)	1.25	1.3
Fibrinogen (340 000)	3.0	8.8

* This list of plasma proteins is incomplete; more than 90 plasma proteins are known. The proteins are listed in order of their electrophoretic mobility (see *Figure 7.1*). Molecular weights are given in parentheses.

The molecular weight (66 400), size and shape (prolate ellipsoid of revolution with axes 14.1 × 4.2 nm) of albumin (Peters and Reed, 1978), while sufficiently large to prevent significant losses in the urine by glomerular filtration, are such that combined with its high concentration in plasma one of its important functions is in the exchange of fluid in the capillary bed (*Figure 7.2*). The Starling equation for calculating the net transcapillary fluid flow can be simplified by writing the net hydrostatic pressure (i.e. $P_c - P_t$) as ΔP and the net oncotic pressure (i.e. $\pi_p - \pi_t$) as $\Delta\pi$ to obtain $J_c = k_f\ (\Delta P - \sigma\Delta\pi)$, in which J_c represents the net transcapillary flow of fluid and the symbols k_f and σ have the same significance as in *Figure 7.2* (Hargens, 1981). By writing the equation in this way, it is easily appreciated that fluid exchange in the capillary bed depends on the net hydrostatic pressure and on the net oncotic pressure. Since both tissue hydrostatic pressure and tissue oncotic pressure have measurable values, especially the latter, it follows that there is little point in determining either capillary hydrostatic pressure alone or the plasma oncotic pressure alone. The importance of the latter is that there is much evidence that the plasma oncotic pressure can be closely approximated by measuring the plasma albumin concentration (Lundsgaard-Hansen, Pappora and Frei, 1981). It can be seen from the complete equation of *Figure 7.2* that a significant fall in albumin concentration will, inevitably, lead to retention of fluid in the tissues and eventually to oedema. The equation, however, indicates that the relation between albumin concentration and oedema formation is not simple, so that the concentration of albumin at which oedema becomes evident is likely to vary among individuals, which has indeed been observed (Keys *et al.*, 1950).

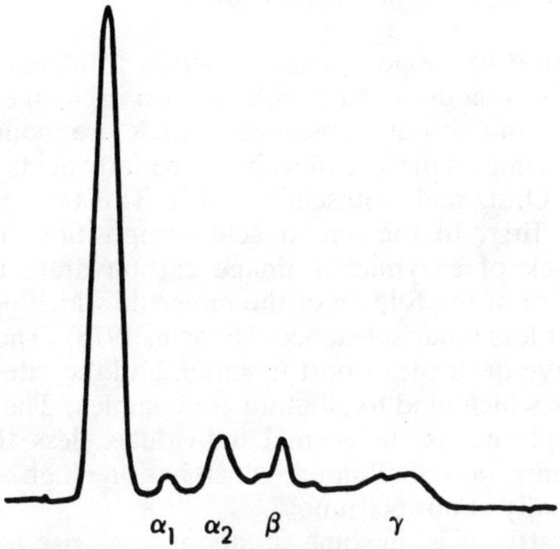

	Albumin	Globulins α1	Globulins α2	Globulins β	Globulins γ
Composition (%)	63.6	3.3	11.2	8.2	13.7
Concentration (g/l)	46.6	2.4	8.2	6.0	10.1

Figure 7.1. Relative concentrations of groups of proteins in plasma. The pattern was obtained by scanning the changes in density of an electrophoretic strip of cellulose acetate membrane on which a small sample of serum from a normal individual had been placed and then subjected to electrophoresis at pH 8.6, 120 V, for 45 min, before being stained with Ponceau S (Varley, *et al.*, 1980)

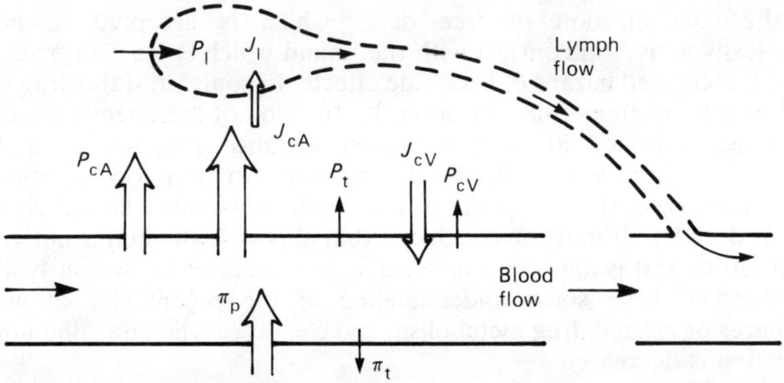

Figure 7.2. Tissue fluid exchange. Representation of the factors influencing the exchange of fluid from the capillaries to the extravascular space and the lymph. The lymph fluid finally returns to the circulating blood via the thoracic duct. The arrows indicate the directions of potential (not actual) fluid flow. The symbols represent the following:

P_c = capillary blood pressure: P_{cA} that at arteriolar end and
P_{cV} that at distal venular end
P_t = tissue fluid pressure
P_l = fluid pressure in tissue lymphatic vessels
π_p = oncotic pressure of plasma protein
π_t = oncotic pressure of protein in tissue spaces
J_l = fluid flow into lymphatics
J_{cA} = potential fluid flow from blood vessels into tissue spaces
J_{cV} = potential fluid flow from tissue spaces into blood

The net capillary fluid transfer (J_c) is obtained from:
$J_c = k_f\{(P_c - P_t) - \sigma_p(\pi_p - \pi_t)\}$ in which k_f is the capillary fluid filtration coefficient and σ_p the capillary membrane reflection coefficient (After Hargens, 1981)

If it were required to assign a single function to albumin it would be 'transport', because in addition to its role in fluid exchange in the tissues, albumin transports numerous substances which are bound to it to a variable extent. Examples include bilirubin, free fatty acids and numerous drugs (Rosenoer, Oratz and Rothschild, 1977). This transport function is probably related, first, to the amino acid composition of the protein, secondly to its lack of enzymically linked carbohydrate molecules and thirdly to the nature of the folding of the molecule which permits binding to it of a variety of less polar substances (Brown, 1978). There is normally considerable reserve of this transport function, and the interactions of the various substances which bind to albumin are complex. The total bilirubin concentration in plasma is, in normal individuals, less than 20 μmol/l, whereas the concentration of albumin, which has one high affinity binding site for it, is normally about 600 μmol/l.

Non-esterified fatty acids, in some situations, may rise to 2 mmol/l, but albumin has six fairly high affinity binding sites for them, so that again there is considerable reserve. However, there is some interaction between the binding of fatty acids and bilirubin, so that high concentrations of the former may reduce the binding of the latter (Brodersen, 1978). Also some drugs, notably sulphonamides, may displace bilirubin from albumin (Sellers and Koch-Weser, 1977). It is clearly possible that when albumin concentration becomes very low (e.g. 20 g/l), combined with jaundice, mobilization of fat and administration of drugs, the binding sites of albumin may become saturated (Sellers and Koch-Weser, 1977). If this occurs the concentration of free drug, which is accepted to be therapeutically active, in contrast with the bound which is inactive, rises, and there is increased hazard of toxic side effects. In contrast, if the drug is excreted mainly by glomerular filtration, its duration of therapeutic effect may be much shortened due to its increased clearance. It is possible that some substances bind less avidly to other proteins for transport, as must have been the case in the rare patients with analbuminaemia who survived for several decades. It must be concluded that although albumin is not an 'essential' protein, it is important in deciding treatment of the seriously ill patient that we have some understanding of the potentially serious consequences of altered drug metabolism and clearance when the albumin concentration is decreased.

Diagnostic aspects

Although it is difficult to think of a satisfactory alternative, the use of the term 'plasma protein' is misleading because few, if any, of the plasma proteins are found only in the plasma of circulating blood. In the case of albumin, more of the total body content is in the extravascular (EV) tissues than in the circulating blood or plasma (P); the ratio EV/P being normally 1.3:1 (Rossing, 1967). This is represented diagrammatically in *Figure 7.3*, in which rounded-off values are given (Rossing, 1967; Ballantyne and Fleck, 1973).

Quantitative aspects of the relationship depicted in *Figure 7.3* can be explored using a simple mathematical method adopted for a digital

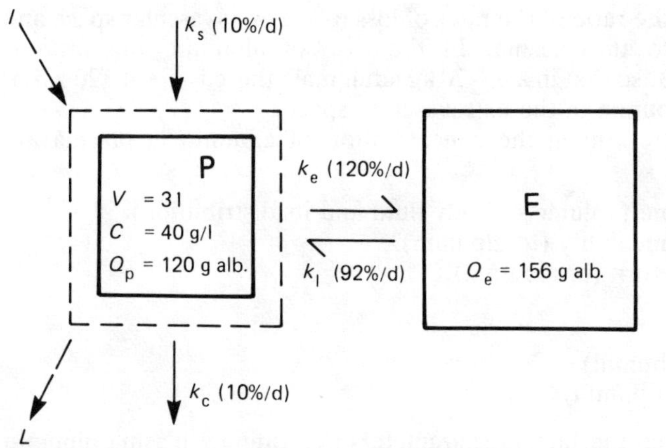

Figure 7.3. Distribution of albumin in the body. The symbols are defined as follows:
P = plasma pool
V = plasma volume ($\simeq$ 3 litres in 70 kg man);
the broken outline indicates that the plasma volume may change rapidly
C = concentration of albumin in plasma ($\simeq$ 40 g/l)
Q_p = quantity of albumin in systemic plasma
$= C \times V (\simeq 120\,g)$
E = extravascular space
Q_e = quantity of albumin in extravascular space ($\simeq$ 156 g)
I = rate of albumin infused intravenously (g/d)
L = rate of albumin lost (e.g. by haemorrhage, in urine, from gut, etc.) (g/d)
k_s = fraction of the intravascular pool (Q_p) of albumin synthesized per day, $\simeq$ 0.1/d or 10%/d
k_c = fraction of the intravascular pool (Q_p) of albumin catabolized per day,
$= k_s \simeq$ 0.1/d or 10%/d
k_e = fractional rate of loss of albumin from the plasma to the extravascular spaces,
= 1.20/d = 120%/d
k_l = fractional rate of return of albumin from the extravascular spaces
to the plasma, = 0.92/d = 92%/d

Note: $k_e \times Q_p = k_l \times Q_e$, i.e. $1.20 \times 120 = 0.92 \times 156 = 144$

computer (Fleck and Clark, 1981; Fleck, 1985). It is also possible to measure most of the factors which determine the concentration of albumin in plasma directly. Plasma volume can be measured in various ways (Wiklander, 1956). Albumin is synthesized by the liver, and the rate of synthesis can be measured using ^{14}C, but the method is tedious (Tavill, Craigie and Rosenoer, 1968). Although the site of catabolism is unknown – it may be the reticulo-endothelial system or a site close to the vascular endothelium (Rossing, Krasilnikoff and Christiansen, 1972) – the rate can be determined using undenatured albumin carefully labelled with radioactive iodine–HISA (McFarlane, 1964). The rate of loss from the body can usually be estimated, including during haemorrhage (Wiklander, 1956), and simple observation gives the rate of intravenous infusion. The rate of loss to the extravascular space can be measured in 1 h as the transvascular escape rate (TER) using radio-iodinated albumin (Rossing, Parving and Lassen, 1976). The rate of lymphatic return (k_l in *Figure 7.3*) of albumin can be determined by calculation in various ways from the data obtained during studies of catabolism using HISA (Fleck, 1984), and the amount of extravascular protein is determined from the ratio k_e/k_l =

Q_e/Q_p, i.e. from the ratio of the rates of loss to the extravascular space and return from it to the plasma. In the case of albumin, the ratio is approximately 1.3, so that in a 65–70 kg adult male there is 1.3 × 120 g, i.e. about 156 g of albumin in the extravascular space.

The factors determining the concentration of albumin in plasma are given below:

(1) Plasma volume (volume of body fluid and its distribution).
(2) Vascular permeability (to albumin).
(3) Lymphatic return (of albumin).
(4) Catabolism.
(5) Synthesis.
(6) Losses (of albumin).
(7) Infusion (of albumin).

The order in which the factors (parameters determining plasma albumin concentration) are given corresponds to the rapidity and magnitude of the effect on albumin concentration induced by sudden change in the parameter (*see* Fleck, 1984). With this background it becomes possible to understand the mechanisms leading to clinically observed changes in albumin concentration, which are frequently misinterpreted.

The concentration of total protein is greater in ambulant than recumbent subjects. This is due to the rapid redistribution of fluid which occurs on changing posture. Plasma protein concentration may change by 15% in 30 min, simply by moving from the erect to the recumbent position (Bohme, 1911).

Any form of injury, trauma or infection is followed by a rapid decrease in albumin concentration, beginning within hours (Myers *et al.*, 1984), to a minimum concentration around the fifth day, followed by a fairly prompt, but partial, recovery for about 2–3 d, then by a much slower recovery towards normal (Fleck, 1976). Concominant with these changes, several other plasma proteins, including fibrinogen and C-reactive protein, show an increase in concentration (Fleck, 1976; Myers *et al.*, 1984). This leads one to question whether the changes in albumin could be due to blood loss, altered fluid dynamics and redistribution of body fluid, or whether any other mechanism is acting. Changes in the rates of catabolism or synthesis of albumin cannot lead to rapid changes (e.g. in less than a few days) in the concentration of albumin because the maximum rate of change is unlikely to be as great as the rates of synthesis and catabolism, which are about 10% of the intravascular pool per day. In contrast, relatively small changes in microvascular permeability could lead to prompt and large changes in albumin concentration, because 120% of the intravascular pool exchanges with the extravascular pool each day (*Figure 7.3*). As mentioned above, loss to the extravascular pool can be measured directly as TER, and it has been reported that TER is increased by more than 100% in septic shock, and within a few hours of cardiopulmonary bypass (Raines *et al.*, 1984). Obviously, intravenous infusion of crystalloid will either expand the blood volume or retain it near its original value, if there has been blood loss; in either case, albumin concentration will fall promptly.

The conclusions are that the decrease in albumin concentration in serious infection is very probably due to increased microvascular permeability and that the prompt fall in albumin concentration after trauma is due to a combination of factors which include increased microvascular permeability, blood loss and intravenous infusion of crystalloid. The relative contribution of each of these varies from patient to patient with the nature and extent of injury and therapy. In addition, changes in the rates of synthesis and catabolism may have a later influence on the rate of recovery of albumin concentration towards its previous value.

The effects of changing nutrition on albumin concentration differ depending on the nature and timing of the change. Complete deprivation of food, but not water, leads to an increase in albumin concentration of approximately 7% in 3 d (Broom *et al.*, 1978). Controlled protein–energy depletion for 24 weeks, which led to the loss of 25% of body weight, was accompanied by a fall of only 7% in albumin concentration and virtually no change in the total quantity of intravascular albumin (Keys *et al.*, 1950). In contrast, when protein depletion is much greater than the deficit in energy intake, the albumin concentration does decrease significantly (Fleck and Munro, 1963). Thus, the response of albumin concentration in nutritional deprivation appears to depend, at least in part, on the ratio of protein to energy intake. Taking these observations with the various factors (*see* list on p. 102) which influence albumin concentration and the possible mechanisms of the fall in albumin concentration during infections and trauma, the use of serum albumin concentration as a nutritional indicator would seem to be ill advised.

It is similarly incorrect to take serum albumin concentration as an index of liver function on the assumption that a low concentration of albumin indicates reduced synthesis and hence impaired hepatocellular function. In general, the opposite holds because the fractional rate of synthesis of albumin is inversely proportional to its concentration (Anderson and Rossing, 1969), so that as the concentration falls, the synthesis rate of albumin should rise. Increased synthesis of albumin occurs in nephrosis (Jensen *et al.*, 1967; Bianchi *et al.*, 1973), protein-losing enteropathy (Wochner *et al.*, 1968) and in some cases of liver disease (Rothschild *et al.*, 1969). Thus, the low albumin concentration in the early stages of liver disease is most likely to be due to fluid retention with consequent increase in plasma volume and is not necessarily due to impaired albumin synthesis (Tavill, 1979). It is only when there has been considerable destruction of hepatocytes that the total amount of albumin synthesized each day is likely to become subnormal.

Consideration of the relation between albumin concentration and the outcome of disease or various procedures has led others to suggest that albumin concentration is a good prognostic indicator: the lower the albumin concentration, the poorer the prognosis (Hay, Whitehead and Spicer, 1975; Anderson *et al.*, 1984). The above discussion is entirely compatible with this, in that the pathological processes are likely to lead to increase in TER, loss of albumin from the gut or urine, etc., or increased breakdown, all of which will reduce the amount of albumin. However, it should be noted that it is not because the concentration of albumin is low that the prognosis is poor, but rather that the magnitude of the fall in albumin concentration is related to the extent of the disease processes.

Therapeutic aspects

The first observation is that albumin cannot make a significant contribution as a source of protein nutrition, since normally only about 14 g are catabolized each day and even twice that quantity would not meet the recommended daily intake of protein (Wretlend, 1972). The second observation is that the effects of intravenous infusion of albumin on increasing plasma albumin concentration are usually disappointing, both in terms of the extent of the increase and the duration of the effect (Conn, 1977). Consideration of the relations depicted in *Figure 7.3* permits an explanation. First, infused albumin is rapidly distributed between the extravascular and intravascular spaces. In a normal individual, more than half the infused albumin will transfer to the extravascular space in less than 24 h, and in patients with serious infections, burn injury or after serious trauma, the loss to the extravascular space will be much greater and more rapid (Schwartzkopff *et al.,* 1981). Consequently, large quantities of albumin have to be given almost continuously to achieve and maintain a significant increase in albumin concentration in seriously ill patients.

There are obviously two ways of achieving an increase in albumin concentration. The most obvious is to infuse albumin, noting that in general (*see Table 7.1*) it is accompanied by fairly large quantities of sodium. This has been done in many cases of acute hypoalbuminaemia, or severely impaired cardiac output with reduced central venous pressure, as seen in severe trauma, or in severe burning injury.

Improvements with this therapy have been described (*see,* for example, Davies, 1982), including increased plasma volume, increased venous return and cardiac output and a fall in peripheral resistance (Schwartzkopff *et al.,* 1981). However, there are those who have advocated that crystalloids alone achieve equally beneficial results, although much larger volumes of fluid were required for resuscitation when crystalloid alone rather than colloid was used (Moss *et al.,* 1971).

In contrast, if it is considered that the plasma volume is already more than adequate, diuretics or fluid restriction can lead to an increase in albumin concentration. It can be argued that in patients in whom microvascular permeability is increased, the loss of infused albumin to the extravascular space may prolong oedema by retaining fluid extravascularly, and that this mechanism might have a deleterious effect in patients with pulmonary oedema.

There have been reports of diuresis following intravenous albumin in cases of oedema associated with very low albumin concentrations (Schreiner, 1971). These observations provide a rationale for using intravenous albumin together with a diuretic to achieve at least transient improvement in pulmonary gas exchange (Skillman, Parikh and Tanenbaum, 1970) and improved cardiac output and glomerular filtration (Davison, 1976). An advantage of giving albumin was that it prevented the fall in plasma volume which occurred when the diuretic was given alone (Davison, 1976).

Conclusions

It is now possible to provide a logical approach to the understanding of the pathophysiological mechanisms leading to hypoalbuminaemia, its clinical investigation and treatment.

The measurement of serum albumin concentration in some situations can provide a useful prognostic indicator, and in many cases it will be of value in monitoring the general response of a patient to treatment. Serum albumin concentration is neither directly related to nutritional status nor is it invariably indicative of the amount synthesized by the liver daily.

The influence of albumin concentration on the pharmacokinetics and therapeutic effects of drugs may be very important in seriously ill patients.

Intravenous albumin can be of value in the treatment of hypovolaemia, although in some instances combination with diuretics has led to even greater benefit to the patient.

One advantage of albumin as a 'plasma volume expander' over artificial high molecular weight substitutes, is its capacity to transport a wide variety of substances, including drugs.

B. Nutritional therapy

J. A. R. Smith

Introduction

The theory behind the use of nutritional support in the postoperative period is sound, but clinical proof is lacking. This section of the chapter will consider the theory, will evaluate the clinical experience to date and will attempt to provide guidelines for the identification of patients at risk. However, this is not always synonymous with selection of patients who will benefit from nutritional therapy and it must be recognized that both the selection process and the actual regimen prescribed are largely empirical.

Basic metabolism

Nutritional physiology is too complex to be considered in detail, but certain facts are of basic importance.

Protein

In contrast to the inactive stores of glycogen and fat, protein is much more dynamic. There is a constant turnover of protein within the body, amounting to between 50% and 60% of the total 300 g of protein metabolized each day. Not all amino acids released by breakdown of endogenous protein are re-utilized, and replacement from other sources is essential. Furthermore, the primary role of protein is functional not storage, including visceral structure, functioning muscle, hormones, carrier proteins, etc. In addition, when trauma has occurred, amino acids are required for repair of damaged tissues.

Protein is an expensive source of energy, but when other sources are deficient and in particular when there is insufficient glucose for the supply of energy to nervous tissue or red blood cells, gluconeogenic amino acids are released for conversion to glucose in the liver.

The main source of amino acids for gluconeogenesis and for other purposes when exogenous supply is reduced is muscle protein, visceral protein being preserved until shortly before death.

Energy

(1) Much has been written about basal metabolic rate and the energy required to ensure preservation of metabolism under specific 'basal' conditions. More helpful is the concept of resting or basal energy expenditure – the energy required to ensure preservation of cardiac, respiratory and cellular activity, including the maintenance of body temperature, i.e. the energy required to stay alive.

(2) To minimize the quantity of protein broken down and used as energy, an alternative source of calories is required. Glycogen from muscle is used up rapidly and while endogenous fat is a valuable store of energy, adaptation to starvation is essential before ketone bodies can be used by nervous tissue. This process takes 2–3 weeks and may be impaired after surgery by elevated levels of insulin which has an anti-lipolytic effect.

(3) In addition to basal energy expenditure, activity energy expenditure is required for mobilization and rehabilitation.

(4) Following major surgery, additional energy (and protein) will be required for the repair of damaged tissue. Such complications as sepsis increase demands for energy yet further. However, sepsis alters the hormonal milieu and may interfere with the response of target cells to the hormones, so that the requirements are far from clear.

(5) Certain tumours, especially those showing rapid growth, may also increase demands for energy. However, there is no evidence that tumours grow proportionally more rapidly than the host itself, merely that the food ingested will not be used entirely by the host.

Fluids and electrolytes

It is common to concentrate on protein and energy. However, without maintenance of the correct fluid and electrolyte balance, not only will the utilization of nutrients be impaired, but their infusion may be positively harmful.

Fluid and electrolyte balance is essential for maintenance of the milieu interieur, without which there will be changes in both the intra- and extracellular compartments, resulting in impaired cell function. While it may be possible to stimulate the entry of nutrients into the cell, for example by the combined use of hypertonic dextrose and insulin, the glucose may not be metabolized. Glucose in the cell will exert an osmotic effect, encouraging the entry of water into the cell, with further derangement of the environment.

By the same token, fluid and electrolyte balance is essential for neuromuscular excitability, myocardial contractility, transmembrane exchange and renal function. Thus, tolerance of infused fluid load and handling of both nutrients and electrolytes will be impaired.

Before any parenteral nutritional therapy is commenced, and throughout the period of support, ensuring fluid and electrolyte balance must take priority over nutritional infusions themselves (*see* Chapter 5).

Albumin

The precise role of albumin has been discussed in Section A of this chapter. Suffice it to say that a serum albumin of under 30 g/l not only indicates a poor prognosis (Simms, Smith and Woods, 1982), but will also result in alterations in colloid osmotic pressure sufficient to interfere with exchange of water, electrolytes and nutrients across the capillary membrane and to encourage the development of oedema.

Even the most successful total parenteral nutritional support will take upwards of 2 weeks to produce significant improvement in albumin levels. Longer periods will be required where both stress and sepsis depress albumin synthesis (Skillman *et al.*, 1976).

Thus, before parenteral nutrition will be utilized satisfactorily, it is essential to deal with such complications as serious sepsis which may depress albumin synthesis, and in the absence of sepsis or increased capillary permeability, artificially to correct low levels of albumin by the infusion of purified plasma fractions (HPPF). Furthermore, it may be necessary to use plasma to supplement the feeding regimen in the first week or more to maintain colloid osmotic pressure.

Responses to surgery

Much attention has been directed to the catabolic responses to surgery, but this can only be considered in the context of the responses relating to fluid and electrolyte balance and to those conditions in which the catabolic response is exaggerated either in time or severity.

Catabolic response

Initially, catabolism is an obligatory protective mechanism aiming to provide both amino acids, nitrogen and energy in response to both accidental and surgical trauma. The duration and the extent of the responses depends on the severity of the trauma, the previous nutritional status of the patient and the development or not of such complications as sepsis.

The response is mediated by a number of hormones including the catecholamines, the glucocorticoids and growth hormone, and results in the following:

(1) Mobilization of glycogen directly from the liver and indirectly from muscle via the Cori cycle to release glucose. In this response, adrenaline is more significant than noradrenaline.

(2) Breakdown of muscle protein to provide the necessary amino acid building blocks for synthesis and repair. The glycogen reserves are exhausted within the first 24 h, following which gluconeogenic amino acids are required to provide glucose as energy for nervous tissue and red blood cell, i.e. the obligatory users of glucose.

(3) The role of endogenous fat in the catabolic response is complex. Growth hormone stimulates fat release, but where stress or sepsis results in elevated levels of insulin, the antilipolytic effect of insulin prevents fat mobilization.

The *extent of the catabolic response* can be monitored crudely by assessment of the nitrogen balance which is most negative in the first 48 h and becomes progressively less negative in the ensuing few days as oral nutrition is resumed.

Both urinary creatinine (arising from muscle phosphocreatinine) and 3-methyl histidine (from muscle myofibrillar protein) have been used to assess the extent of muscle breakdown. The results are influenced by accuracy of collection and meat in the diet in at least the previous 3 d, and so have not proved as valuable as was first hoped.

It must be remembered that the cell breakdown involved will result in release of intracellular potassium.

The *previous nutritional status of the patient* is important in so far as the starved malnourished patient has already utilized much of his muscle protein. Thus, nitrogen losses will be lower than in a normally nourished individual undergoing the same procedure, because of the reduction in available store.

In addition, the longer starvation continues, the more likely is that patient to have adapted to starvation, i.e. to have mobilized body fat, and to have both nervous tissue and red cell capable of using ketone bodies for energy. Three weeks is the required period for full adaptation.

Fluid and electrolyte response

This topic has been covered in Chapter 5. The response is dictated not only by the surgical trauma but by the presence or persistence of any hypovolaemia. The consequent release of antidiuretic hormone, manufactured in the supraoptic nuclei in the hypothalamus and stored in the posterior pituitary, results in increased permeability of the collecting ducts to water so that volume is preserved.

Renin is released from the renal juxtaglomerular apparatus and converts angiotensinogen to angiotensin I. This decapeptide is converted to the active octapeptide angiotensin II by a converting enzyme found especially in the lungs and to a lesser degree in the kidneys. Angiotensin II stimulates the production of aldosterone, which in turn increases the reabsorption of sodium by the distal convoluted tubule. Potassium is lost passively in exchange for sodium – at the very time when increased cell breakdown is occurring.

Hypercatabolism

Hypercatabolism is the term used when the breakdown of body protein continues beyond the first 2–3 postoperative days, where losses are increased by the severity of surgical trauma or where such complications as sepsis exaggerate the losses of nitrogen. In addition, especially in the presence of sepsis, there are other metabolic changes.

The synthesis of protein in general and albumin in particular is depressed, so that low levels represent a combination of increased breakdown and reduced replacement.

There is often a hyperglycaemia, together with elevated levels of serum insulin. This is considered to indicate impaired uptake and metabolism of glucose by the cells and has been named 'insulin resistance'.

Under these circumstances, the tolerance to parenteral nutrition using hypertonic dextrose alone will be impaired. Even if exogenous insulin is used to force glucose into the cells, the failure of metabolism will result in an osmotic effect of the glucose with further reduction in cell function. At the same time, infused nitrogen may not ensure any increase in body protein, especially albumin. Thus, in addition to nutritional therapy, attention must be directed to the cause of the increased catabolism.

Anabolism

Anabolism reverses the tissue losses of catabolism and ensures adequate restoration and the repair of traumatized tissues. The main stimulus to anabolism is the hormonal status – namely insulin and growth hormone – and an adequate supply of amino acids and energy. Anabolic steroids have been used to stimulate the response, but their use in clinical practice is far from clear.

Consequences of malnutrition

As early as 1936 it was reported that preoperative weight loss of 25% of the pre-morbid weight carried a mortality approaching 100%, and that loss of 20% not only increased mortality but also morbidity, as evidenced by an increased risk of anastomosis leakage and wound dehiscence (Studley, 1936). The group studied by Studley were peculiar in so far as they were all patients with chronic peptic ulcer, admitted for medical management, and operated on only if they failed to respond. It is to this particular subset that Studley's data refers.

More recently, the importance of disease-related weight loss has been re-emphasized as a prognostic factor, but the critical value was reported between 10% and 20% (Levenson, Crowley and Seifter, 1975). However, all are agreed that such patients risk an increased incidence of sepsis and of impaired healing of wounds and anastomoses (Geefhuysen *et al.*, 1971; Daly, Vars and Dudrick, 1972; Law, Dudrick and Abdou, 1974).

In a study of patients undergoing surgery for colonic, gastric, oesophageal and bladder tumours, malnutrition was associated with a significant increase in all septic complications, in poor healing and, indeed, in both mortality and long-term survival (Simms, Smith and Woods, 1982).

A number of workers in the USA have linked malnutrition with reduced immunocompetence of cell-mediated type using skin tests to standard recall antigens (Meakins *et al.*, 1977). Surgery itself also reduces cell-mediated immunity (Slade *et al.*, 1975), and if both factors apply additively at the time of surgery, when neoplastic cells are shed into the circulation, the risks of metastatic spread should be high. On the other hand, those are the very patients in whom long-term survival is uncommon, so that data to support or refute the theory is lacking.

By the same token, a number of studies in the UK have failed to confirm a relationship between cell-mediated immunity and prognosis (Brown *et al.*, 1982), except in one small proportion of critically ill, intensive care patients (Bradley, Ledingham and Hamilton, 1981).

It is clear that specific nutritional deficiencies do carry risks of morbidity. Thus, deficiency of zinc or of ascorbic acid will interfere with wound healing. Low levels of essential fatty acids cause skin rashes, and hypophosphataemia may interfere with both energy-rich phosphates and with red cell 2,3-diphosphoglycerate (McLaren, 1981).

While knowledge of the consequences of gross malnutrition and of specific deficiencies is reasonably clear, the relevance of less severe and perhaps more subtle forms of malnutrition is an area largely untouched. Indeed, it may well be that in certain conditions there is an especial sensitivity in malnourished patients.

Causes of malnutrition

In surgical practice, malnutrition is seen most commonly in association with a chronic debilitating disorder such as extensive Crohn's disease or small gut fistula, and with malignant disease especially of the upper gastrointestinal tract. However, any cause of malabsorption may be encountered.

Where there is dysphagia secondary to oesophageal or cardio-oesophageal carcinoma, it is easy to understand the development of malnutrition. Similarly, upper tract neoplasms cause anorexia and studies of voluntary food intake confirm reduction of intake. Attempts have been made to relate anorexia with extent of the tumour, with anorexia, weight loss and prognosis being directly related to the extent of the gastro-oesophageal tumour (Dehn *et al.*, 1984).

An alternative explanation of malnutrition in neoplasia is that the tumour functions as an internal cannibal at the expense of the host. Animal studies have shown that the tumour and the host grow in proportion and that there is no excessive growth of the tumour. However, it is clear that if intake is reduced and a proportion of that is metabolized by the tumour, the share to the host can only be reduced and malnutrition is more likely to develop (Carmichael *et al.*, 1980).

An additional factor in neoplastic disease is that both chemotherapy and radiotherapy also interfere with gastrointestinal function and with appetite (Ota *et al.*, 1979), causing or compounding nutritional deficiency.

The more vascular tumours such as hypernephroma may produce an increase in metabolic rate, so that normal intake of nutrients may be insufficient for increased demands. Furthermore, once liver metastases have developed, there may be impaired ability to metabolize the nutrients ingested.

Methods of nutritional assessment

Clinical

Where the patient is grossly cachectic, clinical diagnosis is easy, but lesser degrees of deficiency prove more difficult to detect. A recent study (Baker *et al.*, 1982) has suggested that an experienced clinician performs at least as well as any other method, but not all clinicians practising nutritional therapy are of equivalent experience.

Anthropometry

Early measurements based on ideal weight or weight for height have been superseded by more sophisticated, but not necessarily more helpful, methods.

Triceps skin fold thickness (TSF), measured by a trained operator with proper Harpenden calipers at the midpoint of the upper arm, gives an index of neutral fat stores. Mid upper arm is defined as the mid-point between the tip of the acromion and the olecranon process. Mid upper arm circumference is measured at the same point, care being taken to keep the measure vertical. From these two measurements it is possible to calculate the mid upper arm *muscle* circumference as an index of muscle protein. These measurements are subject to considerable observer error, which may be compounded by the calculations involved.

Where there is considerable deficiency the prognosis is poor, but lesser degrees of deficit and response to therapy have proved less amenable to anthropometric methods of assessment.

Functional

It is now well established that nutritional therapy is more likely to be effective in restoring muscle protein when the patient is able to resume activity. Thus, it is sound theory to attempt a functional assessment of muscle protein.

The grip strength dynamometer has been claimed to achieve functional assessment. Using the non-dominant hand, impaired grip strength correlates with prognosis and, in contrast with most other methods used to identify poor prognosis or malnutrition, is also effective in monitoring response to therapy (Archer *et al.*, 1982).

Biochemical

Albumin (Alb), and the more acute phase proteins, such as transferrin (measured as total iron binding capacity (TIBC)) or prealbumin, have been used alone and in mathematical combination (*vide infra*). The only readily usable consequence of the studies to date is that a serum albumin level on presentation of under 30 g/l results in a higher rate of complications and identifies some 85% of major complications, i.e. death, major leakage of wounds or anastomoses, or deep sepsis (Simms, Smith and Woods, 1982). However, undernutrition is not the only cause of hypoalbuminaemia and serum albumin is a poor monitor of response to therapy in view of its long half-life (Rothschild, Oratz and Schreiber, 1972).

Cell-mediated immunity

Skin reactivity to the intradermal injection of standard recall antigens or to dinitrochlorobenzene (DNCB) has been widely used in the USA, both to identify patients at risk from surgery and to monitor response to nutritional therapy (Meakins *et al.*, 1977). They have provided evidence that anergy carries a poor prognosis, but those whose reactivity can be restored fare as well as those reacting positively from the start. What is concerning is that this work has not been repeatable in British practice, and that a number of patients initially positive convert to anergy by the time of retesting.

Combination methods

Largely because of dissatisfaction with any one method of assessment, mathematical methods were used to select those parameters of high value and some weighting to allow development of a formula. This was first proposed by Mullens *et al.* (1979) and has since been modified for British practice (Simms, Smith and Woods, 1982). The parameters used in the formula, PI = 150 − 1.66 (ALB) − 0.78 (TSF) − 0.53 (TIBC), are not only influenced by nutritional status, but the formula does help select patients at risk, identifying 65% of all complications and about 80% of major complications. However, not all poor risk patients are helped by full total parenteral nutrition (TPN) – and so the index is now called simply 'prognostic index'. A closer analysis of the formula confirms its value for population studies, but its limited use for the individual (Burton *et al.*, 1983).

Dionigi and others have used cluster analysis which also identifies groups of patients with different degrees of risk, but has the additional benefit of being valuable in assessing response to therapy (Nazari *et al.*, 1982).

Nutritional support

Having identified that malnutrition carries a poor prognosis in surgical practice, it was assumed that repletion of any deficiency would be associated with an improvement in prognosis. This tended to overlook the fact that the primary condition causing the nutritional problem, whether weight loss, hypoalbuminaemia or loss of fat and muscle stores, might well still be active. The initial logic that most humans consume three forms of foodstuffs several times a day and that this ingestion should not be denied surgical patients, was supported by the demonstration that beagle pups could be fed safely intravenously from birth and that they then developed normally into adult dog life (Dudrick, Rhoads and Var, 1967). This was followed by the safe use of total parenteral nutrition in human practice, and it was not long before there was an enormous literature on the subject of parenteral nutrition. However, most papers addressed specific questions, such as energy to nitrogen ratio or the amino acid profile most likely to achieve a positive nitrogen balance, and failed to ask the more thorny question of whether the therapy used was effective or not. Indeed, many of the studies performed were on patients undergoing relatively minor surgery of the cholecystectomy or ulcer type, and while the data obtained was of considerable importance, its direct extrapolation to the critically ill patient following major surgery or who had sustained a major surgical complication could not be justified.

The benefits claimed for adequate nutritional support in the perioperative period have been (a) a reduction in mortality; (b) lower rates of septic complications in the postoperative period (Heatley, Williams and Lewis, 1979); (c) a lower incidence of anastomotic leakage and breakdown (Ward *et al.,* 1982); (d) earlier mobilization and rehabilitation; and (e) improved results in cancer patients where surgical nutrition has been effective in restoring deficiencies in cell-mediated immunity.

As a consequence, nutritional support both by enteral and parenteral routes has become widely established in surgical practice, especially in the Scandinavian countries and in the USA.

Methods of nutritional support

Enteral

Normal diet

Before proceeding to more sophisticated methods of nutritional support, it is important (a) to try to stimulate the patient's appetite, including the use of pre-prandial alcohol, and (b) involving a dietetic system to ensure that the food provided is appetizing and attractive to the individual patient. A correct balance of protein, energy, vitamins, etc., is clearly essential.

Special diet

A normal diet, either minced up or supplied in liquidized form, is often acceptable to individual patients when there are problems not with appetite but rather of dysphagia. However, considerable care is required to present such a diet in an acceptable form and with commercial diets now less expensive, liquidizing has become less common.

Supplements

Supplements are now available to supply extra energy (HiCal) or extra protein (Complan). These are designed as supplements to normal diet, but in certain cases may be acceptable as the basis for a specialized liquid diet.

A variety of commercial preparations are in use. Space does not permit a full consideration of all these, but in general terms it is possible to select a preparation according to the individual needs of patients for energy and protein balance; for supply of nutrients within a given volume; to meet particular requirements for a particular energy source, e.g. carbohydrate, lipid, medium-chain triglycerides, etc., and indeed to minimize the residue resulting from a particular feed, e.g. Vivonex or Flexical.

It must be remembered that patients' acceptability of these diets is very variable (Smith, Coubourgh and Norman, 1979) and while all can theoretically be taken orally, many are better used by tube feeding.

When the oral route is not available or acceptable to the patient, a number of tubes are now available. Fine bore tubes which provide less nasal or pharyngeal irritation than the conventional Ryle's tubes are widely used, and are provided with introducers which make the passage into the stomach relatively safe. In addition, they are radio opaque, so the position can be checked radiologically. Furthermore, more sophisticated coating of both the inside and outside of these tubes by a hydromer reduces the incidence of blockage and allows their life *in situ* to be prolonged, thus avoiding the too frequent replacement of tubes during the course of a patient's nutritional support. The final modification is the use of a weighted fine-bore tube of Dobhof type, although nowadays the weight used tends to be tungsten rather than the potentially toxic mercury of the original tube. This allows the direction of the feeding tube into the duodenum, bypassing the stomach itself (*Figure 7.4*).

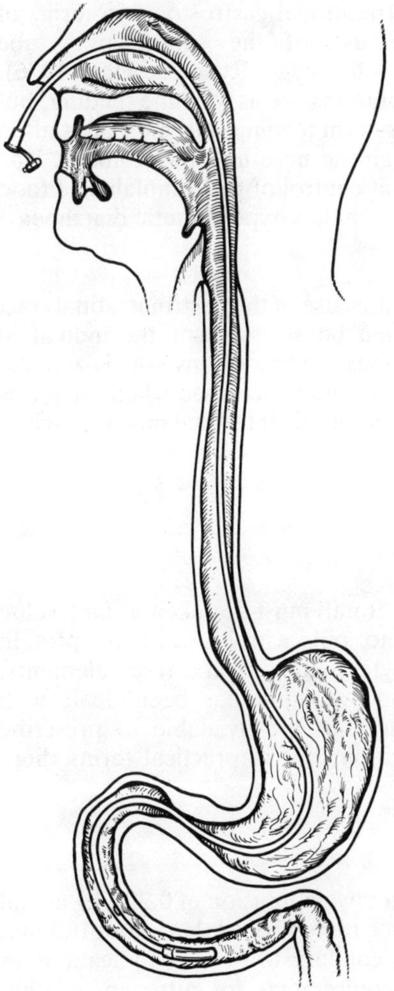

Figure 7.4. The Dobhof weighted tungsten tube. Note that the weighted end allows easy insertion into the duodenum under X-ray control

When using the enteral route for feeding, it is important to remember the principle that the foodstuff should be introduced gradually, at half-strength, for 24 h, being followed by full-strength only if the food is tolerated by the patient. When a tube is used, constant infusion is more satisfactory than bolus feeds and stomach overloading can be avoided.

The food must be provided in sterile form and should be iso-osmotic with plasma as closely as possible. When the stomach osmostat function is bypassed, too rapid infusion of hyperosmolar infusions is much more likely to result in troublesome diarrhoea. By the same token, diarrhoea may result if any of the solutions used become contaminated with bacteria, particularly in situations where there is hypochlorhydria or where the stomach acid protective barrier is bypassed

Jejunostomy

This method has largely replaced the traditional gastrostomy in terms of tube feeding, particularly with the use of the sub-mucosal tube jejunostomy, using a fine-bore feeding tube (Page, Ryan and Haff, 1976). The principles involved in the use of solutions are as for tube feeding, but particularly where there is need for long-term feeding, this method is often to be preferred to tubes passing through the nose into the stomach. The fact that the pylorus is bypassed and that control of the osmolality of food entering the duodenum is therefore lost, makes hyperosmotic diarrhoea a more common problem.

In summary, the methods available to allow use of the gastrointestinal tract are considerable and all of these should be assessed for the individual patient before the question of intravenous feeding of any sort is actually considered. It is clear that safety of use is much increased when the gut is used and, in addition, there are no changes in the intestinal mucosa such as result from parenteral nutritional therapy.

Parenteral

Total parenteral nutrition

It is now well recognized that the term 'total' must be taken at face value and thus the patient must be supplied not only with his needs for protein and energy but also for fluid, electrolytes, vitamins and trace elements. The question of fluid, electrolytes and albumin has been dealt with previously. A number of different methods are available to prescribe requirements for total parenteral nutrition, but in practical terms there seems little to choose between them.

Nitrogen

The basic requirement for nitrogen is met by an infusion of 0.22 g/kg actual body weight per day. However, it must be remembered that major trauma, major surgery and hypercatabolism, secondary to such complications as major sepsis, all produce increased requirements for nitrogen, so that levels of 0.4 g/kg/d or more may be required. In the vast majority of patients, an empirical approach can be adopted, but in a smaller proportion it may be advisable to perform daily nitrogen balance studies and to replace on the subsequent day what has actually been lost in the previous 24 h.

In selecting the solution of choice, a number of important considerations must be made. First, the fluid load to be tolerated by the individual patient may be crucial, but fortunately various commercial preparations available contain different quantities of nitrogen in different units of volume. Secondly, it is vital to ensure that adequate quantities of essential amino acids are infused together with an adequate balance of the so-called semi-essential and the non-essential nitrogen sources. Thirdly, at particular times, for example during growth, there may be an increased requirement for such amino acids as cysteine or histidine, so that these become essential for a limited period in development. Fourthly, there is some evidence that in hepatic disease or in severe sepsis, branch chain enriched amino acid solutions may be of particular benefit. Finally, for patients in renal failure, the most important consideration is to supply the essential amino acids and certain solutions are now being assessed scientifically for this purpose. It is traditional to compare the amino acid profile of the solutions in current use with the amino acid content of egg protein. However, it must be said that initial fears about the toxic effects of solutions containing relatively high amounts of glycine have not now been born out with clinical experience.

Energy

There is no longer any place for the solutions containing sorbitol, fructose and ethanol. The initial advantage claimed of being independent of insulin is now known not to hold true. The former two interfere with adenine nucleotide function in the liver and are associated with elevations in plasma lactic acid levels. These do not reach significance in the majority of patients, but are potential hazards in patients with metabolic acidosis or sepsis in whom more modest elevations may be of particular seriousness.

Thus, in current practice, both hypertonic dextrose and fat emulsions are the solutions of choice. There is considerable debate about the relative proportions to be used. There is agreement that at least 30% of the total energy should be supplied as carbohydrate but, in practice, equi-caloric proportions of fat and carbohydrate tend to be used.

If carbohydrate alone is used (16.8 J/g; 4 cal/g) certain problems are likely to be faced:

(1) To give the same amount of energy, a larger volume of fluid is required compared to a combination of fat and dextrose.
(2) Infusion of insulin would usually be essential, but while this carries certain theoretical advantages in terms of stimulating anabolism, should there be any disparity between the infusion of insulin and that of dextrose, serious hypoglycaemia may result.
(3) In the longer term, fatty infiltration of the liver will result.
(4) The combined use of insulin and dextrose may allow entry of glucose into the cell accompanied by potassium and water, but where there is any cellular dysfunction, this will result only in intracellular oedema as not all the glucose will be metabolized.

Fat alone has been advocated, particularly by the Scandinavian authorities, in the nutritional support of severe burn injury. However, this method also carries certain disadvantages.

Except in those patients who have adapted to starvation, nervous tissue and red cells are obligatory users of glucose for energy and thus the use of fat solutions alone carries a theoretical risk of an increased amount of muscle protein breakdown to supply gluconeogenic amino acids. Once adaptation to starvation has taken place, however, these tissues can use ketone bodies for energy, but first this takes about 21 d of starvation and secondly, in the presence of any degree of catabolism, the anti-lipolytic effect of insulin forbids efficient adaptation. However, fat is a convenient source of energy, providing 37.8 J/g (9 cal/g) and also supplying some of the body needs for essential fatty acids and for phosphate.

In most centres, fat and carbohydrate solutions are used together to supply needs for energy, with an attempt being made to ensure, whenever possible, that all fat emulsions are infused before 2.00 a.m. so that the blood can be cleared of fat droplets before blood is withdrawn in the early morning for Coulter analysis. Providing 50% of energy needs with fat emulsion allows the use of less strong dextrose solutions and, in many patients, no exogenous insulin is required to maintain a plasma glucose of around 10 mmol/l.

Until recently, attempts have been made to relate the quantity of energy according to the amount of nitrogen infused, but energy infusions must be infused at the same time as nitrogen in order to maximize utilization of the infused amino acids and to minimize the amount of amino acids broken down for gluconeogenesis. In patients who are malnourished, an energy to nitrogen ratio of 200:1 may be necessary but, conversely, in the presence of severe sepsis, a ratio of 420 J (100 cal) for each gram of nitrogen will be a maximum tolerated. In normal clinical practice, an energy to nitrogen ratio of 150:1 is usual.

An alternative approach has been to estimate the energy requirements on empirical grounds, usually administering 197.4 J/kg (47 cal/kg) of body weight. However, more sophisticated studies using indirect calorimetry have revealed that very few patients following major surgery have a resting energy expenditure in excess of 8.4 kJ (2000 cal) and it is therefore suggested that any infusion which provides more energy than this is at least unnecessary and may be positively harmful (Hill and Church, 1984).

Trace elements

There is increasing information about both the number of trace elements required and the likely critical value which must be replaced during total parenteral nutritional therapy. Commercial preparations (Addamel) are available and such deficiencies as zinc, copper, magnesium and manganese can be anticipated and prevented. Most difficulty is faced with hypophosphataemia, particularly in a regimen where fat emulsion is not used routinely. This substance must be infused separately. It is to be hoped that, one day, as much information about trace element requirements will be known about man as is currently known about commercially reared farm animals (Kingsnorth, 1984).

Vitamins

Solutions to replace both water- and fat-soluble vitamins are also available. However, it must be remembered that folic acid in particular is sensitive to light and must be protected from exposure by the use of a coloured bag over a container of this solution. In the short term, injections of vitamin B_{12} are seldom required, because body stores last from between 6 months and 8 years, with an average of 2 years. In patients where deficient absorption may already be present, e.g. following massive ileal resection or gastric resection, earlier replacement may be required.

Peripheral infusion of isotonic amino acids

This form of support is based on a concept first elaborated by Blackburn and colleagues in Boston (Blackburn *et al.*, 1973). If, after major surgery, a carbohydrate solution is infused, there is an insulin response. Insulin is anti-lipolytic and thus the only source of amino acids to replenish the pool must come from the breakdown of muscle protein. On the other hand, if no carbohydrate whatsoever is infused, and fluid requirements are met by isotonic amino acid solutions, then there is no insulin response. Endogenous fat is mobilized for energy purposes and this can be monitored both by an increase in free fatty acid concentrations and in the concentration of ketone bodies both in blood and in urine. This allows utilization of the infused amino acids and thus the breakdown of muscle protein is minimal. This phenomenon has been shown to be a fact, provided there is no increase in endogenous insulin levels, for example in association with severe sepsis or in stress such as associated with multiple trauma (Smith and Simms, 1981; Miller *et al.*, 1977).

The method is simple, is not associated with a high incidence of thrombophlebitis, despite the use of the peripheral vein, and can be easily monitored by a simple blood and urine testing. The exact place of this form of therapy in the nutritional armamentarium is not yet clear and is the subject of ongoing study.

Clinical data

Amidst a plethora of papers on the subject of parenteral nutrition, it is very difficult to find any conclusive data that its use can be justified by either metabolic or clinical terms. It seems clear that in the intensive care type of patient, who is usually hypercatabolic, the use of total parenteral nutrition can slow or stop the loss of body weight associated with excessive breakdown of muscle protein and, on the basis that weight loss of greater than 20% of the pre-morbid body weight is of dire prognostic significance, can be considered to be of benefit. Indeed, it is difficult if not impossible to study such patients scientifically in a controlled manner and few clinicians would dare withhold this form of therapy to such patients at the present time.

In other areas, however, data is less convincing. Only Moghissi *et al.* (1977) studying patients undergoing oesophagectomy, Muller *et al.* (1982) studying patients undergoing gastrectomy and Heatley *et al.* (1979) have claimed benefit, and their papers do not stand up well to critical analysis.

In Moghissi's paper, following 10 d of parenteral nutrition, weight gains of 20 lb (9 kg) were claimed, but it is difficult to know from where such weight could be derived, as neither accumulation of protein, nor of glycogen, would explain these changes. Indeed, it seems likely that, despite the fluid balanced results reported, weight gains of this magnitude can only be due to water. In Muller's study, it was rather strange that total parenteral nutrition was only of benefit if the infusion of fat emulsions was totally avoided. This is contrary to conventional thinking and practice and has not been corroborated in other studies. In Heatley's study, the main advantage appeared to be a lower incidence of septic complications and this work has not been substantiated in other centres following controlled trials.

Our own studies considered two groups of patients. The first were those undergoing gastrectomy or oesophagogastrectomy for carcinoma, where the control group were compared with a group who were fed intravenously for 7–10 d before surgery and after operation until normal oral intake was resumed, usually about 10 d. The third group in the study were fed intravenously only for the period after surgery. The use of parenteral nutrition reduced the negative nitrogen balance and the use of pre- and postoperative parenteral nutrition conferred the dubious benefit that, although in this group the number of oesophageal anastomoses was higher and that the incidence of oesophageal leakages was increased, none of these patients actually died. Thus, there was no short-term metabolic or clinical benefit and at follow-up at 1 year, no longer term benefit was obvious that would have suggested improvement in the immunocompetence as a result of nutritional support which might have been of longer term benefit to the patient.

In the second study, patients undergoing radical total cystectomy for carcinoma were the subjects. After examination under anaesthetic, and confirmatory biopsy, patients were subjected to a course of radiotherapy to 4000 rad. After an interval of 4–6 weeks, surgery was performed, diversion usually being by ileal conduit. Up to the time of the study, such patients both in our centre and elsewhere had been fed routinely intravenously and this method of support had been considered to be one explanation of the improvement in fatality which had been seen in the past 10 years. However, in our study, no patient died and no obvious metabolic or clinical benefit could be identified (Smith *et al.*, 1984).

Peripheral amino acids

In our controlled studies, we have first of all compared two groups of patients undergoing colonic resection, one receiving 5% dextrose and normal saline for fluid requirements and the other, isotonic amino acids alone. In the latter group, nitrogen balance was improved and the fall in albumin was less, but there was no obvious clinical benefit in association with these changes. In later studies – patients undergoing colonic, gastric, oesophageal and bladder resection – an alternative amino acid solution was also effective in reducing the negative nitrogen balance, but equally conferred no particular benefit clinically or metabolically on the patients concerned. However, it should be noted that the changes in nitrogen balance produced were very similar to those in the parallel study of total parenteral nutrition.

Conclusions

Thus, there is little evidence to support the routine use of either form of parenteral nutritional therapy in clinical practice, and it is clear that what is desired is a method of selecting a high risk group of patients and of identifying which of those patients is likely to benefit from nutritional therapy. If, in addition, the same method can be used to monitor response to nutrition or to identify benefit and to establish an end point, where therapy will be ineffective or where safe surgery can be undertaken, then an ideal would be achieved.

Complications of parenteral nutrition

In addition to the complications common to any intravenous infusion, parenteral nutrition carries certain specific problems, broadly categorized into mechanical, biochemical and sepsis. However, there is no doubt that prevention is possible for the vast majority to be described.

Mechanical

The route of choice for central venous feeding is the infraclavicular approach to the right subclavian vein. Few anatomical structures in that area have escaped trauma, including subclavian artery, pleura, lung, brachial plexus. On the left, trauma to the thoracic duct is reported.

Displacement of the cannula up to internal jugular vein is relatively common. Catheter emboli have required removal, including lodgement in the heart. Catheter design has reduced but not removed this complication.

Biochemical

One of the principal complications is hyperglycaemia when glucose alone is used for energy, or where excessively hypertonic solutions are used in the presence of insulin resistance. This complication risks a hyperosmolar crisis with intracellular dehydration and an osmotic diuresis.

Hypoglycaemia usually occurs, not as a simple rebound phenomenon but when exogenous insulin is used to maintain a plasma glucose of 10 mmol/l and the insulin continues after the dextrose has been stopped. Hypophosphataemia, hypozincaemia and hypovitaminosis have been discussed. Acid–base disturbance is much less common now that only glucose is used as the carbohydrate source of energy.

The iron contained in Addamel is only 0.65 mg compared with a minimum daily requirement of 1.0 mg. In the longer term, infusion or injection of iron may be necessary if an iron-deficiency anaemia is to be avoided.

Sepsis

Infection is the most serious current complication and is the main indication for the stringency in insisting that all cannulae are inserted with full aseptic standards in theatre. The subcutaneous tunnel route should be used for all but short-term feeding (7–10 d). Nursing care needs to be scrupulous and once inserted the line should be used for *no* purpose other than feeding.

If pyrexia does develop, an alternative cause for fever should be sought in the wound, the urine or the respiratory system. A blood culture is taken from both the central line and a peripheral vein. The TPN solution is replaced by crystalloid fluid and the solutions being used are sent for bacteriological assay. If the pyrexia persists the line is removed and, if clinically indicated, replaced. If the fever settles, TPN is resumed but any rapid return of pyrexia indicates removal of the line. Whenever a line is removed for any purpose, the tip must be submitted to bacteriological investigation. Any proven sepsis is treated with the appropriate antibiotic (*Figure 7.5*).

Monitoring nutritional therapy

On the one hand, monitoring must ensure safety of therapy and on the other, some assessment of efficacy is required. Safety is ensured by maintaining fluid and electrolyte balance, avoiding any anaemia, especially of iron-deficiency type, and ensuring that the plasma glucose does not exceed 10 mmol/l and that glycosuria does not occur.

Monitoring efficacy is much more difficult. In a negative way, if weight loss persists or albumin continues to fall, either TPN is ineffective or some alternative cause such as sepsis must be present. Any improvement in albumin, TIBC or pre-albumin levels indicates improvement, but their absence does not indicate absence of efficacy.

Monitoring cell-mediated immunity has not proved beneficial.

Too much emphasis should not be placed on nitrogen balance or body weight, especially as increase in the latter may only indicate water retention.

Indications for total parenteral nutrition

The list below gives the standard but empirical indications for TPN:

(1) Gastrointestinal tract not available or unable to supply increased requirements.
(2) No oral intake after 5 d – actual or anticipated.
(3) Clinical cachexia – pre- and postoperative.
(4) Short gut syndrome.
(5) Clinical malnutrition – perioperative.
(6) ?Neoplasia ± immunocompetence.

It must be emphasized that these indications are based on theory and 'best buy' rather than on scientific proof. Until there is a better approach, it is safer to err on the side of too much rather than too little nutritional support.

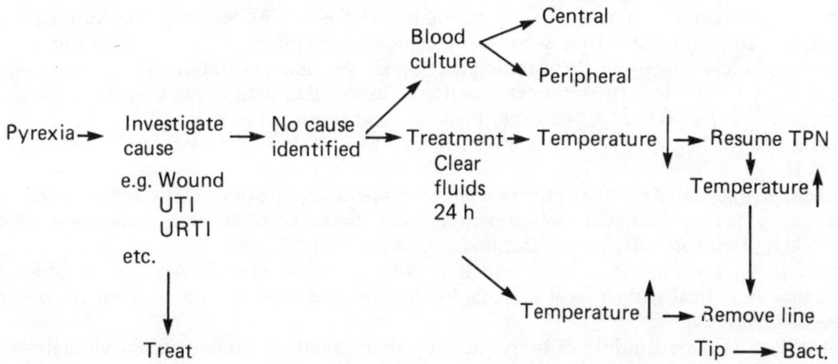

Figure 7.5. Flow chart for the management of pyrexia in patients undergoing total parenteral nutrition

The future

The most important requirement is for a method to identify poor risk patients, to select which of these are likely to benefit from nutritional support, to monitor their progress and to allow recognition of an end point, either of maximal benefit or of when surgery could be more safely undertaken. It would also allow identification of those people unlikely to benefit from therapy or from major surgery.

What is also required is a clearer understanding of how much and of which solution should be used if parenteral therapy is indeed required. In fact, advances in enteral solutions and methods may further reduce the need to use the parenteral route.

It is also likely that there will be a more scientific prescription of nitrogen, calories, minerals, vitamins and even of specific amino acid combinations, tailored for both the individual and his disease process.

Above all, it must be recognized that TPN is expensive, both in terms of finance and morbidity, and every step must be carefully taken to minimize both its use and its complications, without denying other patients a form of therapy which ought to contribute to saving of life.

References

ANDERSON, C. F., MOXNESS, K., MEISTER, J. and BURRITT, M. F. (1984). The sensitivity and specificity of nutrition-related variables in relationship to the duration of hospital stay and the rate of complication. *Mayo Clinic Proceedings,* **59,** 477–483

ANDERSON, S. B. and ROSSING, N. (1969). Metabolism of albumin and G-globulin in man during albumin infusions and during plasmaphoresis. In *Physiology and Pathophysiology of Plasma Protein Metabolism* (Birke, G., Norberg, R. and Plantin, L. O., Eds), pp. 135–142. Oxford; Pergamon Press

ARCHER, T. J., DAWES, R., KLIDJIAN, A. M. and KARRAN, S. J. (1982). Early postoperative fatigue in the prediction of serious postoperative complications. *Clinical Nutrition,* **1,** Special Supplement, 94

BAKER, J. P., DETSKY, A. S., WESSON, D. E., WOLMAN, S. L., STEWART, S., WHITEWELL, J., LANGER, B. and JEEJEEBHOY, K. N. (1982). A comparison of clinical judgement and objective measurements. *New England Journal of Medicine,* **306,** 969–972

BALLANTYNE, F. C. and FLECK, A. (1973). Experience with a commercial preparation of ^{125}I-labelled human albumin for study of albumin metabolism. *Journal of Clinical Pathology,* **26,** 499–502

BIANCHI, R., MARIANI, G., PILO, A., TONI, M. G. and DONATO, L. (1973). Short term determination of plasma protein turnover by a two-tracer technique using plasma only or plasma and urine data. In *Protein Turnover* (Wolstenholme, G. E. W. and O'Connor, M., Eds.), Ciba Foundation Symposia 9 (new series). London; Elsevier/Excerpta Medica/North-Holland

BLACKBURN, G. L., FLATT, J. P., CLOWES, G. H. A., and O'DONNELL, T. E. (1973). Peripheral intravenous feeding with isotonic amino acid solutions. *American Journal of Surgery,* **125,** 447–454

BLOMBÄCK, B. and HANSON, L. A. (1976). *Plasma Proteins.* New York; Wiley Interscience

BOHME, A. (1911). Uber die Schwankungen der Serumkonzentration beim gesunden Menschen. *Deutsches Archiv. für Klinische Medizin,* **103,** 522–562

BRADLEY, J. A., LEDINGHAM, I. MCA. and HAMILTON, D. N. H. (1981). Assessment of host resistance in critically ill surgical patients by the response to recal skin antigens. *Intensive Care Medicine,* **7,** 105

BRODERSEN, F. (1978). Binding of bilirubin and other ligands to human serum albumin. In *Albumin: Structure, Biosynthesis and Function* (Peters, T., Jnr. and Sjöholm, I., Eds), Federation of European Biochemical Societies, Vol. 50, Colloquium B9, pp. 61–70. Oxford; Pergamon Press

BROOM, J., FLECK, A., DAVIDSON, D. F., ROSENBERG, K. and DURNIN, J. V. G. A. (1978). Biochemical adaptations in early starvation: observations on sex difference. *Proceedings of the Nutrition Society,* **37,** 92A

BROWN, J. R. (1978). Structure and evolution of serum albumin. In *Albumin: Structure, Biosynthesis and Function* (Peters, T., Jnr. and Sjöholm, I., Eds.), Federation of European Biochemical Societies, Vol. 50, Colloquium B9, pp. 1–10. Oxford; Pergamon Press

BROWN, R., BANCIEWICZ, J., HAMID, J., PATEL, N. J., WARD, C. A., RARRAND, R. J., PUMPHREY, R. S. H. and IRVING, M. (1982). Failure of delayed hypersensitivity skin testing to predict post operative sepsis and mortality. *British Medical Journal,* **284,** 851–853

BURTON, S., KAY, R., SIMMS, J. M., SMITH, J. A. R. and WOODS, H. F. (1983). Assessing the performance of prognostic nutritional indices. *Clinical Nutrition,* **2,** Special Supplement, 0.92

BUZBY, G. P., MULLEN, J. L., MATTHEWS, D. C., HOBBS, C. L. and ROSATO, E. F. (1980). Prognostic nutritional index in gastrointestinal surgery. *American Journal of Surgery,* **139,** 160–166

CARMICHAEL, M. J., CLAGUE, M. B., KEIR, M. J. and JOHNSTON, L. D. A. (1980). Whole body protein turnover, synthesis and breakdown in patients with colorectal cancer. *British Journal of Surgery,* **67,** 736–739

CONN, H. O. (1977). The use, misuse and abuse of albumin infusions. In *Albumin: Structure, Function and Uses* (Rosenoer, V. M., Oratz, M. and Rothschild, M. A., Eds.), pp. 1–5. Oxford; Pergamon Press

DALY, J. M., VARS, H. M. and DUDRICK, S. J. (1972). Effects of protein depletion on strength of colonic anastomoses. *Surgery, Gynecology and Obstetrics,* **134,** 15–21

DAVIES, J. W. L. (1982). *Physiological Responses to Burning Injury.* London; Academic Press

DAVISON, A. M. (1976). The use of albumin concentrates in hypoproteinaemic states. *Clinics in Haematology,* **5,** 135–148

DEHN, T. C. B., REZNEK, R. H., NOCKLER, I. B. and WHITE, F. E. (1984). The pre-operative assessment of advanced gastric cancer by computed tomography. *British Journal of Surgery,* **71,** 413–417

DUDRICK, S. J., RHOADS, J. E. and VARS, H. M. (1967). Growth of puppies receiving all nutritional requirements by vein. *Fortschritte Parentteralen Ernahrung,* **2,** 16

FLECK, A. (1976). Injury and plasma proteins. In *Metabolism and the Response to Injury* (Wilkinson, A. W. and Cuthbertson, Sir David, Eds.), pp. 229–236. Tunbridge Wells, Kent, UK; Pitman

FLECK, A. (1985). Computer models for plasma protein metabolism studies. *Annals of Clinical Biochemistry* (in press)

FLECK, A. and CLARK, B. (1981). Plasma protein concentration after injury – a simple computer model. In *Homeostasis in Injury and Shock* (Biro, Z., Kovach, A. G. B., Spitzer, J. J. and Stoner, H. B., Eds), *Advances in Physiological Science,* Vol. 26, pp. 81–89. Oxford; Pergamon Press

FLECK, A. and MUNRO, H. N. (1963). Protein metabolism after injury. *Metabolism,* **12,** 783–789

GEEFHUYSEN, J., ROSEN, E. U., KATZ, J., IPP, T. and METZ, J. (1971). Impaired cellular immunity in kwashiorkor with improvement after therapy. *British Medical Journal,* **iv,** 527–529

HARGENS, A. R. (1981). Introduction and historical perspectives. In *Tissue Fluid Pressure and Composition* (Hargens, A. R., Ed.), pp. 1–9. Baltimore; Williams and Wilkins

HAY, R. W., WHITEHEAD, R. G. and SPICER, C. C. (1975). Serum-albumin as a prognostic indicator in oedematous malnutrition. *Lancet,* **ii,** 427–429

HEATLEY, R. V., WILLIAMS, R. H. P. and LEWIS, H. M. (1979). Preoperative intravenous feeding – a controlled trial. *Post-Graduate Medical Journal,* **55,** 541–545

HILL, G. L. and CHURCH, J. (1984). Energy and protein requirements of general surgical patients requiring intravenous nutrition. *British Journal of Surgery,* **71,** 1–9

JENSEN, H., ROSSING, N., ANDERSEN, S. B. T. and JARNUM, S. (1967). Albumin metabolism in the nephrotic syndrome in adults. *Clinical Science,* **33,** 445–457

KEYS, A., BROZEK, J., HENSCHEL, A., MICKELSEN, O. and TAYLOR, H. L. (1950). *The Biology of Human Starvation,* Vols I and II. Minneapolis; University of Minnesota Press

KINGSNORTH, A. N. (1984). Trace elements in adult total parenteral nutrition. *British Journal of Parenteral Therapy,* **5,** 8–22

LAW, D. K., DUDRICK, S. J. and ABDOU, N. I. (1974). The effects of protein calorie malnutrition on immune competence of the surgical patient. *Surgery, Gynecology and Obstetrics,* **139,** 257–266

LEVENSON, S. M., CROWLEY, L. V. and SEIFTER, E. (1975). Starvation. In *Manual of Surgical Nutrition,* pp. 236–264. Philadelphia; Saunders

LUNDSGAARD-HANSEN, P., PAPPORA, E. and FREI, E. (1981). Clinical indications for human serum albumin. In Joint WHO/IABS Symposium on the Standardisation of Albumin and Plasma Substitutes and Plasmaphoresis. *Developments in Biological Standardisation,* Vol. 48, pp. 7–30. Basel; Karger

MCFARLANE, A. S. (1964). Metabolism of plasma proteins. In *Mammalian Protein Metabolism* (Munro, H. N. and Allison, J. B., Eds.), Vol. I, ch. 8, pp. 297–341. New York; Academic Press

MCLAREN, D. S. (1981). Nutritional disorders in surgical patients. In *Nutrition and the Surgical Patient* (G. L. Hill, Ed.), pp. 1–11. Edinburgh; Churchill Livingstone

MEAKINS, J. L., PIETSCH, J. B., RUBENICK, O., KELLY, R., RODE, H., GORDON, J. and MACLEAN, L. D. (1977). Delayed hypersensitivity: indicator of acquired failure of host defences in sepsis and trauma. *Annals of Surgery,* **186,** 241–250

MILLER, J. D. B., BLACKBURN, G. L., BISTRIAN, B. R. *et al.* (1977). Effect of deep surgical sepsis on protein sparing therapies and nitrogen balance. *American Journal of Clinical Nutrition,* **30,** 1528–1532

MOGHISSI, K., HORNSHAW, J., TEASDALE, P. R. and DAWES, E. A. (1977). Parenteral nutrition in carcinoma of the oesophagus treated by surgery: nitrogen balance and clinical studies. *British Journal of Surgery,* **64,** 125–128

MOSS, G. S., SIEGEL, D. C., COCHIN, A. and FRESQUEZ, V. (1971). Effects of saline and colloid solutions on pulmonary function in haemorrhage shock. *Surgery, Gynecology and Obstetrics,* **133,** 53–58

MULLENS, J. L., BUZBY, G. P., WALDMANN, T. F., GERTNER, M. H., HOBBS, C. L. and ROBATO, E. F. (1979). Prediction of operative mortality by preoperative nutritional assessment. *Surgical Forum,* **30,** 80–82

MULLER, J. M., BRENNER, U., DIENST, C. and PICHLMAIER, H. (1982). Preoperative parenteral feeding in patients with gastrointestinal carcinoma. *Lancet,* **1,** 68–71

MYERS, M. A., FLECK, A., SAMPSON, B., COLLEY, C. M., BENT, J. and HALL, G. (1984). Early plasma protein and mineral changes after surgery: a two stage process. *Journal of Clinical Pathology,* **37,** 862–866

NAZARI, S., DIONIGI, R., COMODI, I., DIONIGI, P. and CAMPANI, M. (1982). Preoperative prediction and quantification of septic risk caused by malnutrition. *Archives of Surgery,* **117,** 266–274

OTA, D. M., COPELAND, E. M., CORRIERE, J. M. and DUDRICK, S. J. (1979). The effects of nutrition and treatment of cancer on host immunocompetence. *Surgery, Gynecology and Obstetrics,* **148,** 104

PAGE, C. P., RYAN, J. A. and HAFF, R. C. (1976). Continual catheter administration of an elemental diet. *Surgery, Gynecology and Obstetrics,* **142,** 184

PETERS, T. JNR. (1979). Proteins. In *Chemical Diagnosis of Disease* (Brown, S. S., Mitchell, F. L. and Young, D. S., Eds.), ch. 6, pp. 311–362. Amsterdam; Elsevier/North-Holland

PETERS, T. JNR. and REED, R. G. (1978). Serum albumin conformation and active sites. In *Albumin: Structure, Biosynthesis and Function* (Peters, T. and Sjöholm, I., Eds.), Federation of European Biochemical Societies, Vol. 50, Colloquium B9, pp. 11–20. Oxford; Pergamon Press

PETERS, T. JNR. and SJÖHOLM, I., Eds. (1978). *Albumin: Structure, Biosynthesis and Function.* Federation of European Biochemical Societies, Vol. 50, Colloquium B9. Oxford; Pergamon Press

RAINES, G., FLECK, A., LEDINGHAM, I. MCA. and WALLACE, P. (1984). Increased microvascular permeability to albumin after major surgery, in shock, and in cancer patients. *Scottish Medical Journal,* **29,** 45

ROSENOER, V. M., ORATZ, M. and ROTHSCHILD, M. A. (1977). *Albumin: Structure, Function and Uses.* Oxford; Pergamon Press

ROSSING, N. (1967). The normal metabolism of ^{131}I-labelled albumin in man. *Clinical Science,* **33,** 593–602

ROSSING, N., KRASILNIKOFF, P. A. and CHRISTIANSEN, C. (1972). Plasma protein catabolism in the capillary wall? In *Protides of the Biological Fluids* (Peeters, H., Ed.), Vol. 19, pp. 437–441. Oxford; Pergamon Press

ROSSING, N., PARVING, H. H. and LASSEN, N. A. (1976). Albumin transcapillary escape rate as an approach to microvascular physiology in health and disease. In *Plasma Protein Turnover* (Bianchi, R., Mariani, G. and McFarlane, A. S., Eds.), pp. 357–370. London; Macmillan Press

ROTHSCHILD, M. A., ORATZ, M. and SCHREIBER, S. (1972). Albumin synthesis. *New England Journal of Medicine,* **286,** 748–757

ROTHSCHILD, M. A., ORATZ, M., ZIMMON, D., SCHREIBER, S. S., WEINER, I. and VAN CANEGHEM, A. (1969). Albumin synthesis in arthritic subjects with ascites studied with carbonate-C^{14}. *Journal of Clinical Investigation,* **48,** 344–350

SCHREINER, G. E. (1971). The nephrotic syndrome. In *Diseases of the Kidney* (Strauss, M. B. and Welt, L. G., Eds.), 2nd edn, Vol. 1, pp. 503–636. Boston; Little, Brown

SCHWARTZKOPFF, W., SCHWARTZKOPFF, B., WURM, W. and FRISIUS, H. (1981). Physiological aspects of the role of human albumin in the treatment of chronic and acute blood loss. In Joint WHO/IABS Symposium on the Standardisation of Albumin, Plasma Substitutes and Plasmaphoresis. *Developments in Biological Standardisation,* Vol. 48, pp. 7–30. Basel; Karger

SELLERS, E. M. and KOCH-WESER, J. (1977). Clinical implications of drug–albumin interaction. In *Albumin: Structure, Function and Uses* (Rosenoer, V. M., Oratz, M. and Rothschild, M. A., Eds.), pp. 159–182. Oxford; Pergamon Press

SIMMS, J. M., SMITH, J. A. R. and WOODS, H. F. (1982). A modified prognostic index based upon nutritional measurements. *Clinical Nutrition,* **1,** 71–79

SKILLMAN, J. J., PARIKH, B. M. and TANENBAUM, B. J. (1970). Pulmonary arteriovenous admixture improvement with albumin and diuresis. *American Journal of Surgery,* **119,** 440–447

SKILLMAN, J. J., ROSENOER, V. M., SMITH, P. C. and FANG, M. S. (1976). Improved albumin synthesis in post operative patients by amino acid infusion. *New England Journal of Medicine,* **295,** 1037–1040

SLADE, M. S., SIMMONS, R. L., YUNIS, E. and GREENBERG, L. J. (1975). Immunodepression after major surgery in normal patients. *Surgery,* **78,** 363–372

SMITH, J. A. R., COUBOURGH, H. and NORMAN, J. N. (1979). The problem of patient acceptance of elemental diets in surgical practice. *British Journal of Clinical Practice,* **33,** (2), 43–46

SMITH, J. A. R. and SIMMS, J. M. (1981). A comparison of peripheral and central venous nutrition after total cystectomy. *British Journal of Surgery,* **68,** 809

SMITH, J. A. R., SIMMS, J. M., WILLIAMS, J. L. and WOODS, H. F. (1984). Is total parenteral nutrition necessary after total cystectomy? A pilot study. *Clinical Nutrition,* **3,** 55–58

STUDLEY, H. O. (1936). Percentage of weight loss. A basic indicator of surgical risk in patients with chronic peptic ulcer. *Journal of the American Medical Association,* **106,** 458–460

TAVILL, A. S. (1979). Protein metabolism and the liver. In *Liver and Biliary Disease* (Wright, R., Alberti, K. G. M. M., Karran, S. and Milward-Sadler, G. H., Eds.), ch. 5, pp. 83–107. London; Saunders

TAVILL, A. S., CRAIGIE, A. and ROSENOER, V. M. (1968). The measurement of the synthetic rate of albumin in man. *Clinical Science,* **34,** 1–28

VARLEY, H., GOWENLOCK, A. H. and BELL, M. (1980). *Practical Clinical Chemistry,* Vol. 1, p. 85. London; Heinemann

WARD, M. W. N., DANZI, M., LEWIN, M. R., RENNIE, M. J. and CLARK, C. G. (1982). The effects of subclinical malnutrition and refeeding on the healing of experimental colonic anastomoses. *British Journal of Surgery,* **69,** 308–310

WIKLANDER, O. (1956). Blood volume determinations in surgical practice. *Acta Chirurgica Scandinavica,* **208,** Supplement, 3–136

WOCHNER, R. D., WEISSMAN, S. M., WALDMANN, T. A., HOUSTON, D. and BERLIN, N. I. (1968). Direct measurement of the rates of synthesis of plasma proteins in control subjects and patients with gastrointestinal protein loss. *Journal of Clinical Investigation,* **47,** 971–982

WRETLAND, A. (1972). Complete intravenous nutrition. *Nutrition and Metabolism,* **14,** Supplement, 1–57

Part III

Cardiovascular and pulmonary complications

Chapter 8

Cardiovascular stability in the postoperative patient

K. M. Taylor

Introduction

In the postoperative patient, maintenance of cardiovascular stability is a principal factor in overall recovery and ultimate prognosis. In the post-cardiac surgery patient it assumes prime importance, but even in non-cardiac surgery cases the occurrence of cardiac decompensation or episodes of cardiac arrhythmias may induce cardiac instability with inevitable worsening of the patient's overall condition. In particular, coronary artery disease, present in a very high percentage of the adult population, may result in acute myocardial infarction as a major complicating factor in the clinical course of any patient recovering from major, or even minor, surgery. In addition, patients with known cardiovascular discase require particular attention to this aspect of peri- and postoperative care, if morbidity and even mortality is to be kept to a minimum. An appreciation of the factors influencing haemodynamic stability, and in particular cardiac pumping efficiency, is helpful in understanding the various ways in which cardiovascular stability may be compromised in the postoperative patient.

Factors affecting cardiac pumping efficiency

The heart is a pump and it should never be forgotten that the aim in cardiac care is the achievement and maintenance of optimal pump efficiency. Although a specific problem may exist, for example an arrhythmia, its importance lies in its ability to reduce pumping efficiency and therapy should be directed towards restoration or at least improvement of pumping efficiency. It is also important to remember that pumping is an energy-requiring work and that energy supply–demand inequality should always be considered. It is perfectly possible to increase cardiac output and thus apparently improve cardiac efficiency, but if this rise in output is achieved without a balancing rise in myocardial energy supply, pumping efficiency has not been improved and serious consequences may result, in particular myocardial ischaemia. This unhelpful sequence of events has in the past been associated with the injudicious use of certain inotropic therapy regimens.

When considering cardiac pumping efficiency, the heart may be represented as the left ventricular chamber. The factors affecting pumping efficiency are:

(1) Heart rate.
(2) Heart rhythm disturbance.
(3) Atrial filling pressure.
(4) Peripheral vascular resistance.
(5) Myocardial contractility.

Heart rate

Cardiac output is the product of heart rate times stroke volume, and thus heart rate will directly modify cardiac output. This relationship between change in heart rate and change in cardiac output is not linear, however, since at the upper and lower extremes of heart rate (less than 50–60 beats/min or greater than 120 beats/min), reciprocal changes in stroke volume fail to compensate. It is important to realize that the stroke volume changes depend to a considerable extent on normal left ventricular compliance. Where left ventricular compliance is reduced, for example in myocardial oedema, ischaemia or a cardiomyopathy, increased left ventricular stretch and hence stroke volume cannot be relied upon in slower heart rates. As a general rule, the accepted range for heart rate in the postoperative patient should be 10–20 beats/min above the accepted norms in the resting state, since the obligatory water retention which occurs following surgery will be associated with some impairment in left ventricular compliance.

It is not often appreciated that heart rate must also be considered in relation to pre-existing ventricular size, particularly in patients with long-standing cardiac pathology (Taylor and Bain, 1983). Where cardiac disease has produced a greatly dilated ventricular cavity, such a heart requires a long diastolic filling time and tolerates even relatively fast heart rates less well than a ventricle of normal size. Conversely, the small hypoplastic ventricle tolerates slow heart rates poorly and requires a relatively rapid rate for optimal pumping efficiency. Extremes of heart rate will also affect coronary blood flow. Coronary filling occurs principally in diastole, and the progressive shortening of diastole which accompanies a rise in heart rate will be associated with a corresponding reduction in coronary blood flow. Excessively slow heart rates can also compromise coronary flow, the elevated intramyocardial wall tension towards the end of diastole squeezing the coronary capillary bed and reducing coronary blood flow to the further detriment of the ventricular myocardium.

Heart rhythm disturbance

Disturbance in cardiac rhythm may clearly be life threatening if ventricular tachycardia, ventricular fibrillation or cardiac asystole occur. Less dramatic disturbances in cardiac rhythm may, however, affect cardiac pumping efficiency in one of two ways: (a) by producing a heart rate which is outside the compensated range for that patient; (b) by disturbing or removing the synchronization of normal sinus rhythm, specifically the occurrence of atrial systole less than 0.2 s prior to ventricular systole.

Treatment of such non-life-threatening disturbances in cardiac rhythm may therefore be directed towards restoration of normal sinus rhythm, and this may be possible with either appropriate drug therapy or electrical cardioversion. In certain situations, however, sinus rhythm may not be able to be restored immediately. In this case, improvement may be gained in pumping efficiency by restoring the heart rate to within the normal compensated range. It is important to realize that atrial fibrillation, although well tolerated in patients who are chronic fibrillators, may be very poorly tolerated in terms of haemodynamics when a patient accustomed to sinus rhythm goes into atrial fibrillation acutely in the postoperative period.

Atrial filling pressure

The demonstration by Starling (1918), that the energy of contraction was proportional to the initial length of the cardiac muscle fibres, indicates that atrial filling pressure or preload is an important determinant of cardiac pumping efficiency in relation to the stretch property of myocardial cells. Starling also found that excessive stretching of ventricular muscle led to a reduction in pumping efficiency as occurs with cardiac failure. Left atrial pressure measurement is the most accurate and useful parameter by which to regulate cardiac pumping efficiency, since optimilization of left-sided filling pressure, normally around 10–15 mm Hg, will ensure maximal output efficiency of the ventricle, output, that is the principal cardiac pumping chamber. Although right atrial pressure levels (normally around 5–10 mm Hg) tend to move in parallel with left atrial pressure, this relationship is not always maintained, and in cases of right ventricular dysfunction or if tricuspid valve dysfunction is present, the right atrial filling pressure may be greater than 25 mm Hg, and elevated levels of right atrial filling pressure may be necessary to achieve optimal cardiac function.

There is an increasing trend towards the use of pulmonary artery wedge pressure, using inflatable balloon-tip catheters wedged in the peripheral pulmonary artery to monitor indirectly the left atrial pressure. The initial flow-directed catheters have been further developed to incorporate thermistor sensors and proximal injection orifices to permit thermodilution cardiac output determination. The use of pulmonary artery wedge pressure measurement has been widely introduced in recent years into intensive care practice, and into the postoperative monitoring of patients with actual or potential haemodynamic disturbance, and is likely to become an integral part of haemodynamic monitoring.

Peripheral vascular resistance

The importance of peripheral vascular resistance in the modification of left ventricular performance is increasingly recognized. It is now appreciated that peripheral resistance is a principal determinant of left ventricular performance (Sonnenblick and Downing, 1963). Increasing clinical attention is paid to the state of the peripheral circulation, since mere measurement of arterial blood pressure is not of itself sufficient to make definitive comments regarding the adequacy of the patient's haemodynamic status.

Normal levels of arterial blood pressure may be obtained in patients whose actual cardiac output is extremely low, simply by a balancing increase in peripheral vascular resistance. While this mechanism may be protective in the short term, prolonged periods of increased peripheral resistance are highly dangerous. Many pathophysiological mechanisms are operative in the patient during and after surgery which lead to increases in peripheral resistance, and these will be discussed in greater detail in the section on vasoconstriction.

Myocardial contractility

In addition to the factors affecting cardiac pumping efficiency already discussed, the contractile state of the cardiac muscle fibres themselves is a fundamental determinant of cardiac performance. Reduction in myocardial contractility may be temporary, related to a disturbance of myocardial cell function in which improvement may be anticipated after spontaneous recovery or appropriate therapy. Included in this category are conditions of hypoxia, acidosis, disturbance in the sodium/potassium balance across the cell membrane, increase in myocardial or interstitial water content, and reduced tissue ionized calcium levels. Various cardiopressant drugs, for example beta blockers, calcium antagonists and anti-arrhythmic agents may also produce a temporary disturbance of myocardial contractility.

Permanent reduction in myocardial contractility presents a particular problem. The underlying pathology may be myocardial fibrosis, the result of long-standing myocardial ischaemia or previous acute myocardial infarction, or it may be an idiopathic or toxic cardiomyopathy. The vogue for using stimulating inotropic drugs to increase output from a permanently damaged ventricle is increasingly called into question. It may well have compounded problem cases by increasing myocardial energy demand, with consequent myocardial ischaemic and oxygen debt. Increasingly, where a permanent reduction in myocardial contractility exists in a particular patient, management should rest even more on the accurate maintenance of the other factors influencing cardiac pumping efficiency, i.e. rate, rhythm, filling pressure and vascular resistance.

Vasoconstriction

The importance of vasoconstriction in cardiovascular stability has been increasingly recognized in the past few years. This awareness has been reflected in the increasing use of vasodilator therapy in the management of the failing heart, and of patients with cardiovascular instability. The pathological consequences of vasoconstriction are twofold; first, the peripheral circulation is reduced; secondly, vasoconstriction necessarily increases left ventricular work. Where the elevation of peripheral vascular resistance is modest, and myocardial function is normal, the increased peripheral resistance will be associated with an increase in myocardial performance and in ventricular work. Further elevation in peripheral resistance will, however, impose an increasing after-load on the left ventricle, with eventual reduction in cardiac pumping efficiency and fall in cardiac output. In patients whose ventricular function is already compromised and whose reserve is negligible, even small rises in peripheral vascular resistance may result in significant ventricular dysfunction, thus further impeding left ventricular output.

An appreciation of some of the mechanisms of vasoconstriction indicate that a vicious circle situation may rapidly develop. A reduction in peripheral circulation will be associated with increased release of vasoconstrictive substances, which will further increase vascular resistance and further diminish cardiac output (Taylor *et al.,* 1977).

Vasoconstriction is an almost inevitable accompaniment of cardiac surgery procedures, and may also complicate the postoperative period in a wide variety of clinical situations. The patients exhibit the features of cold peripheries, slow capillary refill, spiky arterial wave forms and a marked core to periphery temperature gradient. The arterial blood pressure levels are not of themselves necessarily helpful. The patients may be normotensive or even hypertensive in absolute terms. The spiky nature of the arterial wave form is helpful in interpreting the absolute levels of blood pressure in vasoconstricted patients.

The aetiology of vasoconstriction is varied, although recent studies have identified particular vasoactive substances as at least major aetiological factors. Among these are activation of the renin/angiotensin system, with production of elevated levels of the vasoconstrictor angiotensin II (Roberts *et al.,* 1978; Taylor *et al.,* 1979a), increased catecholamine activity and elevated levels of the hormone vasopressin (Watkins *et al.,* 1982). In cardiac surgery patients in particular, the principal role of angiotensin II in the occurrence of postoperative vasoconstriction has now clearly been established. Angiotensin II, the end product of renin/angiotensin activation, is a powerful vasoconstrictor and elevated levels have been shown both during and after cardiac surgical procedures, and also following the occurrence of circulatory failure from non-cardiac causes (Taylor, Bain and Morton, 1980). In addition to its peripheral vasoconstrictive action, angiotensin II has also been shown to produce sub-endocardial ischaemia, which may further compromise cardiac pumping efficiency (Gavras *et al.,* 1975). The principal role of angiotensin II in postoperative haemodynamics is seen in relation to the dramatic haemodynamic effects of using specific angiotensin I/angiotensin II conversion inhibitor substances to produce a marked and rapid fall in the elevated level of angiotensin II (*Figures 8.1* and *8.2*). A double haemodynamic effect is seen, namely a rapid fall in elevated levels of peripheral vascular resistance index to normal levels (around 20 index units), and a simultaneous and significant rise in cardiac index as the peripheral resistance levels fall to normal (Taylor *et al.,* 1979b).

The increasing use of vasodilator therapy in vasoconstricted patients, for example with infusion of sodium nitroprusside or of short- or medium-acting nitrate preparation such as GTN, has been associated with significant improvement in cardiac index consequent upon the reduction of peripheral vasoconstriction (Stinson *et al.,* 1977). During the vasoconstricted phase, levels of central venous pressure, pulmonary wedge

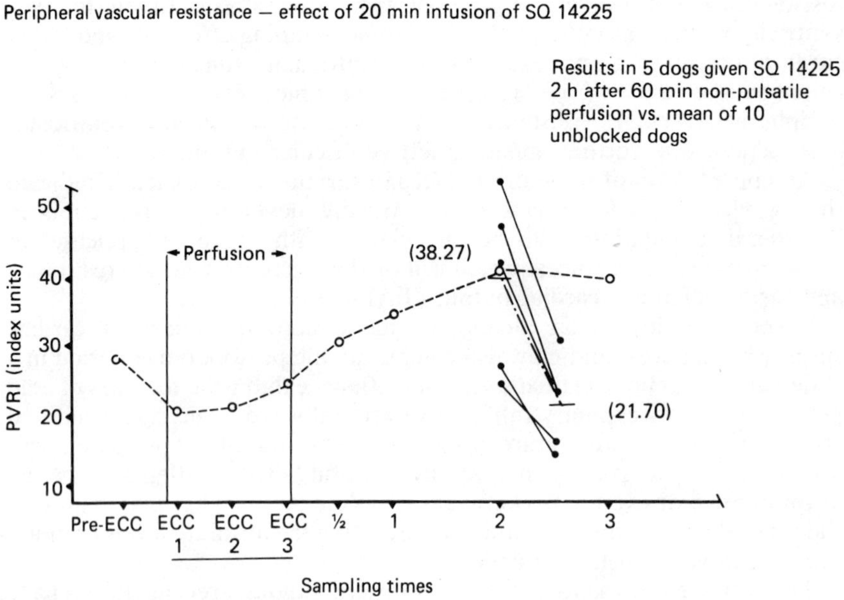

Figure 8.1. Effect of infusion of angiotensin-converting enzyme inhibitor on elevated levels of peripheral vascular resistance index (PVRI) in dogs in the early postoperative period after open-heart surgery. Control dogs' levels of PVRI shown by dotted line (From Taylor *et al.*, 1980, by permission of the publishers)

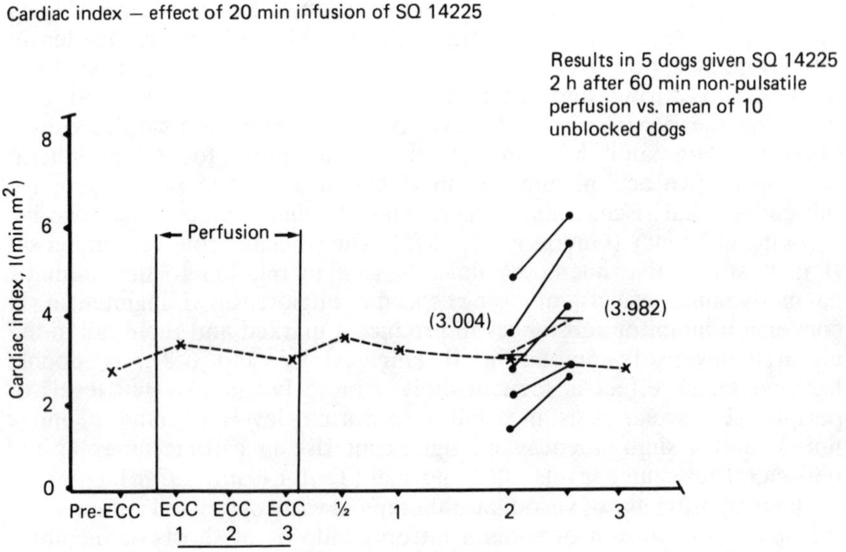

Figure 8.2. Effect of infusion of angiotensin-converting enzyme inhibitor on cardiac index (CI) values in dogs in the early postoperative period after open-heart surgery. Control dogs' levels of CI shown by dotted line (From Taylor *et al.*, 1980, by permission of the publishers)

pressure and left atrial pressure are relatively elevated, despite the fact that most patients are hypovolaemic. As the vasoconstriction recedes and the peripheral circulation opens up, volume replacement is necessary to maintain adequate levels of ventricular filling pressure. Where volume loading is being undertaken, either using blood, colloid or crystalloids, particular care must be exercised in patients who in addition to any cardiac pathology may have increased pulmonary capillary permeability. In patients suffering from adult respiratory distress syndrome, even a small increase in pulmonary capillary pressure will be associated with a marked fluid transit from the vascular compartment into the interstitial space. In these patients, careful monitoring of the pulmonary capillary wedge pressure is therefore of great importance. Although it is not often appreciated, patients in left ventricular failure can endure increases in pulmonary capillary pressure with a much less profound effect in terms of fluid transit.

Water and electrolyte metabolism

It is well known that an overall increase in circulatory volume will be associated with an increase in cardiac chamber stretch and a decrease in cardiac compliance. The cardiac and respiratory effects of excessive water retention and fluid therapy in the postoperative patient have to some extent been overstated. As previously indicated, in a pure cardiac decompensation situation there is a greater capacity to endure increased pulmonary capillary pressure without excessive fluid movement across the pulmonary capillary membrane. The tolerable limits for pulmonary capillary pressure are, however, much tighter in conditions of pulmonary dysfunction, especially those with a permeability defect. It is increasingly appreciated that during certain forms of surgery, in particular open-heart surgery, defects in pulmonary capillary permeability occur in a very high percentage of patients. The most extreme example of this is the full-blown picture of adult respiratory distress syndrome, where avoidance of increase in pulmonary capillary pressure is absolutely mandatory.

Although the details of water and electrolyte metabolism in the postoperative patient are dealt with more fully in other chapters of this book, disturbances of water and electrolyte metabolism have implications for the cardiovascular system in the postoperative patient. There is an obligatory expansion of the extracellular fluid volume following injury. As has been suggested in relation to circulatory overload, over-zealous fluid administration may not seriously disturb cardiovascular stability and, unless the pulmonary capillary membranes are already damaged, may not be associated with gross pulmonary disturbance. The margin for error as far as the cardiovascular system is concerned, in terms of pure fluid excess, is probably greater than has previously been recognized.

There are situations, however, in which underlying pathology may predispose patients to greater cardiovascular and pulmonary dysfunction, if fluid balance is not accurately maintained. Aldosterone is known to be implicated in the water and salt retention following surgery. Continued and increased aldosterone secretion may be a feature of conditions where hepatic metabolism is disordered. Impairment in hepatic metabolism may be a feature of the overall pathological state of the patient, but more particularly where congestive cardiac failure is present hepatic breakdown of aldosterone will be impaired and the overall circulatory problems compounded by a super-added hyperaldosteronism (Flear, 1969). This condition is well recognized in the medical treatment of patients with congestive cardiac failure, in whom water and electrolyte imbalance may at least partly be corrected by aldosterone antagonist therapy, for example with spironolactone.

Of perhaps greater significance than pure water imbalance is the maintenance of normal sodium/potassium balance, particularly in relation to the differential concentrations of these cations across cell membranes. It is now known that reduction in intracellular potassium concentration and simultaneous increase in intracellular sodium concentration may be a feature of many serious illnesses. Extreme degrees of this sodium/potassium reversal have been described in severe burns, in sepsis and in patients with congestive cardiac failure (Hinton, Allison and Farrow, 1972). Minor degrees of this syndrome are also seen in a number of patients undergoing open-heart surgical procedures.

The aetiology of this sodium/potassium imbalance is thought to centre on the sodium pump mechanisms at the cell membrane, and although Flear's concept of the 'sick-cell syndrome' (Flear, 1970) is not widely accepted, there are situations in which this malfunction of the sodium pump mechanism can clearly be demonstrated. Despite the continuing controversy over the frequency and severity of the so-called sick-cell syndrome, there is no question that sodium/potassium imbalance across the myocardial cell has significant implications for cardiovascular stability. Reduction in intracellular potassium concentration in the myocardium is known to be associated with cardiac instability, the appearance of ventricular arrhythmias, an increase in pacing thresholds and an increase in sensitivity to digoxin therapy (Flear and Singh, 1973). If established, this sodium pump malfunction will induce a vicious circle situation, since the failing heart will be further compromised by disturbance of its own sodium/potassium intracellular balance. Mere measurement of the serum electrolytes may not be sufficient to fully alert the surgical team to the existence of this syndrome. The appearance of a falling serum sodium with a parallel rise in serum potassium is suggestive, but should be confirmed by urinary electrolyte measurements. The marked fall in urinary sodium levels and the rise in urinary potassium levels will confirm the existence of this syndrome, so that appropriate intervention therapy can be undertaken. It cannot be stressed enough that the appearance of a low serum sodium level is misleading in this particular clinical situation, and that mistaken administration of intravenous sodium to counteract the hyponatraemia can seriously aggravate the situation and lead to even greater cardiovascular instability.

Therapy in this syndrome should be directed first towards improving cardiac output, and secondly towards providing greater energy supply to the failing sodium pump mechanisms. In this regard, the use of glucose/insulin/potassium infusions has been associated with marked clinical benefit. In severe sodium pump malfunction, 50% dextrose, 100 ml over 2 h, with 40 mmol potassium, and insulin according to Dextrostix, can be used in the initial resuscitation of severe cases. Early detection of a trend to sodium/potassium imbalance in postoperative patients can be dealt with at an earlier stage in its natural history by the simple provision of 20% dextrose infusion.

Vascular permeability and blood cell microaggregates

Cardiovascular instability may also occur in the postoperative patient, in relation not to a primary cardiac source, but in relation to the peripheral vasculature. Vascular permeability is clearly vital in terms of the integrity of the peripheral circulation, and changes in vascular permeability may occur in a variety of clinical situations. It is known that numerous vasoactive substances exert considerable effects in local or general vascular permeability. Such substances include histamine, serotonin, kinins, the end products of complement activation and possibly free superoxide radicals. The release of these vasoactive substances may occur simply as a result of the operative procedure. There is recent evidence which indicates that plasma histamine levels are elevated above 1 ng/ml, that is into the pathological range, during major surgery and furthermore that elevated levels may persist into the early postoperative period (Hosking, Man and Taylor, 1985). In addition, studies have demonstrated the phenomenon of microaggregation of the formed elements of the blood in the circulation of patients during and after surgical procedures. This is obviously of particular importance where the patient's blood is exposed to biomaterials, as happens in insertion of synthetic materials into the vascular system during open-heart surgery where the patient is on total extracorporeal circulation, and also during shunting procedures including haemodialysis (*Figure 8.3*).

In these specific situations, considerable microaggregation occurs, possibly as a result of the primary process of platelet adhesion and aggregation, with resulting incorporation of white and red blood cells and fibrin. It is also known that microaggregates are present in stored blood, and may be introduced into the patient's venous circulation during homologous blood transfusion. Even the use of micropore filtration of stored blood may not wholly prevent the passage of microaggregates or the passage of released vasoactive substances from microaggregates into the patient's circulation. It is not often appreciated that studies have shown that microaggregates are not inert bodies. They are biologically active and have been shown to extrude the contents of mast cell secretory granules, i.e. histamine, serotonin, kinins, etc., from the microaggregate into the vascular or interstitial space.

The lung appears particularly susceptible to microaggregation-related damage with subsequent disturbance of vascular permeability. The lung itself acts as a filter for microaggregates, and recent studies have shown a high incidence of pulmonary capillary permeability defects during and after major surgical procedures. Where a severe degree of pulmonary

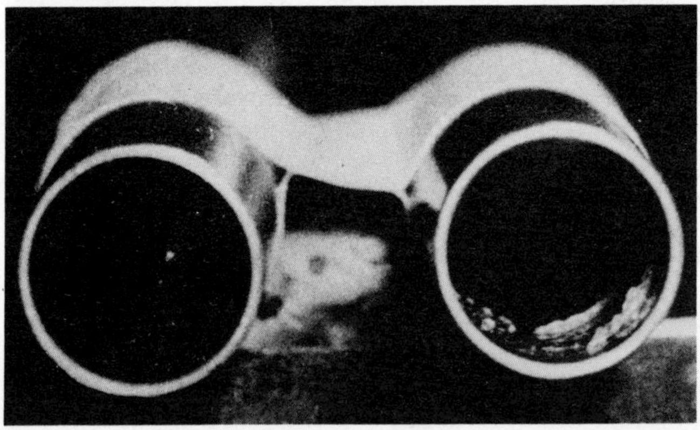

Figure 8.3. Aggregates formed in connector tube in extracorporeal circuit after passage of fully heparinized blood at 4.0 l/min for 90 min. Pre-perfusion connector tube appearance shown for comparison

dysfunction occurs as a result of pulmonary capillary permeability defects, consequent hypoxia may exert a secondary pathological effect on myocardial contractility. The whole area of vascular permeability defect, and the possible roles of substances like histamine and serotonin, require much further investigation. It is striking how little is known at present regarding the patterns of response of these vasoactive substances during even general surgical procedures.

Local vascular vasoactive substances

One of the areas of emerging interest in the field of cardiovascular physiology and pathology is the presence within the blood vessel walls of a spectrum of vasoactive substances. It is now known, for example, that concentration gradients may exist across the vascular endothelial wall, of substances which may exert opposing but balanced haemodynamic effects. Such a situation is known to exist in relation to thromboxane and prostacyclin, with the axis moving towards one or other under different clinical conditions. The recent studies have suggested that impaired perfusion in the central circulation is associated with an increase in the local concentration of thromboxane in the peripheral blood vessels, whereas restoration of adequate circulation moves the axis towards the prostacyclin side. Other substances of current interest are leucotrienes, which are known to exert profound local vascular effects, but have also been shown in recent studies to be pronounced coronary vasocontrictors. Other workers are investigating the presence of an as yet unidentified vasodilator substance present within vascular endothelium.

It is clear from all these pilot studies that many vasoactive substances are present and active in the peripheral circulation, and that disturbance in the physiological balance either by local trauma or by some central pathology may induce marked haemodynamic effects mediated through these locally occurring vasoactive agents. Activation of the complement system continues to be a subject of interest. Complement activation does appear to occur during open-heart surgery, but this may be related to the exposure of the blood to the artificial circuit and complement activating materials such as nylon (Kirklin *et al.*, 1983). Free radical damage is being looked for, particularly in relation to the lung where early results suggest that activation of white cells may be demonstrated together with high levels of lipid peroxidation products.

As might be anticipated, the interest in these particular vasoactive substances is paralleled by a development of potentially therapeutic antagonists. The roles of antihistamine therapy, of serotonin antagonists and of anti-free radical substances such as vitamin C and superoxide dismutase are interesting, but at the present time largely experimental (Dormandy, 1983). There is no doubt, however, that in the course of the next 5–10 years, much information will be obtained in this particular area of locally occurring vasoactive substances and their effects on peripheral vascular permeability.

Conclusions

The central importance of cardiovascular stability in any patient is well recognized. The postoperative patient may be at particular risk, either as a result of underlying and possibly subclinical cardiovascular pathology or because of cardiovascular changes associated with the peri- or postoperative period. The maintenance of cardiovascular stability is relatively straightforward in the vast majority of patients. An appreciation of the factors affecting cardiac pumping efficiency will inevitably lead to the achievement and maintenance of cardiovascular stability throughout the postoperative period. Attention to simple factors such as heart rate, rhythm, atrial filling pressure and peripheral vascular resistance will be sufficient, in the vast majority of cases, to ensure a smooth course from the cardiovascular point of view.

Vasoconstriction is a particularly hazardous haemodynamic environment in which to leave any patient. The inevitable increase in left ventricular work to overcome the increased after-load may induce secondary myocardial ischaemia, and may, in patients with pre-existing coronary artery disease, result in full-blown acute myocardial infarction. The interpretation of absolute levels of blood pressure in relation to the state of the peripheral circulation will prevent many a cardiac mishap. Water and electrolyte disturbances are of importance, particularly where sodium/potassium imbalance occurs. The emerging field of disturbances of vascular permeability, blood cell microaggregation and locally occurring vasoactive substances are all of relevance in the overall picture of cardiovascular stability. Thankfully, in view of the rather limited knowledge which we have at present in these areas, major disturbances in this area of cardiovascular physiology are relatively uncommon and are often the consequence of some other major primary pathology.

References

DORMANDY, T. L. (1983). An approach to free radicals. *Lancet,* **II,** 1010–1016

FLEAR, C. T. G. (1969). Alterations in water and electrolyte distribution in congestive heart failure and their significance. *Annals of the New York Academy of Sciences,* **155,** Article 1, 421–444

FLEAR, C. T. G. (1970). Electrolyte and body water changes after trauma. *Clinical Pathology,* Supplement, **23**(1), 16–31

FLEAR, C. T. G. and SINGH, C. M. (1973). Hyponatraemia and sick cells. *British Journal of Anaesthesia,* **45,** 976–994

GAVRAS, H., KREMER, D., BROWN, J. J., GRAY, B., LEVER, A. F., MACADAM, R. F., MEDINA, A., MORTON, J. J. and ROBERTSON, J. I. S. (1975). Angiotensin and norepinephrine-induced myocardial lesions: experimental and clinical studies in rabbits and man. *American Heart Journal,* **89,** 321

HINTON, P., ALLISON, S. P. and FARROW, S. (1972). Blood volume changes and transfusion requirements of burned patients after the shock phase of injury. *Lancet,* **1,** 913–915

HOSKING, S., MAN, N. and TAYLOR, K. M. (1985). Plasma histamine levels during major surgery (in press)

KIRKLIN, J. K., WESTABY, S., BLACKSTONE, E. H., KIRKLIN, J. W., CHENOWETH, D. E. and PACIFICO, A. D. (1983). Complement and the damaging effects of cardiopulmonary bypass. *Journal of Thoracic and Cardiovascular Surgery,* **86,** 845–857

ROBERTS, A. J., NIARCHOS, A. P., SUBRAMANIAN, V. A., ABEL, R. M., HERMAN, S. D., SCALEY, J. E., CASE, D. B., WHITE, R. P., JOHNSON, G. A., LARAGH, J. H. and GAY, W. A. (1978). Hypertension following coronary artery bypass graft surgery. Comparison of haemodynamic responses to nitroprusside, phentolamine, and converting enzyme inhibitor. *Circulation,* Supplement 1, **58,** 43

SONNENBLICK, E. H. and DOWNING, S. E. (1963). Afterload as a primary determinant of ventricular performance. *American Journal of Physiology,* **204,** 604

STARLING, E. H. (1918). *The Law of the Heart Beat.* New York; Longmans

STINSON, E. B., HOLLOWAY, E. L., DERBY, G. C., COPELAND, J. G., OYER, P. E., BEUHLER, D. L. and GRIEPP, R. B. (1977). Control of myocardial performance early after open-heart operations by vasodilator treatment. *Journal of Thoracic and Cardiovascular Surgery,* **73,** 523

TAYLOR, K. M. and BAIN, W. H. (1983). The cardiovascular system. In *Handbook of Intensive Care* (Bain, W. H. and Taylor, K. M., Eds.). Bristol; John Wright

TAYLOR, K. M., BAIN, W. H. and MORTON, J. J. (1980). The role of angiotensin II in the development of peripheral vasoconstriction during open-heart surgery. 1. *American Heart Journal,* **100,** 935–937

TAYLOR, K. M., BRANNAN, J. J., BAIN, W. H., CAVES, P. K. and MORTON, J. J. (1979a). The role of angiotensin II in the development of peripheral vasoconstriction during cardiopulmonary bypass. *Cardiovascular Research,* **8,** 269

TAYLOR, K. M., CASSALS, J. G., MITTRA, S. M., BRANNAN, J. J. and MORTON, J. J. (1980). Haemodynamic effects of angiotensin converting enzyme inhibition after cardiopulmonary bypass in dogs. *Cardiovascular Research,* **14**(4), 199–205

TAYLOR, K. M., CASSALS, J., MORTON, J. J., MITTRA, S., BRANNAN, J. J. and BAIN, W. H. (1979b). The haemodynamic effects of angiotensin blockade after cardiopulmonary bypass. *British Heart Journal,* **41,** 380

TAYLOR, K. M., MORTON, J. J., BROWN, J. J., BAIN, W. H. and CAVES, P. K. (1977). Hypertension and the renin–angiotensin system following open-heart surgery. *Journal of Thoracic and Cardiovascular Surgery,* **74,** 840

WATKINS, D. W., PETERSON, M. B. KONG, D. L., KONO, K., BUCKLEY, M. J., LEVINE, F. H. and PHILBIN, D. M. (1982). *Journal of Thoracic and Cardiovascular Surgery,* **84,** 250–256

Chapter 9

The role of serotonin in blood pressure regulation

J. Symoens and P. M. Vanhoutte

Introduction by the Editors

Cardiovascular complications are relatively common after major surgery, their incidence increasing with age, type of anaesthesia and pre-existing atherosclerosis. The latter condition becomes more common with advancing years, from 6% at 45 years to 100% over age 80 years. The most serious risk factor is a history of myocardial infarction in the preceding 6 months, where the risk of serious cardiac problems is 55%. Even after 3 years, the risk of further infarct remains 1% (relative to a general risk of 0.6%). However, hypertension in itself is a significant risk factor, yet little is known about the pathogenesis of changes in blood pressure, especially in the postoperative period. A number of clinical mediators have been implicated, including serotonin. This chapter reviews the role of serotonin, with particular reference to experimental data, but provides a basis to improve understanding of a significant clinical problem.

(J.A.R.S. and J.W.)

The idea that serotonin might play a role in hypertension is not new. Page and his co-workers discovered the monoamine during their search for humoral pressor agents which might be held responsible for the increased vascular resistance in hypertension (Rapport, Green and Page, 1948; Page, 1957). The initial enthusiasm regarding the potential role of serotonin in hypertension progressively faded away. There are three main reasons for this scepticism: (a) serotonin injected intravenously into normal animals or man has variable effects on blood pressure; (b) there is no evidence that plasma levels of serotonin are augmented in hypertensive patients; (c) serotonergic antagonists have not been very successful in lowering arterial blood pressure in hypertensive animals and man. However, several recent findings have revived the hypothesis that peripheral serotonin may play a role in hypertension (Vanhoutte, 1982a, 1982b, 1983; Vanhoutte and Cohen, 1983; Vanhoutte, Cohen and Van Nueten, 1984; Vanhoutte *et al.*, 1983).

The fate of serotonin

Most of the serotonin found outside the central nervous system is synthesized from dietary tryptophan in the enterochromaffin cells of the gut. Most of the serotonin overflowing from these cells into the blood is removed by the liver or actively taken up and deaminated by monoamine oxidase (MAO) in endothelial cells, in particular in the lungs, which allow less than 1% of the serotonin contained in portal blood to pass. The principal metabolite, 5-hydroxyindole-acetic acid (5-HIAA) is excreted in the urine at a rate of 2–10 mg/dl in a normal adult human. The serotonin escaping hepatic and endothelial metabolism is avidly taken up by platelets and stored in the dense granules. The concentration of serotonin in normal human blood is 60–400 ng/ml, contained almost exclusively in the platelets. Free circulating serotonin levels are negligible in healthy individuals (±1 ng/ml). The platelets release the monoamine when activated by a variety of agents including serotonin itself (Erspamer, 1961; Thompson, 1971; White, 1971; Zucker, 1975). Once released, serotonin can modulate platelet reactions and affect the contractile behaviour of the blood vessel wall.

Serotonin and platelets

Platelets respond to various stimuli with a uniform sequence of morphological reactions, including: (a) shape change or transformation of a smooth disc to a spiny sphere; (b) reversible aggregation or cohesion of cells without degranulation; (c) degranulation and release-reaction, depending on the nature and the concentration of the inducer. During the release-reaction, the contents of the alpha-granules (including platelet factor 4 and β-thromboglobulin) and of the dense granules (including serotonin) are released. The platelet activation is linked to an increase of free intracellular Ca^{2+} ions which activate the contractile proteins (actomyosin) of the platelets. The Ca^{2+} ions usually are mobilized from intraplatelet stores (Zucker, 1975; De Clerck and David, 1981) and the serotonin-induced rise of free intracellular Ca^{2+} during shape changes of human platelets can be blocked by serotonergic S_2 receptor blockers such as ketanserin (Pletscher and Affolter, 1983).

Serotonin is a relatively weak activator of human platelets, as it induces shape change and reversible aggregation without release-reaction (De Clerck and David, 1981). Biphasic aggregation with degranulation (*Figure 9.1*) occurs occasionally in healthy humans, but is more frequent in patients

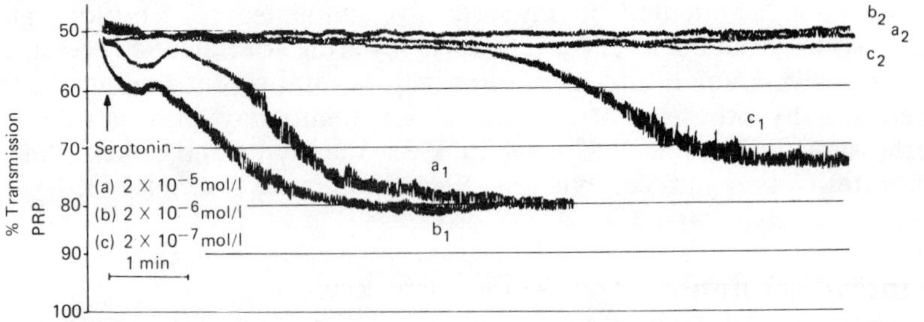

Figure 9.1. Irreversible platelet aggregation with release-reaction induced by various concentrations of serotonin (a_1, b_1, c_1) in platelet-rich plasma (PRP) from a post-myocardial infarction patient. A single oral dose of 60 mg ketanserin taken 1 h before blood sampling prevents the effect of the same concentrations of serotonin (a_2, b_2, c_2) (J. De Crée, unpublished data)

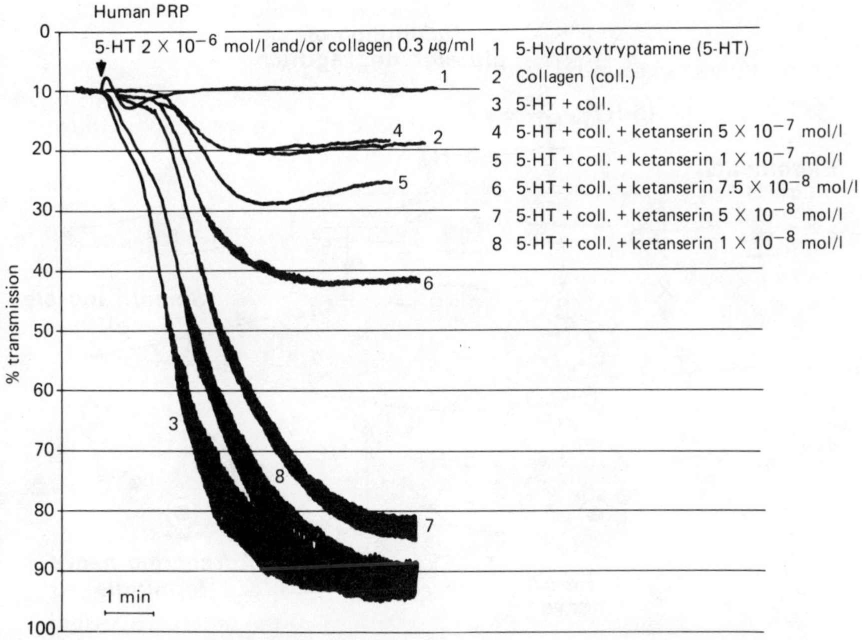

Figure 9.2. Platelet aggregation induced in human platelet-rich plasma (PRP) by serotonin and/or collagen, and dose-dependent inhibition of the effect by ketanserin (From De Clerck, David and Janssen, 1982, by permission of the publishers)

with cardiovascular disease (De Crée *et al.*, 1985). However, serotonin potentiates the platelet reaction to low concentrations of other agonists including adenosine diphosphate (ADP), collagen, epinephrine and norepinephrine (*Figure 9.2*). The direct and amplifying effects of serotonin on platelet aggregation are mediated by activation of S_2-serotonergic receptors on the platelet membrane (De Clerck, David and Janssen, 1982; Pletscher and Affolter, 1983).

Serotonin and blood vessels

Depending on the type of blood vessel, its localization, the species and the integrity of the endothelium, serotonin causes contraction or dilatation (*Figure 9.3*) (Vanhoutte, 1982a, 1982b; Vanhoutte and Cohen, 1983; Vanhoutte, Cohen and Van Nueten, 1984; Vanhoutte *et al.*, 1983).

Serotonin causes dose-dependent contractions of most large blood vessels, with, however, important differences in sensitivity depending on the origin of the tissue studied. At the microcirculatory level, serotonin is a potent constrictor of venules. The constrictor response to serotonin can be augmented by the acute (e.g. local cooling in cutaneous blood vessels, or hypoxia in coronary arteries) or chronic (e.g. aging) conditions to which blood vessels are exposed. In most large arteries and in venules, serotonin evokes contraction by activation of S_2-serotonergic receptors on the cell

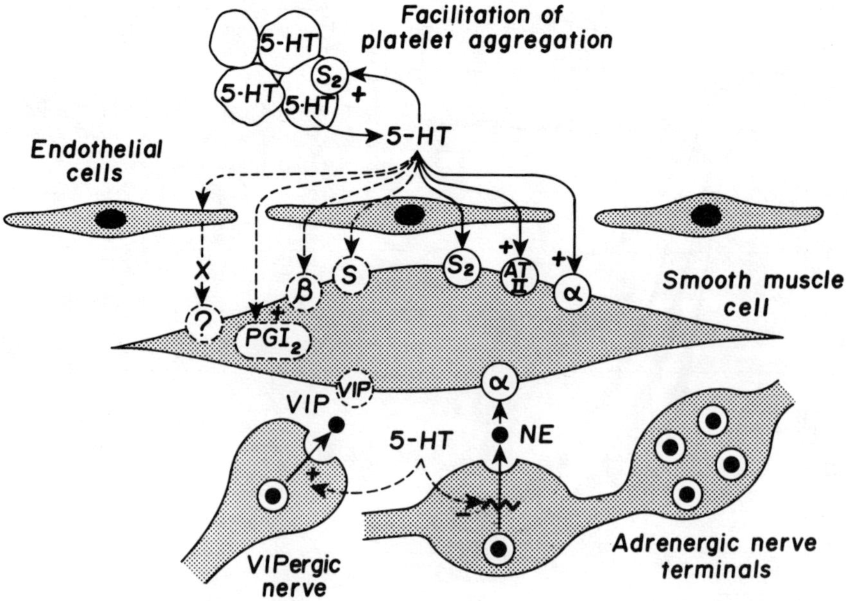

Figure 9.3. Multiple effects of serotonin on the blood vessel wall. Vasoconstriction could be caused by: (1) activation of serotonergic receptors on the smooth muscle cells; (2) amplification of the vasoconstrictor responses of other neurohumoral mediators (e.g. norepinephrine, NE; angiotensin II); (3) activation of post-junctional α-adrenoceptors (α); or (4) an indirect sympathomimetic effect, by displacement of stored norepinephrine from adrenergic nerve terminals. Free serotonin also activates S_2 receptors on platelets causing enhanced release of the stored amine. Vasodilatation could be caused by: (1) inhibition of adrenergic neurotransmission (presumably by activating S_1-serotonergic receptors); (2) activation of inhibitory autonomic nerves (presumably causing release of vasoactive intestinal polypeptide, VIP); (3) activation of inhibitory serotonergic receptors (S) on the smooth muscle cells; (4) activation of the production of prostacyclin (PGI_2); (5) stimulation of β-adrenoceptors (β); and (6) triggering of endothelium-dependent relaxation (presumably mediated by S_1-serotonergic receptors). Not all these effects have been demonstrated in all blood vessels. + = excitatory effect, amplification; − = inhibitory effect (From Vanhoutte and Cohen, 1983, by permission of the publishers)

membrane of vascular smooth muscle cells. Their activation triggers the contractile process mainly by increasing the entry of extracellular Ca^{2+} into the cells. In other blood vessels, e.g. cutaneous blood vessels, serotonin may directly or indirectly activate α_1-adrenoceptors on the vascular smooth muscle cells. In addition to the direct vasoconstrictor effects, the most characteristic feature of serotonin is its ability to amplify the constrictor responses to other neurohumoral mediators, including noradrenaline, thromboxane A_2, angiotensin II, histamine, etc. (*Figure 9.4*). The amplifying effect of serotonin is mediated by serotonergic S_2 receptors on the vascular smooth muscle cells.

The vasodilator (depressor) effect of serotonin has been observed mainly in the intact organism, in particular at the level of the small precapillary vessels (*Figure 9.5*). The effect is most marked when

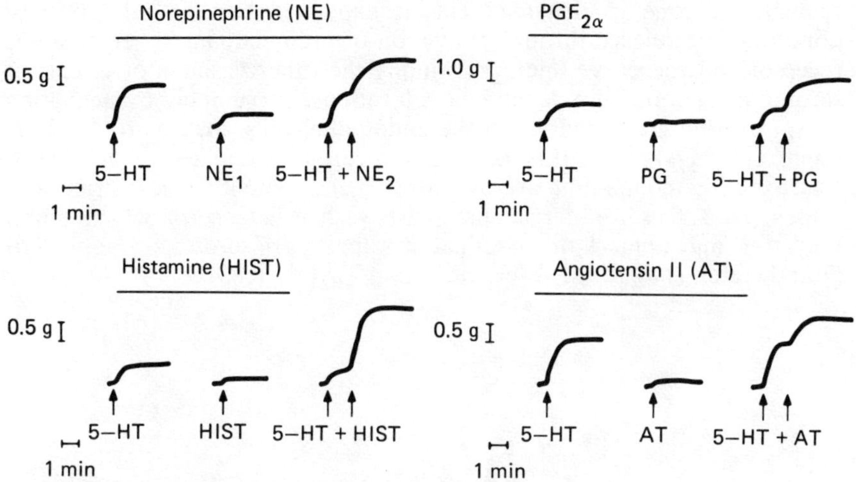

5–HT:2.9 x 10^{-8}mol/l; NE_1:7.4 x 10^{-10}mol/l; $PGF_{2\alpha}$:4.5 x 10^{-7}mol/l;

HIST:2.1 x 10^{-7}mol/l; AT:1.5 x 10^{-10}mol/l

Figure 9.4. Vasoconstriction induced by serotonin (5-HT), norepinephrine, prostaglandin $F_{2\alpha}$, histamine, angiotensin II and amplification of these effects by serotonin (From Van Nueten, 1983, by permission of the publishers)

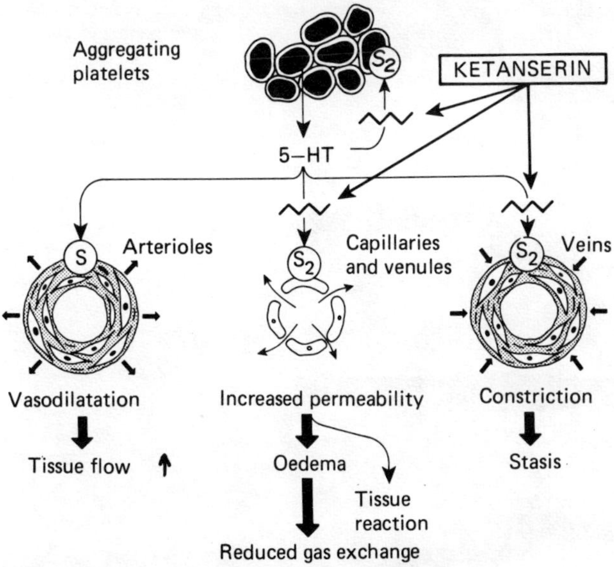

Figure 9.5. Potential role of serotonin at the microcirculatory level. The release of serotonin from aggregating platelets would tend to: cause vasodilatation at the arteriolar level (left); increase capillary and venular permeability (middle); and cause venoconstriction (right). The combination of these effects favours local oedema and stasis. The increased permeability and venoconstriction are mediated by S_2-serotonergic receptors, at which selective antagonists could prevent the response (From Vanhoutte and Cohen, 1983, by permission of the publishers)

sympathetic tone is elevated. This is explained best by inhibition of noradrenaline release through activation of prejunctional S_1-serotonergic receptors on the nerve endings. Among the other vasodilator effects of serotonin, endothelium-dependent relaxations, presumably by activation of S_1-serotonergic receptors on the endothelial cells, may be particularly important (*Figure 9.3*). It is likely that in certain vascular beds the dilator effects of the monoamine are overcome by the potent vasoconstriction it causes. Thus, S_2-serotonergic antagonists such as ketanserin, which inhibit the latter, may unmask the vasodilator properties of serotonin (*Figure 9.6*) (Van Nueten *et al.*, 1981; McLennan and Taylor, 1983).

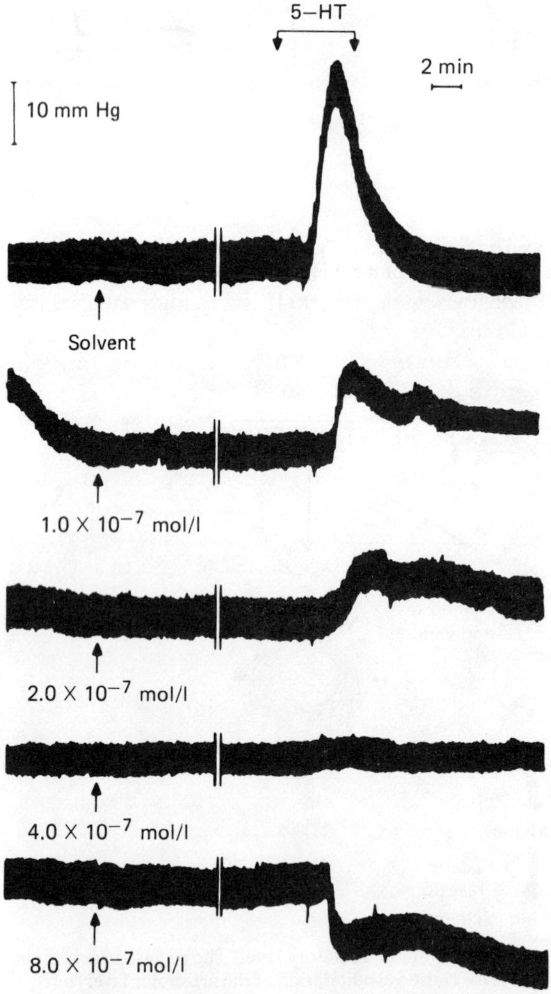

Figure 9.6. Demonstration, in the isolated perfused guinea pig stomach, that increasing concentrations of the S_2-serotonergic antagonist ketanserin inhibit the vasoconstrictor response to serotonin and eventually reverse it to a vasodilator reaction (From Van Nueten *et al.*, 1981, by permission of the publishers)

Serotonin and arterial blood pressure

In animals, after exclusion of the nervous control of blood vessels by pithing, serotonin causes a prompt, uncomplicated rise in blood pressure lasting several minutes. In contrast to the pithed animal, in the intact animal intravenous serotonin causes variable changes in blood pressure. If nervous vasomotor tone is high, the response is predominantly hypotensive and vice versa (Page, 1957).

Serotonin appears to play a minor role in cardiovascular control of healthy animals and man, as it is effectively removed from the plasma by platelets and endothelial cells. To imply that serotonin contributes to the aetiology of disease(s), one must assume that either the mechanisms of uptake, metabolism and release are altered or that the vascular sensitivity to serotonin is increased.

Serotonin and hypertension

The vascular responsiveness to the vasoconstrictor effect of serotonin is specifically increased in aging normotensive rats (De Mey and Vanhoutte, 1981) and, even more, in adult hypertensive rats (McGregor and Smirk, 1970; Haeusler and Finch, 1972; Collis and Vanhoutte, 1977; De Mey and Vanhoutte, 1981; Taylor and McLennan, 1983). It is not increased in very young hypertensive rats (Collis, De Mey and Vanhoutte, 1979). The increased responsiveness to serotonin seen in hypertensive animals probably reflects premature aging of the blood vessel wall exposcd chronically to an abnormal distending pressure. The vasoconstrictor response to serotonin in adult hypertensive rats is markedly more increased than the vasoconstrictor response to other pressor agents, e.g. noradrenaline or angiotensin II (*Figure 9.7*). An increased responsiveness of blood vessels to the vasoconstrictor effects of serotonin has also been observed in atherosclerotic monkeys and rabbits (Yokoyama and Henry, 1979; Lucas, Saffitz and Henry, 1981; Heistad *et al.,* 1984). The rate of development of tachyphylaxis to the vasoconstrictor effect of serotonin is considerably delayed in spontaneously hypertensive rats, compared to normotensive animals. It is also delayed in aging normotensive rats (De Mey and Vanhoutte, 1981). The ability to clear serotonin from the blood in the lungs appears to be reduced in spontaneously hypertensive rats (Roth and Wallace, 1980). Old spontaneously hypertensive rats have excessive amounts of platelet aggregates within the glomeruli characterizing glomerular thrombosis. Heparin treatment reduces the number of glomeruli with platelet aggregates and normalizes mean arterial blood pressure, suggesting a causal relationship between glomerular thrombosis and hypertension in old spontaneously hypertensive rats (Mandal *et al.,* 1978).

In patients with essential hypertension, various abnormalities of platelet function have been described: (a) increased sensitivity of platelets to aggregating agents, including serotonin (Poplawski, Skorulska and Micwiarowski, 1968; Coccheri and Fiorentini, 1971; Vlachakis and Aldedort, 1980; Matsumo *et al.,* 1981; Affolter *et al.,* 1984); (b) increased

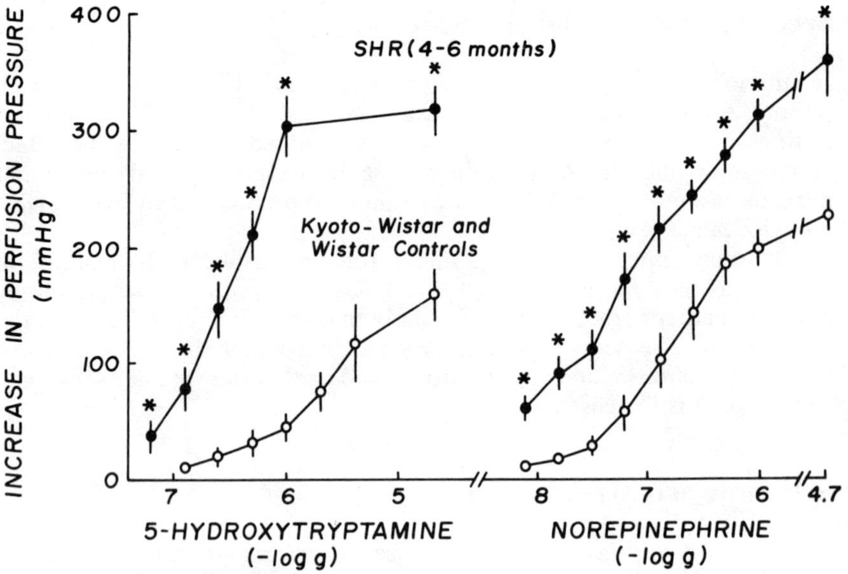

Figure 9.7. Vasoconstrictor response to 5-hydroxytryptamine (left) and norepinephrine (right) in isolated Tyrode-perfused kidneys from normotensive and spontaneously hypertensive (SHR) adult rats (From Vanhoutte, 1982b, by permission of the publishers)

plasma levels of β-thromboglobulin which is indicative of the platelet release reaction (Mehta and Mehta, 1981; Petralito *et al.*, 1982; Kjeldsen *et al.*, 1983); (c) lowered serotonin content of platelets (Bhargava *et al.*, 1979; Baudouin-Legras *et al.*, 1985; Guicheney *et al.*, 1985); (d) reduced uptake of serotonin by platelets (Bhargava *et al.*, 1979; Baudouin-Legros *et al.*, 1985; Guicheney *et al.*, 1985). These observations strongly suggest that, at least in certain patients with essential hypertension, platelet activation occurs which is sufficient to produce intravascular release of serotonin. In addition, the vascular responsiveness to the vasoconstrictor effect of serotonin is augmented in the forearm vessels of hypertensive patients (Doyle, Fraser and Marshall, 1959).

The defects in the handling of serotonin by platelets and endothelial cells and the augmented responsiveness of the vascular smooth muscle could help to explain the increase in peripheral resistance seen in hypertensive patients (*Figure 9.8*). The fact that, in hypertensive patients, free circulating serotonin levels are not elevated is not meaningful because such levels do not necessarily reflect the amounts liberated at the interface between aggregating platelets and the blood vessel wall, nor the amount of vasoconstriction induced by serotonin. The latter depends on the neurogenic vasomotor tone, the (hyper)responsiveness of the blood vessel wall, the integrity of the endothelium and the amplification by serotonin of the responses to other vasopressor agents. Likewise, the free plasma levels of catecholamines do not reflect the degree of adrenergic tone either (Folkow *et al.*, 1983). Page (1957) has stated: 'I personally suspect that it is the minute amounts of serotonin liberated in situ that are important rather than these of the order of magnitude used to demonstrate pharmacological phenomena.'

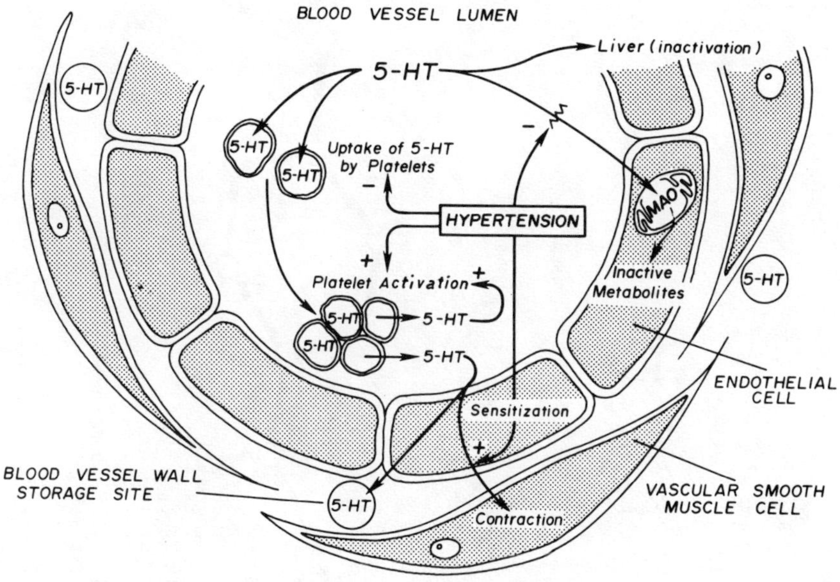

Figure 9.8. The handling of serotonin (5-HT) by platelets and the blood vessel wall in hypertension. MAO = monoamine oxidase; + = activation; − = inhibitory effect (From Vanhoutte, 1982b, by permission of the publishers)

Serotonergic antagonists: ketanserin and the treatment of hypertension

If serotonin plays a role in the maintenance of the augmented peripheral resistance in chronic hypertension, serotonergic antagonists should lower arterial blood pressure in hypertensive animals and man. Early attempts were disappointing, presumably: (a) because the drugs used blocked both the vasodilator and vasoconstrictor effects of serotonin; (b) because they had agonistic properties, which are particularly important in stimulating the hypertensive blood vessels; or (c) because they had serious central side-effects. More recently, ketanserin (*Figure 9.9*) may provide an example of an antihypertensive serotonergic antagonist.

Ketanserin is a selective S_2-serotonergic antagonist. It does not bind to the S_1-binding sites and is devoid of agonistic properties. It has both an α_1-adrenergic and a H_1-histaminergic blocking activity, although these occur at larger concentrations than required to antagonize S_2-serotonergic receptors (Leysen *et al.*, 1981; Van Nueten *et al.*, 1981; De Clerck, David and Janssen, 1982). Ketanserin antagonizes serotonin-induced vasoconstrictions and unmasks serotonin-induced vasodilatation (*Figure 9.6*). It antagonizes serotonin-induced platelet aggregation (*Figure 9.1*); it inhibits the amplifying effects of serotonin on vasoconstriction and platelet aggregation induced by other agonists (*Figures 9.2* and *9.4*); it antagonizes the hypertensive response to serotonin in pithed rats (Fozard, 1982;

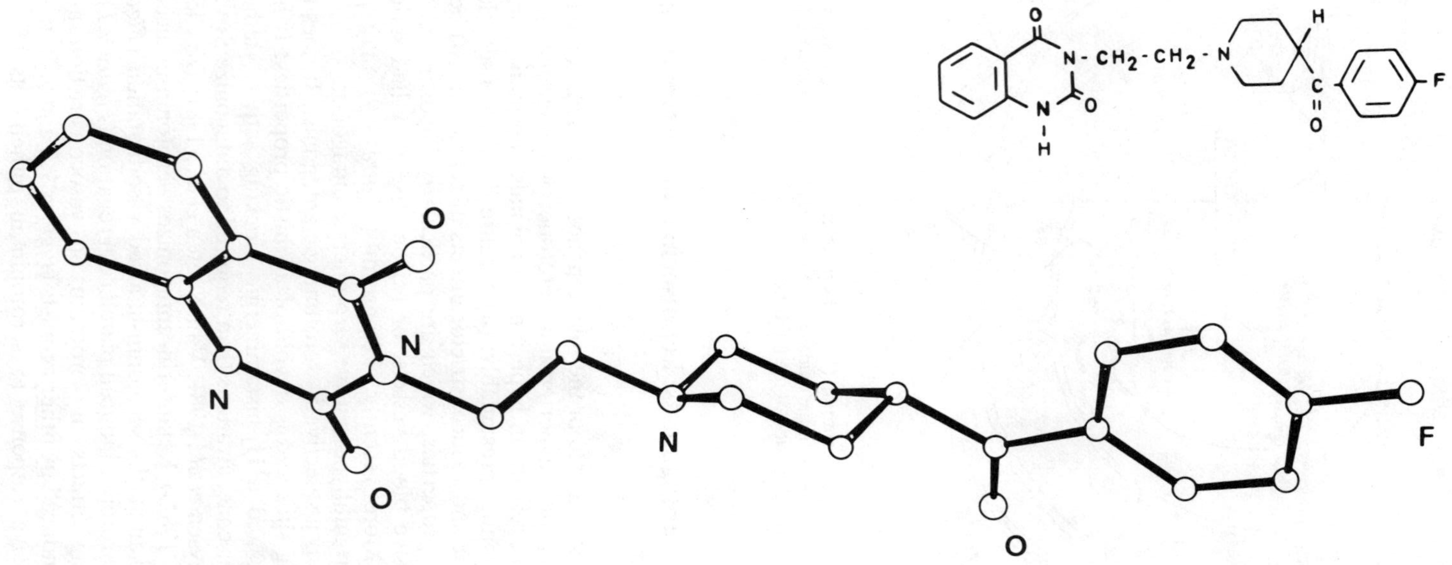

Figure 9.9. Structural formula of ketanserin: 3-[2-[4-(4-fluorobenzoyl)-1-piperidinyl]ethyl]- 2,4 (1*H*, 3*H*)-quinazolinedione

Kalkman, Timmermans and Van Zwieten, 1982; Persson, Hedner and Henning, 1982; Cohen, Fuller and Kurz, 1983) and lowers blood pressure in spontaneously hypertensive rats (*Figure 9.10*) acutely and after chronic oral treatment (Van Nueten *et al.,* 1981; Fozard, 1982; Kalkman, Timmermans and Van Zwieten, 1982; Persson, Hedner and Henning, 1982; Cohen, Fuller and Kurz, 1983; Wright and Angus, 1983; McCall and Schuette, 1984; Pettersson *et al.,* 1984).

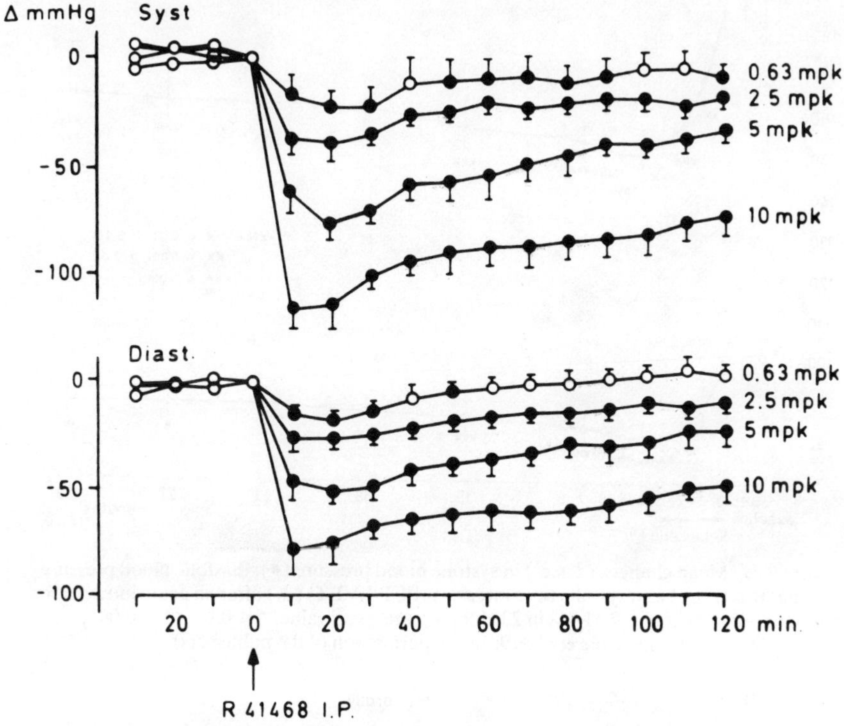

Figure 9.10. Dose-dependent decreases in both systolic and diastolic blood pressure by ketanserin in the unanaesthetized spontaneously hypertensive rat (From Van Nueten *et al.*, 1981, by permission of the publishers)

A single intravenous or oral dose of ketanserin reduces systolic and diastolic blood pressure in patients with essential hypertension (*Figure 9.11*) (De Crée, Verhaegen and Symoens, 1981; Wenting *et al.*, 1984). The effect is maximal within 5 min after intravenous and 1 h after oral treatment. The antihypertensive effect lasts 1–8 h and parallels the plasma levels of ketanserin. Blood pressure is usually not reduced in normotensive individuals (*Figure 9.12*) (Trenk *et al.*, 1983). Chronic oral treatment with ketanserin as sole therapy (20–40 mg b.i.d.) effectively reduces blood pressure in approximately 75% of patients with essential hypertension. The effect is similar to that obtained with β-adrenoceptor blocking agents or with thiazide diuretics (*Figure 9.13*), although the patients responding to either drug are different. Older patients tend to respond better to ketanserin than younger people (*Figure 9.14*). The reduction in blood pressure is proportional to the initial blood pressure (*Figure 9.15*).

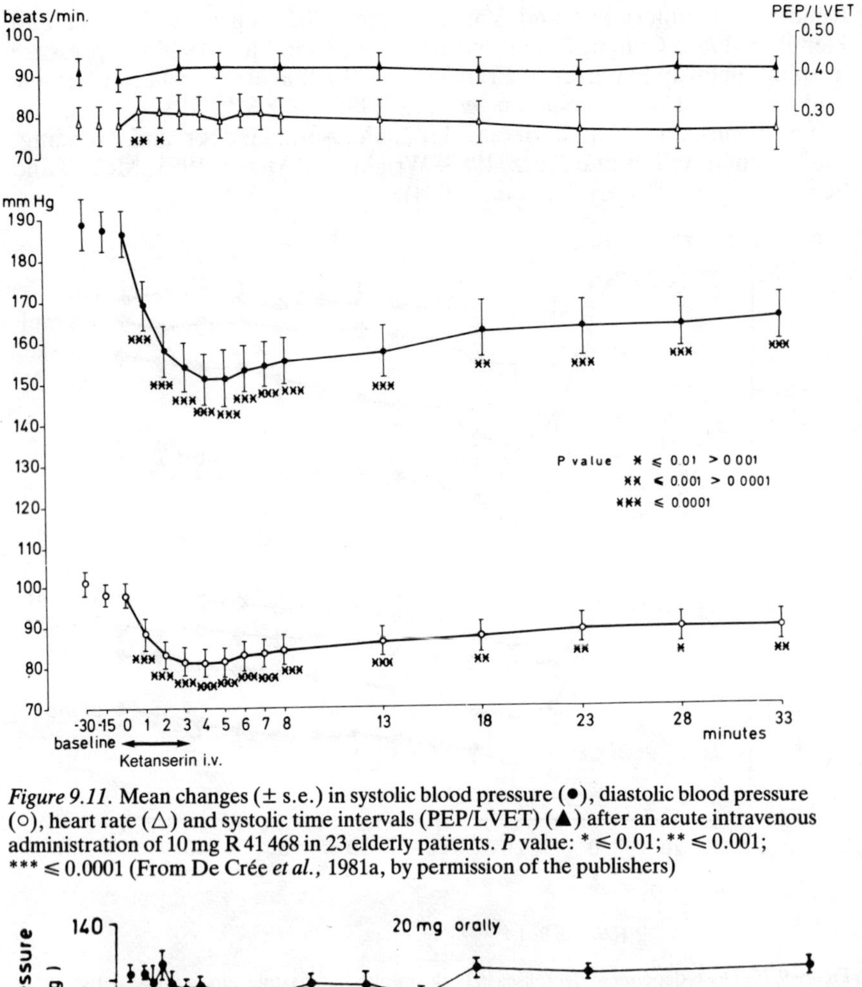

Figure 9.11. Mean changes (± s.e.) in systolic blood pressure (●), diastolic blood pressure (○), heart rate (△) and systolic time intervals (PEP/LVET) (▲) after an acute intravenous administration of 10 mg R 41 468 in 23 elderly patients. *P* value: * ≤ 0.01; ** ≤ 0.001; *** ≤ 0.0001 (From De Crée *et al.*, 1981a, by permission of the publishers)

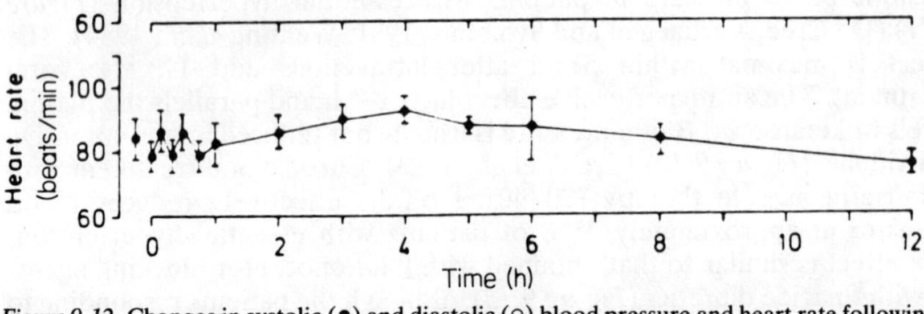

Figure 9.12. Changes in systolic (●) and diastolic (○) blood pressure and heart rate following single intravenous (10 mg) and oral (20 mg) doses of ketanserin in 8 healthy volunteers. Mean ± s.e. (mean) (From Trenk *et al.*, 1983, by permission of the publishers)

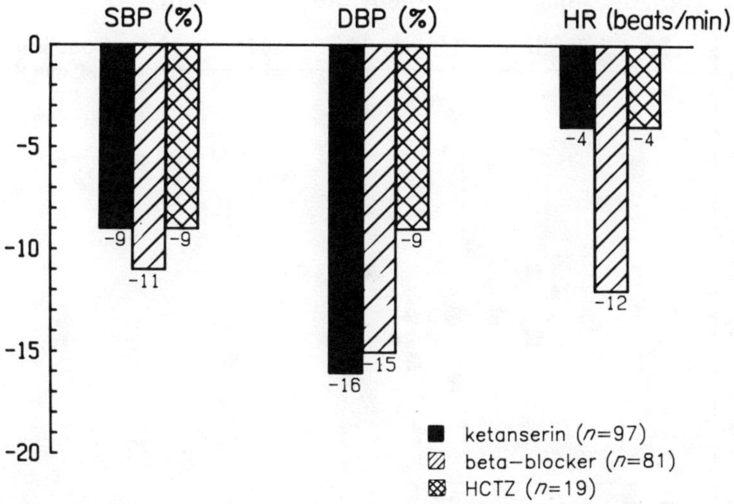

Figure 9.13. Reduction of systolic (SBP) and diastolic (DBP) blood pressure and heart rate (HR) after 3 months of treatment in monotherapy with ketanserin (40 mg b.i.d.), the beta-blockers metoprolol (100 mg b.i.d.), atenolol (100 mg o.d.) and propranolol (80 mg b.i.d.), and hydrochlorothiazide (25 mg b.i.d.) (Pooled data from comparative studies; Janssen Pharmaceutica, unpublished data)

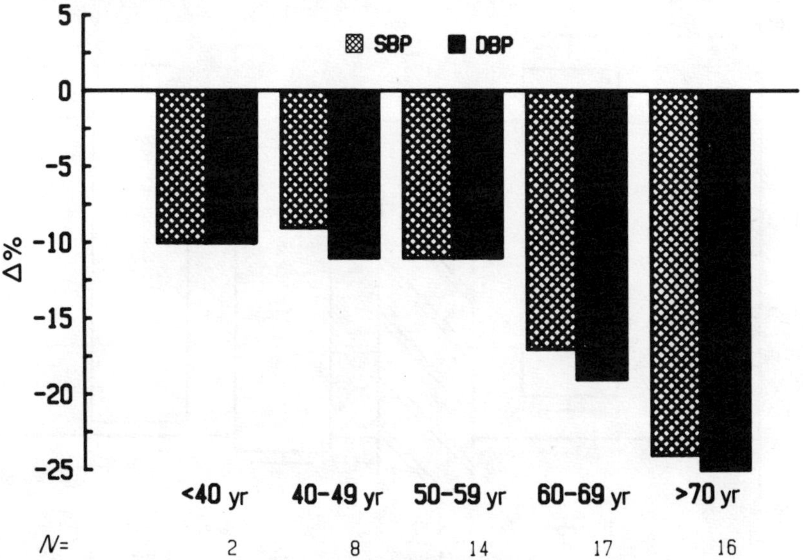

Figure 9.14. Maximal reduction in blood pressure (in %) after a single intravenous dose of 10 mg ketanserin in 57 patients with essential hypertension, in function of age (J. De Crée, unpublished data)

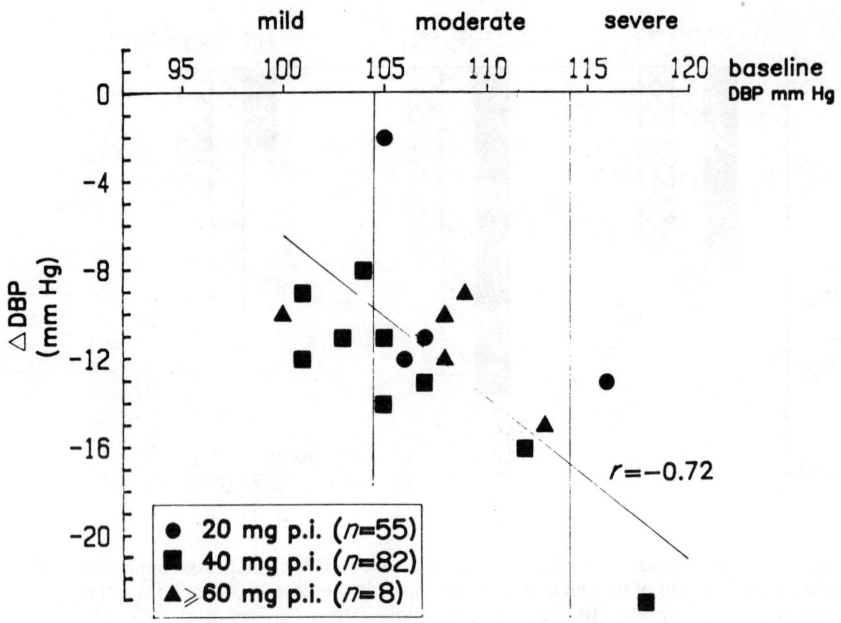

Figure 9.15. Change of diastolic blood pressure (DBP) in function of pretreatment DBP after 1–2 months of treatment with ketanserin in placebo-controlled and dose-finding studies. Each dot represents the end point of one study. The dose of ketanserin is indicated by symbols (Janssen Pharmaceutica, unpublished data)

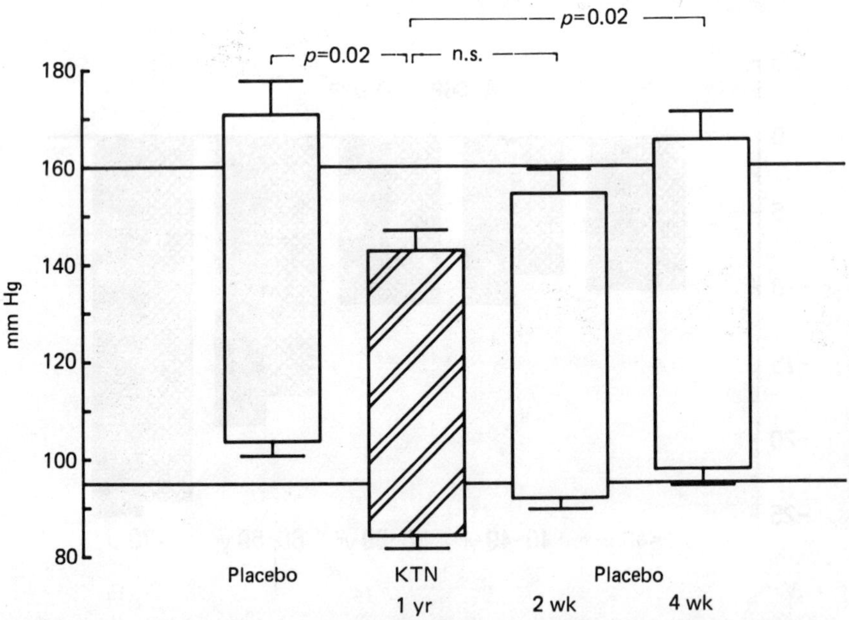

Figure 9.16. Systolic and diastolic blood pressure in 7 patients with essential hypertension at the end of a placebo run-in period, after 1 year of treatment with ketanserin in monotherapy and 2 and 4 weeks after discontinuation of ketanserin (Janssen Pharmaceutica, unpublished data)

Therapeutic doses of ketanserin do not produce postural hypotension. The antihypertensive effect of ketanserin is maintained during prolonged treatment. When treatment is discontinued, blood pressure increases slowly (*Figure 9.16*). There is no rebound hypertension (De Crée *et al.*, 1981a, 1981b; Anderson, Morgan and Dumpys, 1983; Andren *et al.*, 1983; Hedner, Persson and Berglund, 1983; Omvik and Lund-Johansen, 1983; Persson, Hedner and Berglund, 1983; Fagard *et al.*, 1984; Hedner, Persson and Berglund, 1984; Kirch and Ohnhaus, 1984).

Ketanserin reduces blood pressure by reducing systemic vascular resistance. After intravenous injection, heart rate and cardiac output increase slightly and transiently (*Figure 9.17*) (Wenting *et al.*, 1984). After

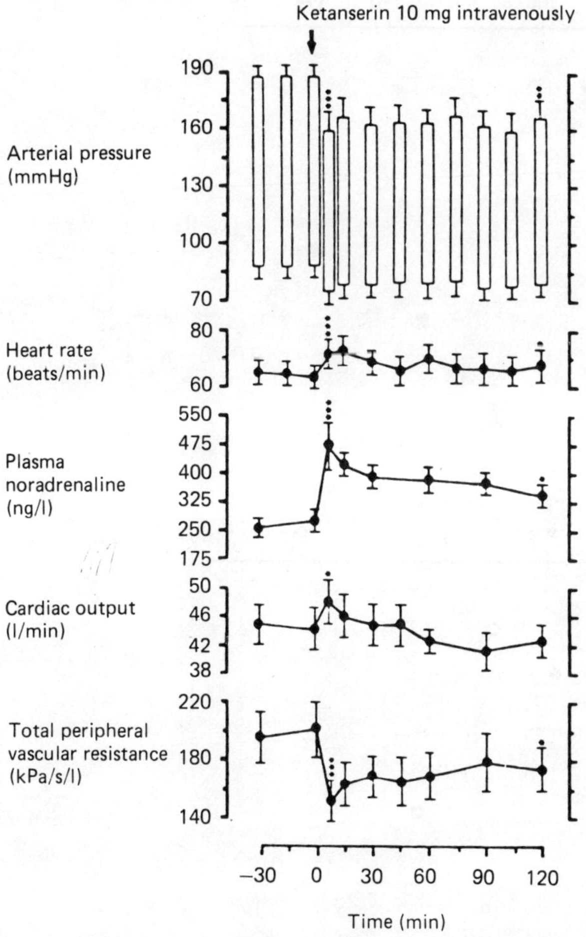

Figure 9.17. Effects of ketanserin on arterial pressure, heart rate, plasma noradrenaline, cardiac output and total peripheral vascular resistance in 12 patients with essential hypertension. $*p < 0.05$; $**p < 0.01$; $***p < 0.001$ (From Wenting *et al.*, 1982, by permission of the publishers)

chronic oral treatment, heart rate slightly decreases (*Figure 9.13*) and cardiac output remains unchanged or increases slightly (Omvik and Lund-Johansen, 1983; Fagard *et al.*, 1984). The sympathetic response to dynamic and isometric exercise is blunted, but the exercise tolerance is unaffected (Persson, Hedner and Berglund, 1983; Fagard *et al.*, 1984). Ketanserin improves the antihypertensive effect of beta blockers or diuretics when the response to these agents alone is insufficient. The effect of ketanserin in combination with these agents is proportional to the initial blood pressure (*Figure 9.18*).

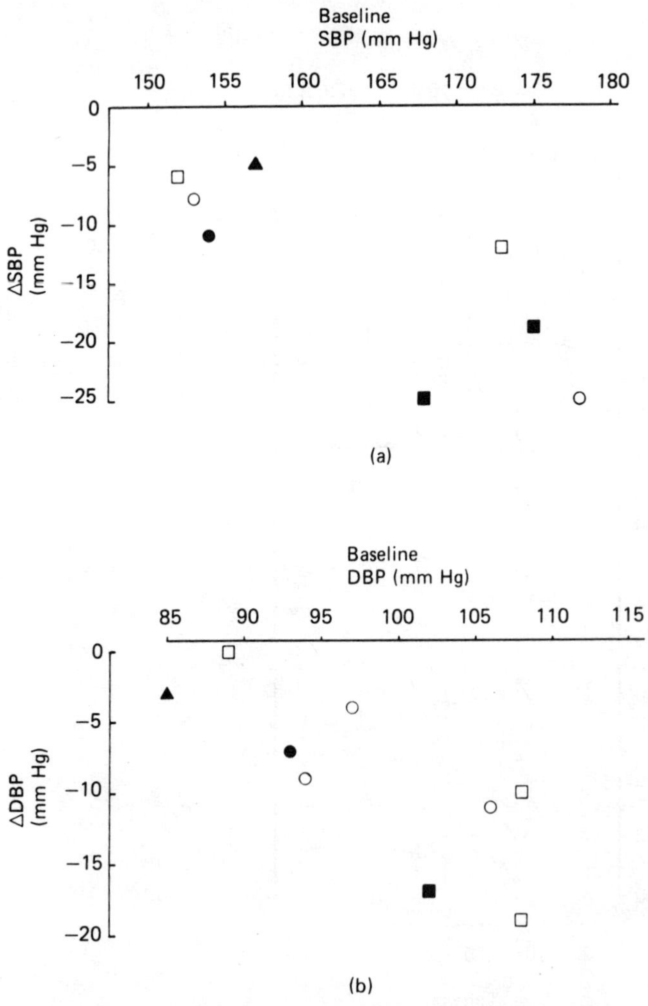

Figure 9.18. Change of systolic (a) and diastolic (b) blood pressure when ketanserin is added to a diuretic (● ○, n=24), a beta blocker (■ □, n=23) or a combination of both (▲, n=6) for 1 month. Baseline refers to the blood pressure before ketanserin is added. Each dot represents the end point of one study. Closed symbols refer to placebo-controlled studies, open symbols to open studies (Janssen Pharmaceutica, unpublished data)

Is the antihypertensive effect of ketanserin due to serotonergic blockade?

In young or adult spontaneously hypertensive rats the acute decrease in blood pressure caused by various serotonergic antagonists, including ketanserin, parallels their α_1-adrenoceptor antagonistic properties rather than their S_2-serotonergic blocking activity (Cohen, Fuller and Kurz, 1983; Kalkman *et al.*, 1983a, 1983b). Although low doses of ketanserin reduce serotonin-induced hypertension in pithed rats, higher α_1-adrenergic blocking concentrations are needed to reduce blood pressure in spontaneously hypertensive rats (Kalkman *et al.*, 1982; Persson, Hedner and Henning, 1982; Cohen, Fuller and Kurz, 1983; Kalkman *et al.*, 1983a, 1983b; Pettersson *et al.*, 1984). Thus, in the spontaneously hypertensive rat, adrenergic rather than serotonergic blockade explains the acute blood pressure lowering effect of ketanserin. Chronic oral treatment with ketanserin attenuates the development of hypertension in the spontaneously hypertensive rat without affecting the sensitivity to phenylephrine (Pettersson *et al.*, 1984). In renal hypertensive rats, tolerance to α_1-adrenergic but not to S_2-serotonergic blockade occurs after a few days of treatment with ketanserin (Criscione and Hedwall, 1984). Thus, it is possible that in the rat reduction in blood pressure seen with chronic treatment with ketanserin depends in part on peripheral S_2-serotonergic blockade, as a central mechanism of action probably does not contribute to the antihypertensive effect of ketanserin in the rat (Persson, Hedner and Henning, 1982; Pettersson *et al.*, 1984).

In hypertensive humans, the acute intravenous injection of ketanserin lowers blood pressure at a dose that does not shift the dose–response curve to phenylephrine (*Figure 9.19*), but that effectively blocks S_2-serotonergic receptors (Wenting *et al.*, 1984). With prolonged intravenous infusion or during chronic oral treatment, ketanserin alters the dose–response curve

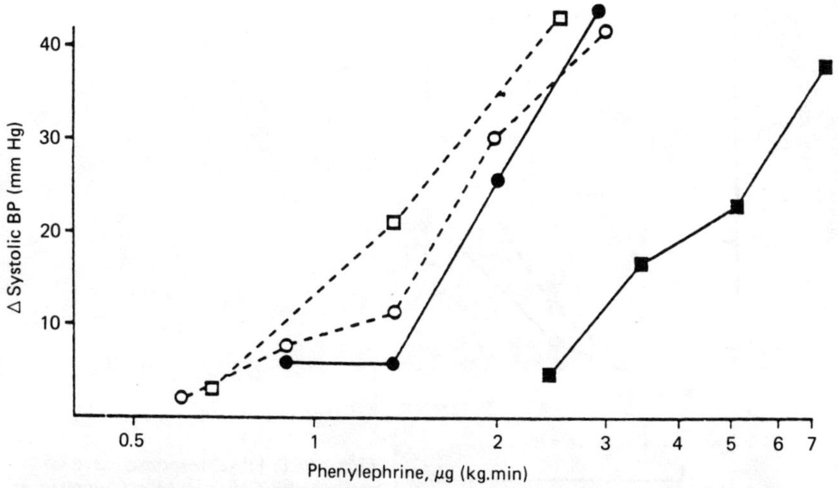

Figure 9.19. Log dose–response curve for phenylephrine following placebo (□---□) and prazosin 1 mg orally (■—■), and for placebo (○---○) and ketanserin 10 mg i.v. (●—●) (J. I. S. Robertson, unpublished data, by permission)

to methoxamine or phenylephrine (*Figure 9.20*). Ketanserin only depresses the responses to the highest doses of the agonists, in contrast to the selective α_1-adrenergic antagonist prazosin which shifts the whole curve to the right (*Figure 9.19*). The partial shift of the dose–response curve to methoxamine and phenylephrine may illustrate a partial, non-competitive, α_1-adrenoceptor antagonism exerted by ketanserin, as well as non-specific antagonism of the response to pressor agents in general. Certainly, the pattern of blood pressure reduction with ketanserin differs from that observed with prazosin or other selective α_1-adrenoceptor blocking agents, in that ketanserin has a more pronounced effect on supine than on standing diastolic blood pressure, does not evoke orthostatic hypotension (first-dose effect) and does not cause tolerance when given chronically as sole therapy (Andren *et al.*, 1983; Hedner, Persson and Berglund, 1984).

Since ketanserin reduces blood pressure in patients with autonomic insufficiency who are unresponsive to phentolamine (Wenting *et al.*, 1984), it can reduce blood pressure independently of α_1-adrenoceptor blockade. On the other hand, in patients with essential hypertension, the antihypertensive effect of ketanserin is blunted by treatment with prazosin (Wenting *et al.*, 1984). Thus, a certain degree of α_1-adrenergic tone may be required for the full antihypertensive action of the compound. One possibility is that, in man, S_2-serotonergic receptor stimulation acts mainly by amplifying the α_1-adrenergic component of the pressor response to noradrenaline.

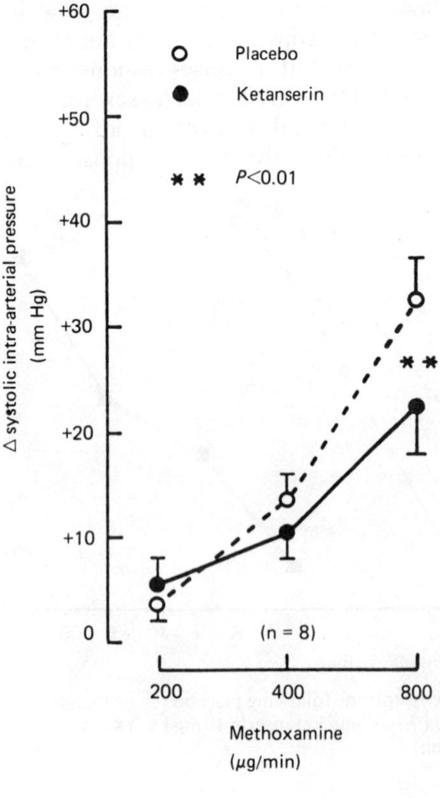

Figure 9.20. Dose–response curve for methoxamine after placebo (○) and after 6 weeks oral ketanserin (40 mg b.i.d.) (●) treatment (From Fagard *et al.*, 1984, by permission of the publishers)

Hypertension, ketanserin and age

Ketanserin tends to be more effective in older than in young patients (*Figure 9.14*). In hypertensives over 50 years of age, the efficiency of the adrenergic and the renin–angiotensin system tend to decrease. There is an age-related reduction in responsiveness to β-adrenoceptor activation and probably also, although to a lesser extent, to α-adrenoceptor activation (Bühler *et al.*, 1980, 1982; Ito *et al.*, 1981; Noguchi, Whitsett and Dickman, 1981; Elliott *et al.*, 1982; Partilla *et al.*, 1982). Stroke volume decreases and total peripheral and renal vascular resistance increase (Birkenhäger and de Leeuw, 1980). With increasing age the serotonin content of platelets decreases (Shuttleworth and O'Brien, 1981), the platelet-release reaction augments and the platelet-survival time shortens (Zahavi *et al.*, 1980). The increased platelet activation may be due primarily to haemodynamic shear stresses in regions of turbulence, such as atherosclerotic narrowing of the vessels (Schmid-Schönbein *et al.*, 1981). Aging, atherosclerotic and hypertensive blood vessels are hypersensitive to serotonin (Doyle, Fraser and Marshall, 1959; Collis and Vanhoutte, 1977; Yokoyama and Henry, 1979; De Mey and Vanhoutte, 1981; Heistad *et al.*, 1984).

Thus, it is conceivable that in older atherosclerotic patients (and animals) platelets are continuously activated to release serotonin and to secrete other vasoactive substances such as thromboxane A_2. The serotonin released from platelets may: (a) facilitate further activation of hypersensitive platelets; (b) constrict the hypersensitive blood vessel wall, which would help to maintain an elevated peripheral vascular resistance – since not all atherosclerotic patients have hypertension, serotonin probably contributes to maintenance of an elevated vascular resistance rather than causing it; and (c) reduce red blood cell deformability and increase blood viscosity (De Crée *et al.*, 1982). There is a direct correlation between blood viscosity and the systolic and diastolic blood pressures (Letcher *et al.*, 1983).

The changes observed in hypertensive patients after treatment with ketanserin are in accordance with this concept. In these patients, ketanserin: (a) decreases peripheral vascular resistance and blood pressure when elevated but not when normal (Hoing, Janssens and Symoens, 1984); (b) appears to be a better antihypertensive agent in older patients, in whom platelet abnormalities are more likely to occur; (c) reduces the sodium content (De Crée *et al.*, 1984) and improves the deformability of red blood cells (De Crée *et al.*, 1982; Waal-Manning*et al.*, 1985; Zannad *et al.*, 1985); (d) inhibits serotonin-induced platelet aggregation, reduces serotonin uptake but does not change the serotonin content of the platelets (Kirch and Ohnhaus, 1984; Baudouin-Legros *et al.*, 1985; Zannad *et al.*, 1985); and (e) reduces the urinary excretion of 5-HIAA (Dzurik *et al.*, 1985; T. Morgan, personal communication) and plasma levels of β-thromboglobulin (Zannad *et al.*, 1985). These phenomena suggest reduced release of serotonin by platelets. Inhibition by ketanserin of the release of serotonin from platelets was also observed in healthy volunteers during isometric exercise (Mara *et al.*, 1983).

In conclusion, the profile of ketanserin suggests a major role for serotonin in older individuals, especially those likely to have atherosclerosis as a complicating condition.

References

AFFOLTER, H., ERNE, P., BUHLER, F. R. and PLETSCHER, A. (1984). Increased sensitivity of blood platelets to 5-hydroxytryptamine in essential hypertension. Submitted for publication

ANDERSON, A., MORGAN, T. and DUMPYS, R. (1983). The effect of ketanserin in essential hypertension. *Clinical and Experimental Pharmacology and Physiology,* **10,** 331–333

ANDREN, L., SVENSSON, A., DAHLOF, B., EGGERTSEN, R. and HANSSON, L. (1983). Ketanserin in hypertension. Early clinical evaluation and dose finding study of a new 5-HT_2 receptor antagonist. *Acta Medica Scandinavica,* **214,** 125–130

BAUDOUIN-LEGRAS, M., LE QUAN-BUI, K. H., GUICHENEY, P., KAMAL, L. A. and MEYER, P. (1985). Platelet serotonin in essential hypertension and in mental depression. *Journal of Cardiovascular Pharmacology* (in press)

BHARGAVA, K. P., RAINA, N., MISRA, N., SHANKER, K. and VRAT, S. (1979). Uptake of serotonin by human platelets and its relevance to CNS involvement in hypertension. *Life Sciences,* **25,** 195–200

BIRKENHAGER, W. H. and DE LEEUW, P. W. (1980). Therapeutic approach to hypertension in the elderly. In *Hypertension in the Young and the Old* (Onesti, G. and Kim, K. E., Eds.). New York; Grune and Stratton, pp. 309–313

BÜHLER, F. R., AMANN, F. W., BOLLI, P., HULTHEN, L., KIOWSKI, W., LANDMANN, R. and BURGISSER, E. (1982). Elevated adrenaline and increased alpha-adrenoceptor-mediated vasoconstriction in essential hypertension. *Journal of Cardiovascular Pharmacology,* **4,** Supplement 1, S134–S138

BÜHLER, F. R., KIOWSKI, W., VAN BRUMMELEN, P., AMANN, F. W., BERTEL, O., LANDMANN, R., LUTOLD, B. E. and BOLLI, P. (1980). Plasma catecholamines and cardiac, renal and peripheral vascular adrenoceptor-mediated responses in different age groups of normal and hypertensive subjects. *Clinical Experimental Hypertension,* **2**(3–4), 409–426

COCCHERI, S. and FIORENTINI, P. (1971). Platelet adhesiveness and aggregation in hypertensive patients. *Acta Medica Scandinavica,* Supplement 525, 273–275

COHEN, M. L., FULLER, R. W. and KURZ, K. D. (1983). Evidence that blood pressure reduction by serotonin antagonists is related to alpha receptor blockade in spontaneously hypertensive rats. *Hypertension,* **5,** 676–681

COLLIS, M. G., DE MEY, C. and VANHOUTTE, P. M. (1979). Renal vascular reactivity in the young spontaneously hypertensive rat. *Hypertension,* **2,** 45–52

COLLIS, M. G. and VANHOUTTE, P. M. (1977). Vascular reactivity of isolated perfused kidneys from male and female spontaneously hypertensive rats. *Circulation Research,* **41,** 759–767

CRISCIONE, L. and HEDWALL, P. R. (1984). The antihypertensive effect of ketanserin is attributable to a α-receptor blockade. *Naunyn-Schmiedebergs' Archives of Pharmacology,* Supplement to Vols 3–5, R.55

DE CLERCK, F. and DAVID, J. L. (1981). Pharmacological control of platelet and red blood cell function in the microcirculation. *Journal of Cardiovascular Pharmacology,* **3,** 1388–1412

DE CLERCK, F., DAVID, J. L. and JANSSEN, P. A. J. (1982). Inhibition of 5-hydroxy-tryptamine-induced and -amplified human platelet aggregation by ketanserin (R 41 468), a selective 5-HT_2-receptor antagonist. *Agents and Actions,* **12,** 388–397

DE CRÉE, J., LEEMPOELS, J., DE COCK, W., GEUKENS, H. and VERHAEGEN, H. (1981a). The antihypertensive effects of a pure and selective serotonin-receptor blocking agent (R 41 468) in elderly patients. *Angiology,* **32**(2), 137–144

DE CRÉE, J., LEEMPOELS, J., DEMOEN, B., ROELS, V. and VERHAEGEN, H. (1985). The effect of ketanserin on 5-HT-induced irreversible platelet aggregation in patients with cardiovascular diseases. *Agents and Actions,* in press

DE CRÉE, J., LEEMPOELS, J., DEMOEN, B. and VERHAEGEN, H. (1984). Possible interaction of 5-hydroxytryptamine with Na^+/K^+ ATPase activity: influence of ketanserin, a 5-HT_2-receptor antagonist. Symposium on Serotonergic Mechanisms in the Cardiovascular System, Zurich, Switzerland, 14–15 June

DE CRÉE, J., LEEMPOELS, J., GEUKENS, H., DE COCK, W. and VERHAEGEN, H. (1981b). The antihypertensive effects of ketanserin (R 41 468), a novel 5-hydroxy-tryptamine-blocking agent, in patients with essential hypertension. *Clinical Science,* **61,** 473S–476S

DE CRÉE, J., LEEMPOELS, J., GEUKENS, H., DE COCK, W. and VERHAEGEN, H. (1982). Are serotonergic mechanisms involved in high blood pressure? In *5-Hydroxytryptamine in Peripheral Reactions* (De Clerck, F and Vanhoutte, P. M., Eds.), New York; Raven Press, pp. 183–192

DE CRÉE, J., VERHAEGEN, H. and SYMOENS, J. (1981). Acute blood-pressure-lowering effect of ketanserin. *Lancet,* **i,** 1161–1162

DE MEY, CH. and VANHOUTTE, P. M. (1981). Effect of age and spontaneous hypertension on the tachyphylaxis to 5-hydroxytryptamine and angiotensin II in the isolated rat kidney. *Hypertension,* **3,** 718–724

DOYLE, A. E., FRASER, J. R. E. and MARSHALL, R. J. (1959). Reactivity of forearm vessels to vasoconstrictor substances in hypertensive and normotensive subjects. *Clinical Science,* **18,** 441–454

DZURIK, R., FETKOVSKA, N., BRIMICHOVA, G. and TISON, P. (1984). Blood pressure, 5-OH indolacetic acid (HIAA) and vanilmandelic acid (VMA) excretion and blood platelet aggregation in hypertensive patients treated with ketanserin. *Journal of Cardiovascular Pharmacology* (in press)

ELLIOTT, H. L., SUMMER, D. J., MCLEAN, K. and REID, J. L. (1982). Effect of age on the responsiveness of vascular· alpha-adrenoceptors in man. *Journal of Cardiovascular Pharmacology,* **4**(3), 388–392

ERSPAMER, V. (1961). Recent research in the field of 5-hydroxytryptamine and related indolalkylamines. In *Progress in Drug Research,* Vol. 3 (Jucker, E., Ed.). Basle; Birkhauser Verlag, pp. 154–331

FAGARD, R., FIOCCHI, R., LIJNEN, P., STAESSEN, J., MOERMAN, E., DE SCHAEPDRYVER, A. and AMERY, A. (1984). Haemodynamic and humoral responses to chronic ketanserin treatment in essential hypertension. *British Heart Journal,* **51,** 149–156

FOLKOW, B., DI BORRA, G. F., HJEMDAHL, P., TOREN, P. H. and WALLIN, B. G. (1983). Measurements of plasma norepinephrine concentrations in human primary hypertension. *Hypertension,* **5,** 399–403

FOZARD, J. R. (1982). Mechanism of the hypotensive effect of ketanserin. *Journal of Cardiovascular Pharmacology,* **4**(5), 829–838

GUICHENEY, P., FINOT, M. F., BAUDOUIN-LEGROS, M., KAMAL, L. A., LE QUAN-BUI, K. H. and MEYER, P. (1985). Platelet serotonin content and uptake in essential hypertensives: effect of ketanserin. *Journal of Cardiovascular Pharmacology* (in press)

HAEUSLER, G. and FINCH, L. (1972). Vascular reactivity to 5-hydroxytryptamine and hypertension in the rat. *Naunyn-Schmiedebergs Archives of Pharmacology,* **272,** 101–110

HEDNER, T., PERSSON, B. and BERGLUND, G. (1983). Ketanserin, a novel 5-hydroxy-triptamine antagonist: monotherapy in essential hypertension. *British Journal of Clinical Pharmacology,* **16,** 121–125

HEDNER, T., PERSSON, B. and BERGLUND, G. (1984). Experience with ketanserin, a serotonin (S_2) antagonist, in longterm treatment of essential hypertension. *Clinical and Experimental Hypertension – Theory and Practice,* **A6**(3), 743–751

HEISTAD, D. D., ARMSTRONG, M. L., MARCUS, M. L., PIEGORS, D. J. and MARK, A. L. (1984). Augmented responses to vasoconstrictor stimuli in hypercholesterolemic and atherosclotic monkeys. *Circularion Research*, **54,** 711–718

HOING, M., JANSSENS, M. and SYMOENS, J. (1984). The hemodynamic profile of ketanserin. Symposium on serotonergic mechanisms in the cardiovascular system, Zurich, Switzerland, 14–15 June

ITO, H., HOOPES, M. T., ROTH, G. S. and BAUM, B. J. (1981). Adrenergic and cholinergic mediated glucose oxidation by rat parotid gland acinar cells during aging. *Biochemical Biophysical Research Communication,* **98**(1), 275–282

KALKMAN, H. O., BATINK, H. D., MARTIN, J. M. C., THOOLEN, H., TIMMERMANS, P. B. M. W. M. and VAN ZWIETEN, P. A. (1983a). Correlation between the affinity for (3H) mianserin-labelled receptors in brain and antagonism of the serotonin pressor response in pithed rats. *Biochemical Pharmacology,* **32**(13), 2111–2113

KALKMAN, H. O., HARMS, Y. M., VAN GELDEREN, E. M., BATINK, H. D., TIMMERMANS, P. B. M. W. M. and VAN ZWIETEN, P. A. (1983b). Hyptensive activity of serotonin antagonists; correlation with α_1-adrenoceptor and serotonin receptor blockade. *Life Sciences,* **32,** 1499–1505

KALKMAN, H. O., TIMMERMANS, P. B. M. W. M. and VAN ZWIETEN, P. A. (1982). Characterization of the antihypertensive properties of ketanserin (R 41 468) in rats. *Journal of Pharmacology and Experimental Therapeutics,* **222**(1), 227–231

KIRCH, W. and OHNHAUS, E. E. (1984). Ketanserin versus atenolol. Double blind comparison of their antihypertensive activity. (in manuscript)

KJELDSEN, S. E., GJESDAL, K., EIDE, I., AAKESSON, I., AMUNDSEN, R., FOSS, O. P. and LEREN, P. (1983). Increased beta-thromboglobulin in essential hypertension; interactions between arterial plasma adrenaline, platelet function and blood lipids. *Acta Medica Scandinavica,* **214,** 369–373

LETCHER, R. L., CHIEN, S., PICKERING, T. G. and LARAGH, J. H. (1983). Elevated blood viscosity in patients with borderline essential hypertension. *Hypertension,* **5,** 757–762

LEYSEN, J. E., AWOUTERS, F., KENNIS, L., LADURON, P. M., VANDENBERK, J. and JANSSEN, P. A. J. (1981). Receptor binding profile of R 41 468, a novel antagonist at 5-HT_2-receptors. *Life Sciences,* **28,** 1015–1022

LUCAS, C., SAFFITZ, J. E. and HENRY, P. D. (1981). Monoaminergic receptor shift in atherosclerotic rabbit aorta. *Circulation,* **64,** Supplement IV, IV–286

MANDAL, A. K., OLEINICK, S. R., JAMES, T. M., WISE, W., LONG, H., NORDQUIST, J. A., BELL, R. D., YUNICE, A. A. and PARKER, D. (1978). Glomerular thrombosis in spontaneously hypertensive rat. II. Immunofluorescence microscopy. III. Effect of heparin. *Microvascular Research,* **16,** 371–390

MARA, G., CONSTANTINI, C., PALERMO, A., SONCINI, M., VITALI, E. and LIBRETTI, A. (1983). Evaluation of a new antiserotoninergic agent (ketanserin R 41 468) on 5HT platelet release. First European Meeting on Hypertension, Milan, Italy, 29 May–1 June

MATSUMO, M., KUSUNOKI, M., UYAMA, O., FUJISAWA, A., MATSUYAMA, T., YONEDA, S., KIMURA, K. and ABE, H. (1981). Platelet aggregation induced by arachidonic acid and thromboxane generation in patients with hypertension or cerebrovascular disease. *Prostaglandins and Medicine,* **7,** 553–562

MCCALL, R. B. and SCHUETTE, M. R. (1984). Evidence for an alpha-1 receptor mediated central sympathoinhibitory action of ketanserin. *Journal of Pharmacology and Experimental Therapeutics,* **228**(3), 704–710

MCGREGOR, D. D. and SMIRK, F. H. (1970). Vascular responses of 5 hydroxytryptamine in genetic and renal hypertensive rats. *American Journal of Physiology,* **219,** 687–690

MCLENNAN, P. L. and TAYLOR, D. A. (1983). Ketanserin, a serotonin-2 antagonist, inhibits the vasoconstriction but not the vasodilatation produced by serotonin. *Clinical and Experimental Pharmacology and Physiology,* **10,** 644

MEHTA, J. and MEHTA, P. (1981). Platelet function in hypertension and effect of therapy. *American Journal of Cardiology,* **47,** 331–334

NOGUCHI, A., WHITSETT, J. A. and DICKMAN, L. (1981). Ontogency of myocardial alpha 1-adrenergic receptor in the rat. *Developmental Pharmacology and Therapeutics,* **3**(3), 179–188

OMVIK, P. and LUND-JOHANSEN, P. (1983). Long-term effects on central haemodynamics and body fluid volumes of ketanserin in essential hypertension. Studies at rest and during dynamic exercise. *Journal of Hypertension,* **1,** 405–412

PAGE, I. H. (1957). Cardiovascular actions of serotonin (5-hydroxytryptamine). In *5-Hydroxytryptamine* (Lewis, G. P., Ed.). London; Pergamon Press, pp. 93–108

PARTILLA, J. S., HOOPES, M. T., ITO, H., DASE, E. M. and ROTH, G. S. (1982). Loss of rat ventricular alpha 1-adrenergic receptors during aging. *Life Sciences,* **31**(22), 2507–2512

PERSSON, B., HEDNER, T. and BERGLUND, G. (1983). Ketanserin in essential hypertension. Effects during rest and exercise. *European Journal of Clinical Pharmacology,* **25,** 307–312

PERSSON, B., HEDNER, TH. and HENNING, M. (1982). Cardiovascular effects in the rat of ketanserin, a novel 5-hydroxytryptamine receptor blocking agent. *Journal of Pharmacy and Pharmacology,* **34,** 442–445

PETRALITO, A., FIORE, C. E., MANGIAFICO, R. A. and MALATINO, L. S. (1982). Beta thromboglobulin plasma levels in different stages of arterial hypertension. *Thrombosis and Haemostasis,* **48,** 241

PETTERSSON, A., PERSSON, B., HENNING, M. and HEDNER, TH. (1984). Antihypertensive effects of chronic 5-hydroxytryptamine (5-HT_2) receptor blockade with ketanserin in the spontaneously hypertensive rat. *Naunyn-Schmeidebergs' Archives of Pharmacology,* **327,** 43–47

PLETSCHER, A. and AFFOLTER, H. (1983). The 5-hydroxytryptamine receptor of blood platelets. *Journal of Neural Transmission,* **57,** 233–242

POPLAWSKI, A., SKORULSKA, M. and MICWIAROWSKI, S. (1968). Increased platelet adhesiveness in hypertensive cardiovascular disease. *Journal of Atherosclerosis Research,* **8,** 721–723

RAPPORT, M. M., GREEN, A. A. and PAGE, I. H. (1948). Crystalline serotonin. *Science,* **108,** 329–330

ROTH, R. A. and WALLACE, K. B. (1980). Disposition of biogenic amines and angiotensin I by lungs of spontaneously hypertensive rats. *American Journal of Physiology,* **239,** H736–H741

SCHMID-SCHÖNBEIN, H., BORN, G. V. R., RICHARDSON, P. P., CUSACK, N., RIEJER, H., FORST, R., ROHLING-WINBEL, I., BLASBERG, P. and WEHMEYER, A. (1981). Rheology of thrombotic processes in flow: the interaction of erythrocytes and thrombocytes subjected to high flow forces. *Biorheology,* **18,** 415–444

SHUTTLEWORTH, R. D. and O'BRIEN, J. R. (1981). Intraplatelet serotonin and plasma 5-hydroxyindoles in health and disease. *Blood,* **57,** 505–509

TAYLOR, D. A. and MCLENNAN, P. L. (1983). Mesenteric vessels from hypertensive rats exhibit an increased responsiveness to serotonin that is inhibited by ketanserin. *Clinical Experimental Pharmacological Physiology,* **10,** 699–700

THOMPSON, J. H. (1971). Serotonin and the alimentary tract. *Research Communication Chemical Pathology Pharmacology,* **2,** 687–781

TRENK, D., MOSLER, A., KIRCH, W., MEINERTZ, T. and JAHNCHEN, E. (1983). Pharmacokinetics and pharmacodynamics of the 5-HT_2-receptor antagonist ketanserin in man. *Journal of Cardiovascular Pharmacology,* **5,** 1034–1039

VAN NUETEN, J. M. (1983). 5-Hydroxytryptamine and precapillary vessels. *Federation Proceedings,* **42,** 223–227

VAN NUETEN, J. M., JANSSEN, P. A. J., VAN BEEK, J., XHONNEUX, R., VERBEUREN, T. J. and VANHOUTTE, P. M. (1981). Vascular effects of ketanserin (R 41 468), a novel antagonist of 5-HT_2 serotonergic receptors. *Journal of Pharmacology and Experimental Therapeutics,* **218,** 217–230

VANHOUTTE, P. M. (1982a). 5-Hydroxytryptamine, vasospasm and hypertension. In *5-Hydroxytryptamine and Peripheral Reactions* (De Clerck, F. and Vanhoutte, P. M., Eds). New York; Raven Press, pp. 163–174

VANHOUTTE, P. M. (1982b). Does 5-hydroxytryptamine play a role in hypertension? *Trends in Pharmacological Sciences,* **3,** 370–373

VANHOUTTE, P. M. (1983). 5-Hydroxytryptamine and vascular disease. *Federation Proceedings,* **42,** 233–237

VANHOUTTE, P. M. and COHEN, R. A. (1983). The elusory role of serotonin in vascular function and disease. *Biochemical Pharmacology,* **32,** 3671–3674

VANHOUTTE, P. M., COHEN, R. A. and VAN NUETEN, J. M. (1984). Serotonin and arterial vessels. *Journal of Cardiovascular Pharmacology,* **6** (Suppl. 2), S241–S248

VANHOUTTE, P. M., VAN NUETEN, J. M., SYMOENS, J. and JANSSEN, P. A. J. (1983). Antihypertensive properties of ketanserin (R 41468). *Federation Proceedings,* **42,** 182–185

VLACHAKIS, N. D. and ALDEDORT, L. (1980). Hypertension and propranolol therapy: effect on blood pressure, plasma catecholamines, and platelet aggregation. *American Journal of Cardiology,* **45,** 321–324

WAAL-MANNING, H. J., BROWN, S. A., SPEARS, G. F. and SIMPSON, F. O. (1985) Clinical studies with ketanserin in hypertension. *Journal of Cardiovascular Pharmacology* (in press)

WENTING, G. J., MAN INT'VELD, A. J., WOITTIEZ, A. J., BOOMSMA, F. and SCHALEKAMP, M. A. D. H. (1982). Treatment of hypertension with ketanserin, a new selective 5-HT_2 receptor antagonist. *British Medical Journal,* **284,** 537–539

WENTING, G. J., WOITTIEZ, A. J. J., MAN INT'VELD, A. J. and SCHALEKAMP, M. A. D. H. (1984). 5-HT, alpha-adrenoceptors and blood pressure. Effects of ketanserin in essential hypertension and autonomic insufficiency. *Hypertension,* **6**(1), 100–109

WHITE, J. (1971). Plate morphology. In *The Circulating Platelet* (Johnson, S. A., Ed.). New York; Academic Press, pp. 46–122

WRIGHT, C. E. and ANGUS, J. A. (1983). Haemodynamic response to ketanserin in rabbits with page hypertension: comparison with prazosin. *Journal of Hypertension,* **1,** 183–190

YOKOYAMA, M. and HENRY, P. D. (1979). Supersensitivity of atherosclerotic arteries to ergonovin partially mediated by a serotonergic mechanism. *Circulation,* **59**(60), Supplement II, 100

ZAHAVI, J., JONES, N. A. G., LEYTON, J., DUBIEL, M. and KAKKAR, V. V. (1980). Enhanced *in vivo* platelet release reaction in old healthy individuals. *Thrombosis Research,* **17,** 329–336

ZANNAD, F., VOISIN, P. H., POINTEL, J. P., SCHMITT, C., FREITAG, B. and STOLTRA, J. F. (1985). Effects of ketanserin on platelet function and red cell filterability in hypertension and peripheral vascular disease. *Journal of Cardiovascular Pharmacology* (in press)
ZUCKER, M. B. (1975). The platelet release reaction. In *Platelets, Drugs and Thrombosis* (Hirsch, J., Cade, J. F., Gallers, A. S. and Schonbaum, E., Eds). Basel; Karger, pp. 27–34

Chapter 10

Respiratory complications of sepsis

T. E. Woodcock and I. McA. Ledingham

Introduction

The respiratory complications of sepsis are numerous and present themselves in various ways. Their consequences may be of minimal inconvenience to the patient or, at the other extreme, may cause life-threatening illness, either alone or as part of a multiple organ failure. The early recognition and appropriate treatment of sepsis and its associated respiratory disorders are important if patient morbidity and mortality are to be minimized. The clinician's task is made more difficult in the post-surgical patient, as the normal response to stress and trauma may mimic the early response to sepsis, and derangements of pulmonary function may be seen even in the 'uncomplicated' post-surgical patient.

This chapter considers the factors that predispose to postoperative sepsis and respiratory complications, and discusses the metabolic and respiratory changes seen in the 'uncomplicated' post-surgical patient. The respiratory complications of sepsis are considered in two parts; first, pulmonary infections and their management and, secondly, the adult respiratory distress syndrome (ARDS). The principles of management of septic shock and ARDS in current practice will be outlined.

Predisposing factors

An awareness of the factors that predispose to postoperative sepsis and pulmonary complications of surgery enables the clinician to identify the patient at particular risk. He may then formulate a rational plan for the preoperative, perioperative and postoperative management of his patient with regard to the prevention of sepsis and the preservation of optimal pulmonary function.

Age

The normal arterial oxygen tension falls progressively with age as the closing volume rises and approximates to, or even exceeds, the functional residual capacity (FRC) (Leblanc, Ruff and Milic-Emili, 1970). In children, the closing volume may exceed the FRC in the supine position up to the age of 6 yr (Mansell, Bryan and Levison, 1972). Hypoxaemia due to a fall in the FRC is therefore more pronounced in the very young and in the elderly. Postoperative respiratory complications are seen more frequently in the older age groups, although this association may be almost entirely accounted for by the higher incidence of pre-existing lung disease in the elderly population.

Obesity

The special problems of the perioperative management of morbidly obese patients have been well reviewed (Fisher, Waterhouse and Adams, 1975; Buckley *et al.,* 1983), although may not be widely appreciated. In particular, the clinician must look for evidence of the Pickwickian syndrome, with sleep apnoea and pulmonary hypertension. There may be a place for the use of regional analgesia or elective intermittent positive pressure ventilation in selected patients.

Malnutrition

In the western world this is a less common problem than obesity. An association between malnutrition and postoperative pneumonia has been demonstrated (Garribaldi *et al.*, 1981). Intensive preoperative nutritional support may reduce the incidence of post-surgical sepsis (*British Medical Journal*, 1979).

Smoking

The association between smoking and chronic bronchitis is irrefutable. In cigarette smokers mucus is thick and tenacious, the normal ciliary clearance is impaired, and defects in alveolocapillary permeability have been demonstrated (Jones *et al.,* 1980). Whether this latter observation has any relevance to the development of non-cardiogenic pulmonary oedema (as in ARDS) is unclear.

Pre-existing lung disease

There can be no doubt that patients with chronic lung disease, in particular chronic bronchitis and asthma, are prone to postoperative pulmonary complications. This single fact may account in large part for the association between advanced age or smoking, and the incidence of postoperative complications (Garribaldi *et al.,* 1981).

Seasonal variations are often seen in cases of chronic bronchitis and asthma, and there may be some advantage in planning non-urgent surgery for the time of year when respiratory function is optimal. Preparation of the patient with respiratory disease begins at the first consultation, when the patient is exhorted to stop or reduce his smoking, or to lose weight, as indicated. The clinician must not be deterred by the knowledge that most patients will choose to disregard this sound advice. Investigation and treatment of these patients follows established medical practice. Particular attention should be paid to the eradication of pulmonary and dental sepsis.

Medication, including steroids, should be continued until the time of induction of anaesthesia and should be resumed as soon as possible thereafter. If unexplained perioperative haemodynamic instability is seen in the patient on long-term steroid medication, the possibility of adrenocortical insufficiency should be considered and, if appropriate, tested by the administration of hydrocortisone. These patients may also be immunocompromised and therefore at particular risk of postoperative sepsis.

Prophylactic cotrimoxazole has been shown to reduce the incidence of postoperative pulmonary complications in patients with chronic obstructive pulmonary disease (Morran and McArdle, 1980), but the routine use of antibiotics cannot be recommended.

A common problem is the patient who presents for elective surgery with a 'cold'. Although general anaesthesia can be conducted uneventfully in the patient with coryza, it is best to postpone non-urgent procedures, particularly surgery of the respiratory tract, chest and abdomen.

Surgery

The assessment of patients for lung surgery is a special problem which will not be considered here. Respiratory complications are very common after surgery of the thorax and upper abdomen, less common after lower abdominal surgery, and rare after minor surgery in ambulatory patients. Systemic sepsis is most frequently associated with gastrointestinal and genito-urinary sources of infection, and is particularly associated with urgent and semi-elective surgical procedures (Ledingham, McArdle and Macdonald, 1980). In some defined circumstances the value of prophylactic antibiotics is widely accepted (*Table 10.1*).

Anaesthesia

Anaesthetic, analgesic and anticholinergic agents all tend to suppress ciliary activity in the respiratory tract and thereby reduce the clearance of secretions. This problem is compounded by the use of unwarmed, unhumidified anaesthetic gases. Nitrous oxide is a more soluble gas than

Table 10.1. Policy of short-term antibiotic prophylaxis (after Keighley, 1983)

Type of surgery	*Antibiotic therapy*
Clean or general surgery	None
Implant surgery	Cloxacillin
Urological surgery (open operations)*	Mecillinam for patients with bacteriuria
Gynaecological surgery*	Cephalosporin or metronidazole for hysterectomy
Gastrointestinal surgery:	
Gastric*	Cephazolin and metronidazole for carcinoma and reconstructive surgery
Biliary*	Cephazolin for choledocholithiasis, repeat operations, jaundiced patients and patients over 70 yr
Appendicectomy	Metronidazole
Colorectal	Metronidazole (+ gentamicin?)
Special considerations:	
Trauma*	Tetanus toxoid: penicillin
Amputation	Penicillin

* Selective.

nitrogen, and pulmonary collapse distal to a bronchial obstruction will occur more readily when it is used. However, the conduct of the anaesthetic procedure is more important than the specific effects of any one anaesthetic agent. The anaesthetist must take steps to avoid provoking bronchospasm by the injudicious use of histamine-releasing anaesthetic agents, and ensure adequate depth of anaesthesia. Pulmonary ventilation, whether controlled or spontaneous, must be adequate during and after the procedure. The airway should be protected from infected foreign material, especially pus and vomit. Postoperative analgesia must be adequate without unduly obtunding the cough reflex or depressing respiration. In this respect, the use of regional analgesia is advocated by some.

The uncomplicated patient

In order to diagnose sepsis and respiratory complications in the early stages of their development, the clinician must have an understanding of the systemic response to stress and trauma, and of the pulmonary consequences of surgery and anaesthesia. The magnitude of these changes will vary from patient to patient but, in general, will be proportional to the extent of trauma inflicted and the duration of anaesthesia. Other factors, most notably the type of anaesthesia used and the adequacy of postoperative analgesia, may modify these responses.

Body temperature

Under general anaesthesia, thermoregulation is modified leading to redistribution of body heat and increased heat loss. In young adult patients, core temperature falls by about 0.3°C/h under normal operating theatre conditions. In elderly patients, the fall in core temperature may be as high as 1.1°C/h and, in children, the high body surface area to body weight ratio predisposes to enhanced heat loss (Holdcroft, 1980). For these reasons, many patients are somewhat hypothermic in the immediate postoperative period.

Pyrexia is usual after significant injury, and is related to the increased metabolic rate and oxygen consumption associated with the endocrine response to stress. The pyrexia of injury does not usually exceed 38°C and rarely lasts for more than 72 h. Pyrexia which exceeds these limits demands investigation.

Leucocytosis

The peripheral white cell count is usually raised within a few hours of significant injury and is another consequence of the endocrine response to stress. In the first 4 days, the white cell count may be as high as $22\,000 \times 10^9$/l. A secondary rise may be seen on or about the seventh day, particularly in patients who have received a blood transfusion. Despite the abundance of white cells, immunocompetence, both cellular and humoral, is compromised after significant injury and is probably further compromised by anaesthesia (Walton, 1979).

Pulmonary function

Derangements of pulmonary function are not infrequently seen following anaesthesia and surgery. The most commonly performed tests (arterial blood gases, forced expiratory volume and forced vital capacity) will not reveal clinically important changes in the respiratory pattern, but are simple to perform at the bedside. When interpreting the results of respiratory function tests, it is important to know the expected values with regard to age, sex and build.

Postoperative respiratory changes may be considered to occur in two phases, early and late (Craig, 1981). They may also be broadly divided into two categories of hypoxaemia and respiratory depression.

Early hypoxaemia

This is a continuation of the disordered gas exchange which occurs during anaesthesia. While the causes are not entirely clear, changes in the FRC and pulmonary vascular autoregulation have been implicated. Derangements of chest wall tone and movement may adversely affect regional ventilation (Jones, 1982). Diffusion hypoxaemia, due to nitrous oxide washout, can be prevented by giving 100% oxygen for a few minutes after discontinuation of nitrous oxide. Hypoxaemia is exacerbated by respiratory depression.

Early respiratory depression

This is a consequence of the anaesthetic technique and may be due to several factors including depletion of total body carbon dioxide stores, together with the central depressant effects of inhalational and systemically administered anaesthetic and analgesic agents. Inadequate reversal of neuromuscular block should always be considered as a potential cause of postoperative respiratory insufficiency in the early phase. It should be remembered that certain antibiotics, in particular the aminoglycosides, may potentiate neuromuscular blockade. For obvious reasons, respiratory obstruction must be differentiated from respiratory depression.

Late phase hypoxaemia

This is more commonly seen in older patients and in patients who have undergone thoracic or upper abdominal surgery. It is associated with a reduced FRC which may be due to chest wall and diaphragmatic changes or pulmonary changes or a combination of both. The expiratory reserve volume (ERV) falls with a reduction in the FRC and may, in fact, be the more appropriate variable to monitor (Jones, 1982). Attempts at ameliorating late phase hypoxaemia have concentrated on provision of adequate systemic or regional analgesia and the use of physiotherapy, breathing exercises and intermittent positive pressure breathing. Although none of these measures has yet been demonstrated to prevent late phase hypoxaemia, their implementation should not be neglected. Judicious use of added inspired oxygen may be necessary if hypoxaemia is severe. Late phase hypoxaemia may last for several days after anaesthesia and surgery.

Late phase respiratory depression

This is usually an expression of the depressant effects of the analgesic agents used and must be distinguished from ventilatory failure due to other pulmonary and extrapulmonary complications. Recently, the use of continuous respiratory monitoring techniques has revealed some alarming disturbances of the respiratory pattern, particularly during sleep, in patients receiving opiate analgesics (Catley *et al.*, 1982).

Pulmonary infection

The commonest pulmonary complications of sepsis in the post-surgical patient are the pulmonary parenchymal infections. Postoperative atelectasis will also be considered, as this may be a fundamental step in the development of the classical respiratory disorders.

Atelectasis

Whether the collapse of lung units in postoperative patients is a primary event in the reduction of the FRC or a result of FRC changes is not known. Partial or complete obstruction of the airway may be caused by accumulation of viscous secretions, and will lead to collapse of the distal airways. If atelectasis is extensive enough to produce clinical features, then a degree of tachypnoea, tachycardia and pyrexia will be seen. The chest radiograph may show patchy atelectasis. If atelectatic areas become confluent or larger airway obstruction leads to segmental or lobar collapse, the classic signs of pulmonary collapse will be evident on clinical examination. Treatment at this stage is primarily aimed at re-expanding the collapsed airways by physiotherapy and controlled breathing exercises. Fire-optic bronchoscopy may sometimes be necessary.

Secondary infection of atelectatic areas may mimic pneumonia; the differentiation is probably not important.

Bronchitis

Exacerbation of chronic bronchitis is not infrequently seen postoperatively, and the responsible organisms will commonly be *Haemophilus influenzae* or *Streptococcus pneumoniae*. In the postoperative patient, sputum samples must be sent to the laboratory, although it would be reasonable to start treatment with cotrimoxazole or ampicillin without awaiting bacteriological confirmation. Physiotherapy and bronchodilators should also be prescribed.

Pneumonia

Postoperative bronchitis may progress to pneumonia, with malaise, pyrexia and tachypnoea. Examination of the chest usually reveals scattered coarse crepitations and sometimes bronchial breathing and dullness to percussion associated with pulmonary consolidation. Hypoxaemia often necessitates supplementation of the inspired oxygen concentration.

Organisms are again likely to be *H.influenzae* and *S.pneumoniae*. Sputum samples and blood cultures must be sent to the laboratory, and treatment started with parenteral cotrimoxazole or ampicillin. Frequent physiotherapy is essential. Potential complications include lung abscess, pleural effusion and empyema.

Classic lobar pneumonia, and the 'atypical' pneumonias, are rare in the post-surgical patient. In the severely immunocompromised patient (e.g. after transplant surgery), opportunistic infections may be life threatening. Isolation of the pathogenic organism may be difficult. Potential causative agents include Gram-negative bacilli, fungi, viruses and *Pneumocystis carinii* (Tobin and Grenvik, 1984).

Aspiration

Inhalation of oropharyngeal or gastric contents may lead to pneumonia, atelectasis and lung abscess. In fit patients, aspiration is only likely to occur when the laryngeal reflexes are obtunded by heavy sedation, anaesthesia or local anaesthetics, but in debilitated patients aspiration may occur preoperatively.

The most florid pulmonary sequela of aspiration of gastric contents is aspiration pneumonitis, a form of ARDS which is known by the eponym Mendelson's syndrome (Mendelson, 1946) when seen in obstetric practice. Treatment is as for ARDS. There is a case for the use of ampicillin and metronidazole to prevent pulmonary infection with upper gastrointestinal tract flora. Steroids have not been shown to be effective in clinical practice (Wolfe and Ruth, 1977; Flick and Murray, 1984).

Sepsis and ARDS

In 1967, Ashbaugh and colleagues described a syndrome of acute respiratory distress associated with the stigmata of pulmonary oedema in 12 adult patients with no evidence of prior lung disease or congestive cardiac failure (Ashbaugh *et al.*, 1967). Since that time much clinical and laboratory research effort has been directed towards elucidating the underlying pathophysiological mechanisms of lung injury and repair in ARDS (Rinaldo and Rogers, 1982) and, although our knowledge remains incomplete, we are currently able to define a number of possible therapeutic objectives. However, 15 years after the first description of the syndrome, there have been no major therapeutic advances in clinical practice and the mortality remains high (Petty and Fowler, 1982).

ARDS is not a specific clinical entity, but there are several strict criteria which must be fulfilled for its confident diagnosis. These may be summarized as follows (Petty and Fowler, 1982):

(1) Pre-existing chronic pulmonary disease or left ventricular failure must be excluded.
(2) There must be a clear history of a catastrophic pulmonary or systemic insult.

(3) Clinical respiratory distress must be evident, defined as a respiratory rate >20 breaths/min, with laboured breathing.
(4) The chest radiograph must show diffuse pulmonary infiltrates which are interstitial in the early stages and alveolar later.
(5) Physiological measurements must confirm hypoxaemia ($PaO_2 < 50$ mm Hg, $FIO_2 > 0.6$), reduced total thoracic compliance (< 50 ml/cm H_2O), increased shunt fraction and increased dead space ventilation. The exclusion of fluid overload or cardiogenic pulmonary oedema may necessitate the placement of a pulmonary artery balloon catheter in some patients.

This definition does not suggest that patients with chronic pulmonary disease, left ventricular failure or fluid overload cannot develop ARDS, but it does mean that the diagnosis in such patients must be presumptive rather than definitive.

In all cases, the accuracy of diagnosis depends upon the care taken to exclude other conditions. Pulmonary oedema must be distinguished from bronchopneumonia and the rarer causes of diffuse opacification on the chest radiograph.

Whether the initial insult is to the epithelial or endothelial surface of the alveolocapillary membrane, the primary abnormality of ARDS is widespread increased permeability of the membrane to larger molecules such as albumen and other proteins; this causes greatly increased fluid flux and, when the compensatory mechanisms are exceeded, flooding of the interstitial and alveolar spaces occurs (Demling, 1980). The oedema fluid is of high protein content, and may also be haemorrhagic. This early capillary permeability defect is not associated with microscopic evidence of capillary injury. The normal alveolar stabilizing properties of surfactant are impaired by the alveolar flooding. Within a few hours of injury, coagulation of intra-alveolar protein begins and necrosis of the alveolar epithelial cells (type I pneumocytes) becomes evident. This is followed by hyperplasia of the surfactant-producing type II pneumocytes and the accumulation of interstitial inflammatory cells, including fibroblasts. Fibrosis, which tends to focus on the alveolar ducts, begins within 7 d of the onset of ARDS. Within the pulmonary microcirculation, thrombotic and/or microembolic occlusion may occur in association with vasoconstriction, interstitial compression and leucocyte aggregation. In severe ARDS, this process may be radiologically demonstrable as pulmonary vascular occlusive lesions on segmental angiography (Greene *et al.*, 1981).

The potential mechanisms of lung injury in ARDS may be as diverse as the physiological insults which can initiate it. Further, the clinician must appreciate that ARDS is often only the pulmonary manifestation of a systemic disorder and that treatment is unlikely to succeed while the primary insult remains unresolved.

It is not the intention here to give a comprehensive review of ARDS in all its forms; instead, discussion is limited to ARDS seen as a complication of surgical sepsis.

Septic shock, or sepsis syndrome (Pepe *et al.*, 1982), is by no means uncommon in hospital practice. The diagnosis is not always obvious, particularly in the elderly postoperative patient, and requires both a high index of suspicion and a knowledge of the circumstances under which septicaemia is likely to occur.

Sepsis syndrome is most frequently seen in general surgical practice, but is by no means exclusive to it. The source of infection is most often situated in the gastrointestinal tract or in the genito-urinary system. The clinical picture is extremely variable. Typically, the patient has undergone emergency or semi-elective abdominal surgery and the early features of sepsis may be concealed, missed or misinterpreted. These early features are fever, tachycardia, hyperventilation and a degree of hypotension with warm extremities, known as the hyperdynamic phase. Not uncommonly, the first indication of serious clinical deterioration is the progression to cyanosis, vasoconstriction, oliguria and confusion with more marked hypotension, the hypodynamic phase. If left untreated, shock soon becomes irreversible. Prompt fluid resuscitation will usually improve the

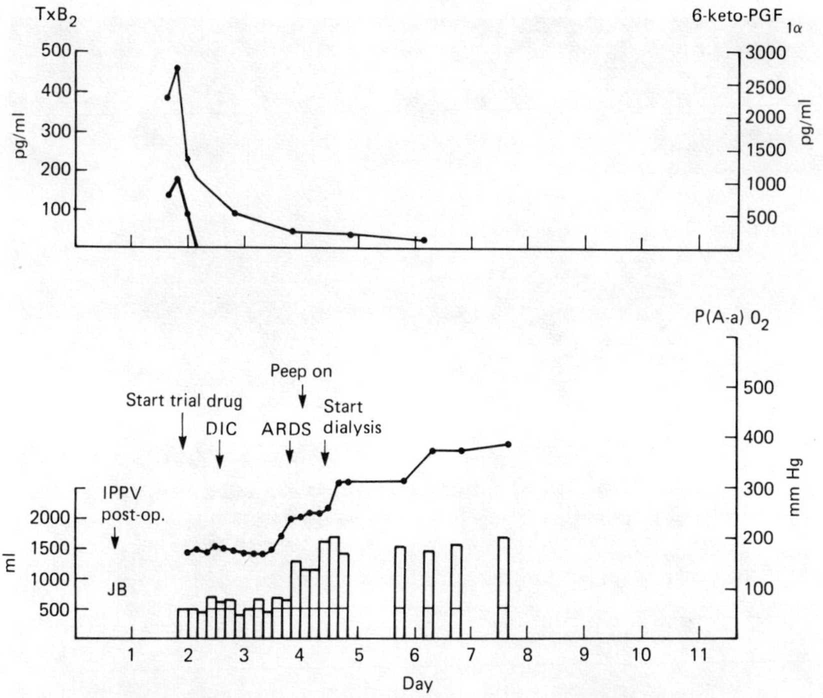

Figure 10.1. Clinical course of a typical post-surgical septicaemia progressing to ARDS. An open prostatectomy was complicated by rectal perforation and haemorrhage; intermittent positive pressure ventilation was continued postoperatively, and septic shock (streptococcal) was diagnosed a few hours later. Antibiotics were started immediately. A trial drug, dazoxiben, was used to inhibit thromboxane synthesis, but this did not prevent development of disseminated intravascular coagulation, ARDS and renal failure. Death occurred on the eleventh day. The upper panel shows arterial levels of thromboxane B_2, which fell to unmeasurable levels soon after dazoxiben was given, and 6-keto-$PGF_{1\alpha}$ (metabolite of prostacyclin) which fell over the next few days. The lower panel shows lung water (columns; measured by the thermal/green dye double indicator dilution technique) which rose abruptly from normal on the third postoperative day with the onset of ARDS. The degree of hypoxaemia is measured by the alveolar–arterial oxygen gradient $P(A-a)O_2$

haemodynamic problem temporarily, but if the source of sepsis remains unresolved progression to multiple organ failure may occur. A degree of hypoxaemia is usually present and hyperventilation leads to a fall in arterial CO_2 tension, which may or may not be a compensatory response to the metabolic acidosis seen in profound shock. The chest X-ray remains clear until the sudden onset of non-cardiogenic pulmonary oedema (*Figures 10.1* and *10.2*) which is a cardinal feature of ARDS. At this point, the high work of breathing and extreme hypoxaemia usually necessitate the institution of intermittent positive pressure ventilation (IPPV).

Other complications of septic shock must be anticipated and sought by regular clinical and laboratory investigation. These include thrombocytopenia (which is occasionally associated with disseminated intravascular coagulation (DIC)), renal failure, gastrointestinal bleeding, hepatic

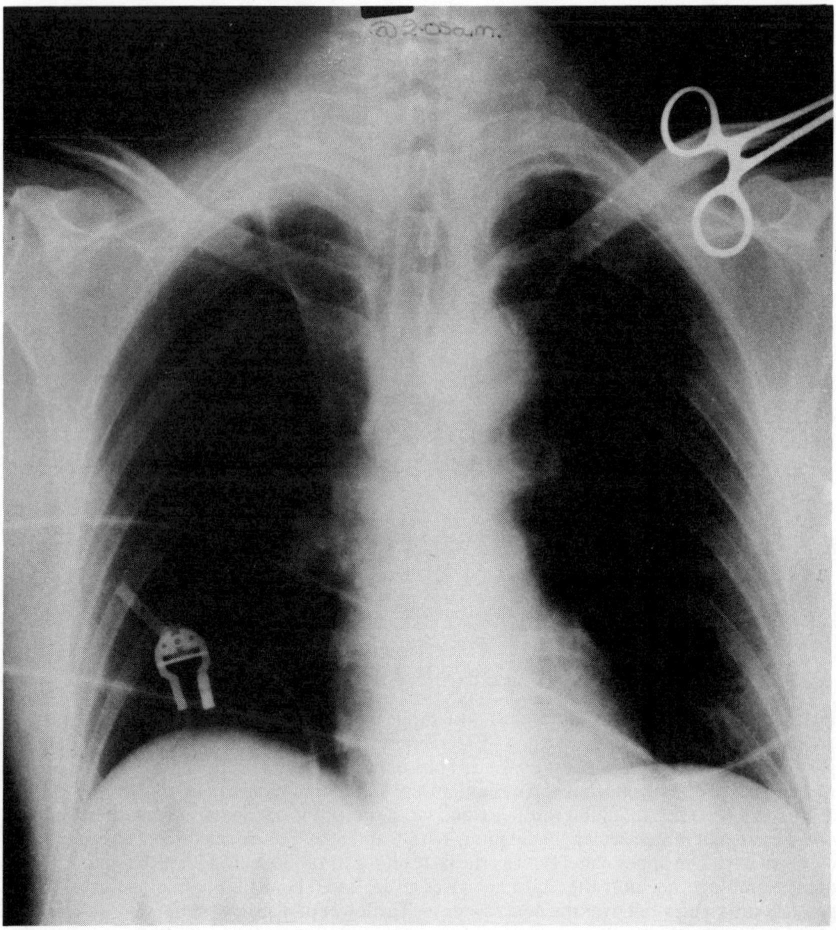

Figure 10.2(a). ARDS–radiographic features. Same patient as in *Figure 10.1*. Chest radiograph taken on day 2 shows no evidence of pulmonary oedema (lung water 480 ml)

dysfunction, and central nervous system abnormalities (Ledingham, McArdle and Macdonald, 1980).

The clinical course of a fairly typical case of postoperative sepsis and ARDS is illustrated in *Figure 10.1*. Portable chest radiographs are shown in *Figure 10.2*.

In patients who survive septic shock and ARDS there may be detectable sequelae of the disease processes, but these are usually not significant. Impairment of respiratory function and cerebral function have been reported. Chronic renal failure is rare among survivors of septic shock complicated by acute renal failure.

The pathophysiological mechanisms of systemic sepsis and its pulmonary complications have been the subject of extensive research and will be summarized here.

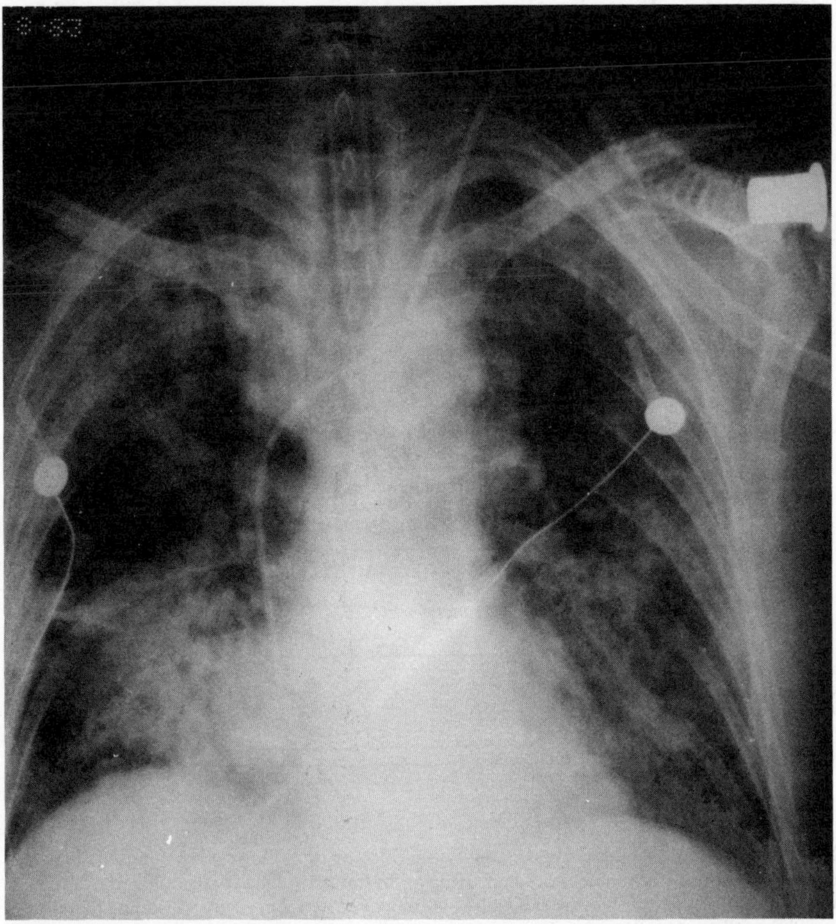

Figure 10.2(b). ARDS–radiographic features. Same patient as in *Figure 10.1*. Chest radiograph taken on day 4 shows typical bilateral infiltrates of ARDS (lung water 1200 ml)

Bacteraemia

It has been estimated that Gram-negative organisms are responsible for about two-thirds of the cases of septic shock, with Gram-positive organisms accounting for the remainder. The two forms of shock are largely indistinguishable at the bedside, although some specific conditions are described, such as meningococcal septicaemia and the toxic shock syndrome.

There are a significant number of patients from whose blood organisms cannot be isolated, even though the sepsis syndrome is fully developed, and a focus of sepsis is obvious. The importance of the role of chemical mediators in the sepsis syndrome is suggested by these observations.

Endotoxin

Endotoxin is the lipopolysaccharide molecule found in the cell wall of Gram-negative bacteria. When infused into animal models it produces

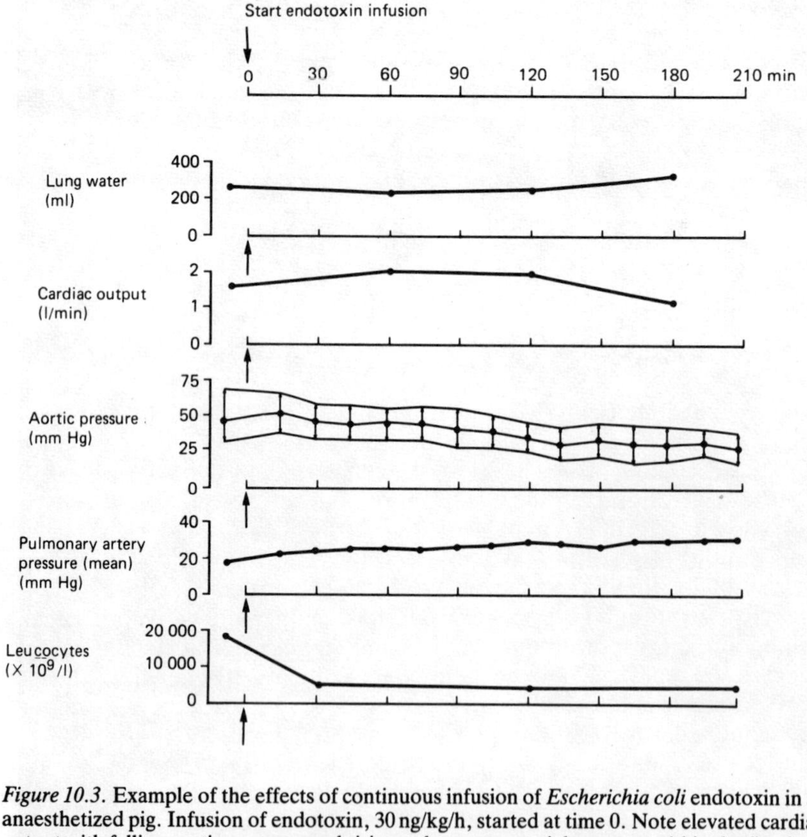

Figure 10.3. Example of the effects of continuous infusion of *Escherichia coli* endotoxin in an anaesthetized pig. Infusion of endotoxin, 30 ng/kg/h, started at time 0. Note elevated cardiac output with falling aortic pressure and rising pulmonary arterial pressure within the first hour. The white cell count falls within 20 min of the start of infusion. During the third hour, cardiac output begins to fall, but the pulmonary arterial pressure continues to rise and lung water increases as pulmonary oedema accumulates. Death occurred in the fourth hour at 220 min

reactions similar to those produced by the infusion of live organisms, most importantly pulmonary arterial hypertension, systemic hypotension, and pulmonary oedema due to a capillary permeability defect (*Figure 10.3*). Such models may be relevant to human septic shock and ARDS. Endotoxin is normally found in the lumen of the large intestine, and enters the portal venous circulation on occasions, but is efficiently removed by the hepatic Kupffer cells which are an important part of the reticulo-endothelial system. Saturation of this clearance system probably occurs in overwhelming sepsis, and may facilitate the progression of endotoxaemia (Bradfield, 1974). The limulus amoebocyte lysate assay may demonstrate the presence of endotoxaemia even in patients with negative blood cultures or Gram-positive bacteraemia (McCartney *et al.,* 1983). Low levels of plasma fibronectin, an opsonic glycoprotein, may be associated with impaired Kupffer cell function (Richards, Scovill and Shin, 1983).

Endorphins

The role of endogenous opioids in septic shock has been the subject of much research. High circulating levels of β-endorphin have been demonstrated in experimental and clinical septic shock and appear to be at least partly responsible for systemic hypotension. Whether the endogenous opioids have any direct effect on the pulmonary consequences of shock is not known.

The complement cascade

Evidence of complement activation (*Figure 10.4*) has been demonstrated in cases of human septic shock. In particular, it has been suggested that, in at-risk patients, high plasma levels of the complement fragment C5a, which promotes activation and aggregation of leucocytes, are predictive of progression to ARDS (Hammerschmidt *et al.,* 1980). Later work has failed to confirm this observation (Weinberg *et al.,* 1983; Schonfeld *et al.,* 1983), and it is likely that other factors yet to be identified may also initiate leucocyte activation (Hallgren *et al.,* 1984). Complement activation occurs when endotoxin is infused into animals, and appears to be responsible for leucocyte aggregation and the pulmonary capillary permeability defect. Putative local mediators of microvascular injury include the arachidonic acid metabolites (eicosanoids), plasma or phagocyte-derived proteases, fibrinogen degradation products (particularly the fibrin D monomer), and toxic oxygen radicles released by activated leucocytes. The well-known autocoids, serotonin and histamine, may play a secondary role in the pulmonary response to sepsis.

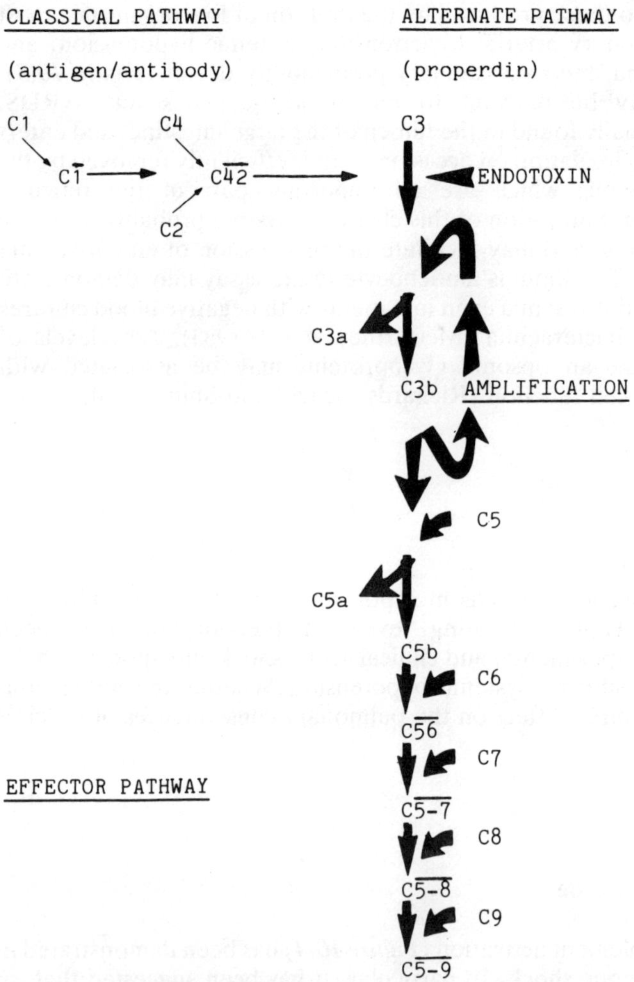

Figure 10.4. Endotoxin-induced complement activation. Note that the alternate pathway is activated. There is consumption of C3 and production of C3a and C5a, the latter being an important factor in granulocyte aggregation. The biological results of complement activation include release of anaphylotoxins, chemotaxis, enhanced immune adherence and cell lysis

The eicosanoids

The ubiquitous prostaglandins and leucotrienes (*Figure 10.5*) may be an important part of the final common pathway in the pulmonary response to shock. Both are metabolites of arachadonic acid which is a phospholipase degradation product of the tissue phospholipids.

The prostaglandins are the cyclo-oxygenase products of arachidonic acid metabolism and can be produced by platelets, leucocytes and many other tissues. In the pathophysiology of sepsis, the important prostaglandins appear to be $PGF_{2\alpha}$ and thromboxane A_2 (Parratt *et al.*, 1982), both powerful vasoconstrictors with a major role in pulmonary vasoconstriction.

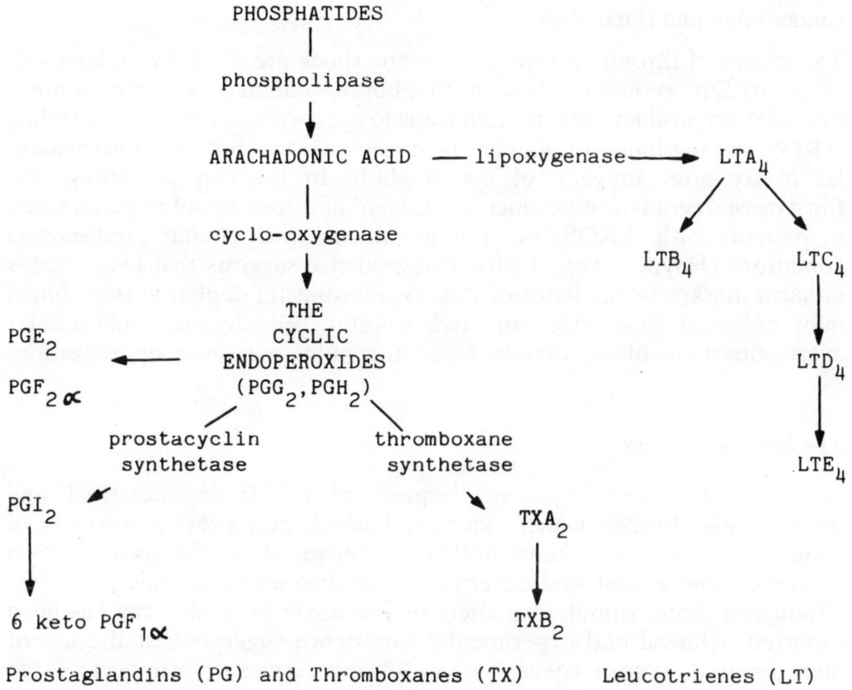

Figure 10.5. The eicosanoids – an outline of the metabolic pathways of arachidonic acid

Prostacyclin (PGI_2) is a vasodilator and platelet anti-aggregator. The stable metabolites of thromboxane A_2 and prostacyclin are thromboxane B_2 and 6-keto-$PGF_{1\alpha}$ which can be measured by radioimmunoassay.

The leucotrienes are derived from arachidonic acid by the action of the enzyme lipoxygenase. One of their outstanding physiological effects is to promote the microvascular exudation of protein, and the leucotrienes LTC_4 and LTD_4 are particularly potent (Piper, 1983).

It has been reported that plasma levels of thromboxane B_2 are elevated in patients dying from septic shock (Reines *et al.*, 1982), although our own experience to date has not consistently confirmed this observation. In some experimental models of endotoxin shock, thromboxane has been demonstrated to mediate the acute pulmonary hypertension which precedes the permeability defect. The leucotrienes have been implicated in the microvascular protein leak which leads to pulmonary oedema (Seeger *et al.*, 1982).

Proteases and oxygen radicals

Activated neutrophils release proteases and toxic oxygen radicals. The proteases are capable of damaging structural proteins and can cleave circulating proteins including the Hageman factor, fibrinogen, complement and fibronectin. The toxic oxygen radicals include superoxides and peroxides, which are themselves cytotoxic, and enhance protease activity by inhibiting antiproteases such as α_1-antitrypsin.

Coagulation and fibrinolysis

The causes of thrombocytopenia in septic shock are not fully understood, but overt DIC is only rarely seen. In laboratory animals, infusion of fibrin degradation products or thrombin leads to microvascular injury resembling ARDS, but depletion of platelets or fibrinogen does not alter microvascular injury after infusion of microemboli. In the clinical setting, the fibrinogen degradation product 'D antigen' has been found to be elevated in patients with ARDS, but not in patients with similar predisposing conditions (Haynes *et al.*, 1980). This evidence suggests that D antigen is either a marker or mediator of ARDS. Fibronectin depletion (*see above*) may be associated with impaired Kupffer cell clearance of cellular aggregates in the blood, thereby facilitating pulmonary microembolization.

The fibrotic process

Arguably the most important sequela of ARDS is interstitial and intra-alveolar fibrosis which, once established, may prevent recovery of respiratory function. Almost nothing is known about the factors which determine the extent and severity of the disordered fibrotic response, although a direct stimulatory effect of endotoxin on fibroblasts has been reported. Clinical and experimental experience suggests that the use of high inspired oxygen concentrations during respiratory support of the injured lung worsens pulmonary parenchymal damage and accelerates fibrosis. Several mechanisms have been proposed.

Host defence

Although there exists no adequate laboratory test to assess accurately a patient's immune status, there is good reason to assume that the immune competence of critically ill patients is severely compromised. Various abnormalities of cellular and humoral defence mechanisms have been demonstrated in critically ill patients (*Table 10.2*), and the normal physical barriers to bacterial contamination are defeated by invasive instrumentation with endotracheal tube, vascular catheters, urinary catheter and, often, a surgical wound. In ARDS, the respiratory tract epithelium is disrupted. It has been shown that the majority of critically ill patients are anergic to common skin recall antigens (Bradley, Ledingham and Hamilton, 1981) and these patients are highly susceptible to secondary infection with the bacteria which predominate in the hospital environment (Tobin and Grenvik, 1984), most notably *Pseudomonas* species.

Summary

The preceding synopsis of pathophysiological mechanisms in sepsis and ARDS cannot adequately reflect the recent profusion of research in this area. The interrelationships between any or all of these factors will, of course, be complex and currently are incompletely understood.

Table 10.2. Abnormalities in cellular and humoral host defence which have variously been detected in critically ill patients. Not all these findings have been confirmed

	Abnormality
Cellular	
Neutrophil:	
numbers	Increased or decreased
chemotaxis	Decreased
adherence	Decreased
phagocytosis	Decreased
Skin graft rejection	Delayed
Recall skin antigen response	Decreased or absent (anergy)
T-lymphocyte:	
numbers	Decreased
mitogen response	Decreased
K-cell activity	Decreased
Humoral	
B-lymphocyte:	
numbers	Decreased
mitogen response	Decreased
Immunoglobulin levels	Decreased
Complement levels	Decreased
Opsonic fibronectin levels	Decreased
Serum inhibitors of cellular function	Present

Therapeutic goals

Although our knowledge of the pathophysiology of septic shock and ARDS remains, at best, incomplete we are currently able to identify a number of potential specific therapeutic goals whose value remains to be established. It is to be hoped that some of these measures may eventually be found to improve the prognosis for patients with sepsis and ARDS.

Endorphins

In experimental models of septic shock, naloxone has an impressive pressor effect. Clinical reports are largely anecdotal (Groeger, Carlon and Howland, 1983), and an autonomic response to sudden arousal cannot be excluded. A potent opiate antagonist with non-opiate analgesic and sedative properties might be of value in clinical practice. Meptazinol is currently under investigation.

Complement activation

The use of 'pharmacological' doses of glucocorticosteroids in septic shock, ARDS, and indeed in many other conditions, has been widely advocated but remains controversial (Bihari, 1984; Sibbald, 1984). The physiological effects of steroids in massive doses are legion, but attention is usually focused upon their effects on the complement system, leucocyte aggregation and capillary permeability. It has been demonstrated that steroids inhibit the leucocyte aggregation caused by C5a and, in even higher doses, can promote disaggregation of leucocytes. Further, amelioration of the microvascular permeability defect has been demonstrated in animal models and in responsive patients with septic ARDS (Sibbald *et al.*, 1981). The effect of steroids on the ultimate outcome from septic shock and ARDS is not known, and until this is established the routine use of steroids cannot be recommended (Bihari and Tinker, 1982; Flick and Murray, 1984).

Eicosanoid effects

It is possible pharmacologically to manipulate the arachidonic acid metabolic pathways in biological systems, and so studies to assess the importance of the role of the eicosanoids in clinical sepsis and ARDS are in progress.

Cyclo-oxygenase is effectively inhibited by many drugs, including the non-steroidal anti-inflammatory agents. Thromboxane synthetase can be specifically inhibited by imidazole and some of its derivatives, including dazoxiben which has been used in clinical research. Prostacyclin opposes the effects of thromboxane A_2, dilating pulmonary vessels and inhibiting platelet agregation. Lipoxygenase inhibitors are under investigation, and prevent formation of the leucotrienes (Higgs and Vane, 1983). Finally, steroids inhibit phospholipase and may thereby be capable of modulating eicosanoid production.

Proteases

Antagonism of neutrophil proteases may be found to be of value in the prevention or treatment of ARDS. Danazol augments serum α_1-antitrypsin levels in individuals with depletion of this protein (Gadek *et al.*, 1980).

Coagulation and fibrinolysis

To date, manipulation of the coagulation system to prevent or reverse capillary plugging has not proved of consistent value in sepsis or ARDS, but may yet find a role in certain defined circumstances such as pulmonary hypertension due to vascular occlusion.

Host defence

Pharmacological stimulation of the immune response is possible with agents such as levimasole (Meakins *et al.*, 1979). Fibronectin deficiency may be treated by administration of cryoprecipitate (Scovill *et al.*, 1978). Passive immunization with *Escherichia coli* antiserum (Zeigler *et al.*, 1982), and removal of endotoxin by plasmaphaeresis (Schwartmann *et al.*, 1979) have been reported in the treatment of endotoxaemia. Activated leucocytes may be removed by leucophaeresis or exchange transfusion (Bjorratn *et al.*, 1984).

Pulmonary fibrosis

A diverse number of agents, including steroids, indomethacin, urokinase and proline analogues, have been shown to be effective inhibitors of experimental pulmonary fibrosis. Amelioration of pulmonary parenchymal structural damage may prove to be important in improving the prognosis of ARDS.

Improvement of gas exchange

By minimizing the need for high inspired oxygen concentrations, the pulmonary toxicity of hyperoxia may be avoidable. Positive end-expiratory pressure (PEEP) up to 30 cm H_2O has been advocated (Shapiro, Cane and Harrison, 1984). Unconventional respiratory modes, such as high frequency ventilation (Sjostrand, 1983) and use of reversed I/E ratios have been investigated. Intrapulmonary administration of surfactant improves gas exchange experimentally. In profound hypoxaemia, extracorporeal membrane oxygenation has been used but does not improve outcome (Zapol and Snider, 1980). Extracorporeal carbon dioxide extraction allows the use of small minute volumes to maintain adequate gas exchange (Gattinoni *et al.*, 1980).

Management

Our rapidly expanding knowledge of the pathogenesis of septic shock and ARDS has unfortunately failed to provide rewarding changes in the principles of management in clinical practice. It is, however, worth reiterating that anticipation and prompt recognition of septic shock and its complications is the cornerstone of good clinical management. The aims of treatment will be considered here in three parts: (a) elimination of the shock state; (b) eradication of sepsis; (c) intensive respiratory, cardiovascular, renal and nutritional support. All three aims are clearly interdependent and require careful integration into clinical practice. In all but the simplest cases the patient will usually require transfer to an intensive care unit after initial resuscitation.

Elimination of the shock state

Defining shock as a state of inadequate oxygen delivery to the tissues, it is clear that attention must be paid to restoring both adequate arterial oxygenation and cardiac output. In the first instance, oxygen should be administered and hypovolaemia adequately corrected. There is controversy concerning the fluid of choice in resuscitation from shock (Lucas and Ledgerwood, 1983), particularly in respect of the pulmonary consequences. In the initial management we feel it is logical to use colloidal solutions to restore the circulating blood volume, attempting to maintain a haematocrit of about 0.3 (haemoglobin 10–11 g/dl). If a clinically adequate circulation is not rapidly achieved, central venous pressure (CVP) should be measured and restored to at least 5 cm H_2O. In the presence of right ventricular dysfunction, central venous pressure is meaningless as an index of left ventricular preload, and pulmonary artery catheterization may be necessary to permit pulmonary artery wedge pressure (PAWP) measurement. Wedge pressure should be restored to at least 9.5 mm Hg and may be pushed to 18 mm Hg. If, at this stage, circulation is still inadequate, the use of inotropes, with or without vasodilators, is indicated. The choice of vasoactive drugs is probably unimportant as long as an adequate circulation is restored. Dopamine is often used. The efficacy of dobutamine in septic shock is being evaluated.

It has been shown that, in the management of critically ill post-surgical patients, therapy is best aimed at restoring 'optimal' rather than 'normal' cardiorespiratory parameters (Shoemaker, Appel and Bland, 1983).

Eradication of sepsis

This vital aspect of the management of surgical sepsis and septic ARDS may be considered under three headings – antibiotic treatment, surgical drainage and prevention of secondary infection. To be effective, the appropriate antibiotics must be administered early in the course of systemic sepsis, and in sufficient dose to achieve good tissue penetration. In practice, having made the diagnosis, the clinician must take samples of blood, drainage fluid, urine and sputum for microbiological examination before prescribing 'best guess' antibiotics while awaiting the results of cultures and sensitivities. Immediate microscopic examination of Gram-stained preparations may sometimes provide useful information and should not be neglected. The choice of antibiotics will depend upon the identification of the likely source of sepsis and, therefore, the likely pathogens (Bradley and Ledingham, 1984). Ideally, the antibiotics prescribed should conform to current hospital protocol, decided in consultation between clinical and laboratory departments.

Sources of sepsis amenable to surgical drainage must be sought and treated early. The patient's condition must be regularly reappraised and, when indicated, surgical intervention must be undertaken as a matter of urgency. The precise timing will depend upon the adequacy of resuscitation from shock, and must be decided in consultation with the anaesthetist. In addition to regular clinical and radiological examination of the patient, other imaging techniques may be of value in detecting septic foci (Driedger *et al.*, 1983). Ultrasound examination can easily be performed at the bedside in critically ill patients if portable equipment is available. Radio-isotope imaging may be valuable.

Patients with septic shock and ARDS are very susceptible to secondary infections. Attending staff must be careful to avoid causing cross-infection. Simple measures such as frequent hand washing, and minimizing movement of nursing staff between patients, are effective. Staff with cutaneous or respiratory tract infections should not come in contact with these patients.

Intensive supportive therapy

After resuscitation from shock, continuous monitoring of the patient is necessary to maintain adequate homeostasis. Adequacy of the circulation is most readily judged by clinical examination and measurement of urine output and the core–peripheral temperature gradient. If more sophisticated facilities are available, therapy should aim to achieve the preferred values of haemodynamic variables which have been estimated for critically ill postoperative patients. In particular, it is desirable to maintain the cardiac output at about 50% above normal and oxygen delivery in excess of 550 ml/min/m^2.

Inspired oxygen concentration should be adjusted to maintain about 95% oxygen saturation (PaO_2 about 10 kPa). Recent work has focused on the importance of respiratory muscle fatigue in critically ill patients (Cohen *et al.*, 1982). In those who develop progressive respiratory distress or in whom hypoxaemia is severe, IPPV should be instituted early. Use of inspired oxygen concentrations greater than 50% should, as far as possible, be avoided by use of PEEP. If PEEP is found to compromise cardiac output, it can usually be restored by judicious use of volume expanders and inotropes. When ARDS is developed, IPPV with PEEP is virtually always necessary.

Maintenance fluids should be prescribed to support a urine output in excess of 0.5 ml/kg/h and normal serum electrolyte concentrations. Fluid overload must be avoided by monitoring fluid balance (with allowances for insensible losses), body weight and PAWP. Fluid restriction alone cannot be expected to eradicate interstitial oedema due to microvascular injury, and if used indiscriminately may accelerate renal failure. There is probably no advantage in trying to restore low serum albumen levels by infusion of plasma. Low serum sodium concentrations are frequently seen and most often reflect overhydration rather than total body sodium depletion. In the absence of excessive sodium losses, it should not be necessary to give more than about 100 mmol Na^+/d.

It is better to prevent renal failure than to treat it. Once renal failure is established, dialysis must be started and, because of the high metabolic rate, will usually need to be performed daily. Between dialyses, continuous ultrafiltration may be of value in maintaining optimal fluid balance. In rare cases, charcoal haemoperfusion may be necessary to treat hepatic failure.

Nutritional support is always required and should be started within 72 h. Parenteral nutrition is usually necessary in the first instance, but enteral nutrition should be instituted as soon as possible. Use of parenteral nutrition demands careful laboratory monitoring if serious complications are to be avoided.

Humane considerations demand attention to the treatment of pain and anxiety. Analgesic agents and anxiolytics are therefore indicated, but must be used sensibly (*Lancet*, 1984). Occasionally, muscle relaxants will be required to facilitate ventilation and to minimize oxygen consumption. There is no evidence that a state of prolonged anaesthesia is beneficial to the patient.

References

ASHBAUGH, D. G., BIGELOW, D. B., PETTY, T. L. and LEVINE, B. E. (1967). Acute respiratory distress in adults. *Lancet,* **2,** 319–323

BIHARI, D. J. (1984). The case for steroids. *Intensive Care Medicine,* **10,** 113–114

BIHARI, D. J. and TINKER, J. (1982). Steroids in intensive care. *British Journal of Hospital Medicine,* **28,** 323–330

BJORRATN, B., BJERTNES, L., FADNES, H. O., FLAEGSTAD, T., GUTTERBERG, T. J., KRISTIANSEN, B. E., PAPE, J., REKVIG, O. P., OSTERUD, B. and AANDERUD, L. (1984). Meningococcal septicaemia treated with combined plasmapheresis and leucopheresis or with blood exchange. *British Medical Journal,* **288,** 439–441

BRADFIELD, J. W. B. (1974). Control of spillover: the importance of Kupffer-cell function in clinical medicine. *Lancet,* **2,** 883–886

BRADLEY, J. A. and LEDINGHAM, I. MCA. (1984). London; Heinemann (in press)

BRADLEY, J. A., LEDINGHAM, I. MCA. and HAMILTON, D. N. H. (1981). Assessment of host resistance in critically ill surgical patients by the response to recall skin antigens. *Intensive Care Medicine,* **7,** 105–108

BRITISH MEDICAL JOURNAL (1979). Leading Article: Parenteral nutrition before surgery? *British Medical Journal,* **2,** 1529

BUCKLEY, F. P., ROBINSON, N. B., SIMONOWITZ, D. A. and DELLINGER, E. P. (1983). Anaesthesia in the morbidly obese. *Anaesthesia,* **38,** 840–851

CATLEY, D. M., THORNTON, C., JORDAN, C.., ROYSTON, D., LEHANE, J. R. and JONES, J. G. (1982). Post-operative respiratory depression associated with continuous morphine infusion. *British Journal of Anaesthesia,* **54,** 235P

COHEN, C. A., ZAGELBAUM, G., GROSS, D., ROUSSOS, C. H. and MACKLEM, P. T. (1982). Clinical manifestations of inspiratory muscle fatigue. *American Journal of Medicine,* **73,** 308–316

CRAIG, D. B. (1981). Post-operative recovery of pulmonary function. *Anesthesia and Analgesia,* **60,** 46–52

DEMLING, R. H. (1980). The pathogenesis of respiratory failure after trauma and sepsis. *Surgical Clinics of North America,* **60,** 1373–1390

DRIEDGER, A. A., SIBBALD, W. J., LEFCOE, M. and MCCALLUM, J. (1983). Diagnostic imaging in the critically ill. In *Recent Advances in Critical Care Medicine,* Vol. 2 (Ledingham, I. McA. and Hanning, C. D., Eds). Edinburgh; Churchill Livingstone, pp. 211–287

FISHER, A., WATERHOUSE, T. D. and ADAMS, A. P. (1975). Obesity: its relation to anaesthesia. *Anaesthesia,* **30,** 633–647

FLICK, M. R. and MURRAY, J. F. (1984). High-dose corticosteroid therapy in the adult respiratory distress syndrome. *Journal of the American Medical Association,* **251,** 1054–1056

GADEK, J. E., FULMER, J. D., GELFAND, J. A., FRANK, M. M., PETTY, T. L. and CRYSTAL, R. G. (1980). Danazol-induced augmentation of serum α_1-antitrypsin levels in individuals with marked deficiency of this antiprotease. *Journal of Clinical Investigation,* **66,** 82–87

GARRIBALDI, R. A., BRITT, M. R., COLEMAN, M. L., READING, J. C. and PACE, N. L. (1981). Risk factors for postoperative pneumonia. *American Journal of Medicine,* **70,** 677–680

GATTINONI, L., AGOSTONI, A., PESENTI, A., PELIZZOLA, A., ROSSI, G. P., LANGER, M., VESCONI, S., UZIEL, L., FOX, U., LONGONI, F., KOLOBOW, T. and DAMIA, G. (1980). Treatment of acute respiratory failure with low frequency positive pressure ventilation and extracorporeal CO_2 removal. *Lancet,* **2,** 2928

GREENE, R., ZAPOL, W. M., SNIDER, M. T., REID, L., SNOW, R., O'CONNELL, R. S. and NOVELLINE, R. A. (1981). Early bedside detection of pulmonary vascular occlusion during Acute Respiratory Failure. *American Review of Respiratory Diseases,* **124,** 593–601

GROEGER, J. S., CARLON, G. C. and HOWLAND, W. J. (1983). Naloxone in septic shock. *Critical Care Medicine,* **11,** 650–654

HALLGREN, R., BORG, T., VENGE, P. and MODIG, J. (1984). Signs of neutrophil and eosinophil activation in adult respiratory distress syndrome. *Critical Care Medicine,* **12,** 14–18

HAMMERSCHMIDT, D. E., WEAVER, L. J., HUDSON, L. D., CRADDOCK, P. R. and JACOB, H. S. (1980). Association of complement activation and elevated plasma C5a with adult respiratory distress syndrome: pathophysiological relevance and possible prognostic value. *Lancet,* **1,** 947–949

HAYNES, J. B., HYERS, T. M., GICLAS, P. C., FRANKS, J. J. and PETTY, T. L. (1980). Elevated fibrin(ogen) degradation products in adult respiratory distress syndrome. *American Review of Respiratory Diseases,* **122,** 841–847

HIGGS, G. A. and VANE, J. R. (1983). Inhibition of cyclo-oxygenase and lipoxygenase. *British Medical Bulletin,* **39,** 265–270

HOLDCROFT, A. (1980). Maintenance of body temperature. In *Body Temperature Control in Anaesthesia, Surgery and Intensive Care.* London; Baillière Tindall, pp. 106–146

JONES, J. G. (1982). Closing volume. In *Anaesthesia Review I* (Kaufman, L., Ed.). Edinburgh; Churchill Livingstone, pp. 43–54

JONES, J. G., MINTY, B. D., LAWLER, P., HULANDS, G., CRAWLEY, J. C. W. and VEALL, N. (1980). Increased alveolar epithelial permeability in cigarette smokers. *Lancet,* **1,** 66–67

KEIGHLEY, M. R. G. (1983). Perioperative antibiotics. *British Medical Journal,* **286,** 1844–1846

LANCET (1984). Editorial: Sedation in the intensive-care unit. *Lancet,* **1,** 1388–1389

LEBLANC, P., RUFF, F. and MILIC-EMILI, J. (1970). Effects of age and body position on airway closure in man. *Journal of Applied Physiology,* **39,** 390–394

LEDINGHAM, I. MCA., MCARDLE, C. S. and MACDONALD, R. C. (1980). Septic shock. In *Recent Advances in Surgery* (Selwyn Taylor, Ed.). Edinburgh; Churchill Livingstone, pp. 161–199

LUCAS, C. E. and LEDGERWOOD, A. M. (1983). The fluid problem in the critically ill. *Surgical Clinics of North America,* **63**(2), 439–454

MCCARTNEY, A. C., BANKS, J. G., CLEMENTS, J. D., SLEIGH, J. D., TEHRANI, M. and LEDINGHAM, I. MCA. (1983). Endotoxaemia in septic shock: clinical and post mortem correlations. *Intensive Care Medicine,* **9,** 117–122

MANSELL, A., BRYAN, A. C. and LEVISON, H. (1972). Airway closure in children. *Journal of Applied Physiology,* **33,** 711–714

MEAKINS, J. L., CHRISTOU, N. V., SHIZGAL, H. M. and MACLEAN, L. D. (1979). Therapeutic approaches to anergy in surgical patients. *Annals of Surgery,* **190,** 286–296

MENDELSON, C. L. (1946). Aspiration of stomach contents into lungs during obstetric anaesthesia. *American Journal of Obstetrics and Gynecology,* **52,** 193

MORRAN, C. and MCARDLE, C. S. (1980). The reduction of post-operative chest infection by prophylactic cotrimoxazole. *British Journal of Surgery,* **67,** 464–466

PARRATT, J. R., COKER, S. J., HUGHES, B., MACDONALD, A., LEDINGHAM, I. MCA., RODGER, I. W. and ZEITLIN, I. J. (1982). The possible role of prostaglandins and thromboxanes in the pulmonary consequences of experimental endotoxin shock and clinical sepsis. In *The Role of Chemical Mediators in the Pathophysiology of Acute Illness and Injury* (McConn, R., Ed.). New York; Raven Press, pp. 195–218

PEPE, P. E., POTKIN, R. T., REUS, D. H., HUDSON, C. D. and CARRICO, C. J. (1982). Clinical predictors of the adult respiratory distress syndrome. *American Journal of Surgery,* **144,** 124–130

PETTY, T. L. and FOWLER, A. A. (1982). Another look at ARDS. *Chest,* **82,** 98–104

PIPER, P. J. (1983). Pharmacology of leukotrienes. *British Medical Bulletin,* **39,** 255–259

REINES, H. D., HALUSHKA, R., COOK, J. A., WISE, W. C. and RAMBO, W. (1982). Plasma thromboxane concentrations are raised in patients dying with septic shock. *Lancet,* **2,** 174–175

RICHARDS, W. O., SCOVILL, W. A. and SHIN, B. (1983). Opsonic fibronectin deficiency in patients with intra-abdominal sepsis. *Surgery,* **94,** 210–217

RINALDO, J. E. and ROGERS, R. M. (1982). Adult respiratory distress syndrome: changing concepts of lung injury and repair. *New England Journal of Medicine,* **306,** 900–909

SCHONFELD, S. A., PLOYSONGSANG, Y., DILISIO, R., CRISSMAN, J. D., MILLER, E., HAMMERSCHMIDT, D. E. and JACOB, H. S. (1983). Fat embolism prophylaxis with corticosteroids. A prospective study in high-risk patients. *Annals of Internal Medicine,* **99,** 438–443

SCHWARTMANN, W. B., TILLOTSON, J. R., TAFT, E. G. and WRIGHT, E. (1979). Plasmapheresis for meningococcaemia with disseminated intravascular coagulation. *New England Journal of Medicine,* **300,** 1277

SCOVILL, W. A., SABA, T. M., BLUMENSTOCK, F. A., BERNARD, H. and POWERS, S. R. (1978). Opsonic α_2 surface binding glycoprotein therapy during sepsis. *Annals of Surgery,* **188,** 521–529

SEEGER, W., WOLF, H., STAHLER, G., NEUHOF, H. and ROKA, L. (1982). Increased pulmonary vascular resistance and permeability due to arachadonate metabolism in isolated rabbit lungs. *Prostaglandins,* **23,** 157–173

SHAPIRO, B. A., CANE, R. D. and HARRISON, R. A. (1984). Positive end-expiratory pressure therapy in adults with special reference to acute lung injury. *Critical Care Medicine,* **12,** 127–141

SHOEMAKER, W. C., APPEL, P. A. and BLAND, R. (1983). Use of physiological monitoring to predict outcome and to assist in clinical decisions in critically ill postoperative patients. *American Journal of Surgery,* **146,** 43–50

SIBBALD, W. J. (1984). The case for steroids – another viewpoint. *Intensive Care Medicine,* **10,** 115–117

SIBBALD, W. J., ANDERSON, R. R., REID, B., HOLLIDAY, R. L. and DRIEDGER, A. A. (1981). Alveolo-capillary permeability in human septic ARDS. *Chest,* **2,** 133–141

SJOSTRAND, U. H. (1983). High frequency positive pressure ventilation. *International Anesthesiology Clinics,* **21**(2), 59–81

TOBIN, M. J. and GRENVIK, A. (1984). Nosocomial lung infection and its diagnosis. *Critical Care Medicine,* **12,** 191–199

WALTON, B. (1979). Effects of anaesthesia and surgery on immune status. *British Journal of Anaesthesia,* **51,** 37–43

WEINBERG, P. F., MATTHAY, M. A., WEBSTER, R., RUSSELL, J., ROSKOS, C., GOLDSTEIN, I. M., HOPEWELL, P. C. and MURRAY, J. F. (1983). Lack of relationship between complement activation and acute lung injury (Abstract). *American Review of Respiratory Diseases,* **127,** Supplement, 95

WOLFE, J. E., BONE, R. C. and RUTH, W. E. (1977). Effects of corticosteroids in the treatment of patients with gastric aspiration. *American Journal of Medicine,* **63,** 719–722

ZAPOL, W. M. and SNIDER, M. T. (1980). Membrane lungs for acute respiratory failure: current status. *American Review of Respiratory Diseases,* **121,** 907–909

ZEIGLER, E. J., MCCUTCHAN, J. A., FIERER, J., GLAUSER, M. P., SADOLT, J. C., DOUGLAS, H. and BRAUDE, A. I. (1982). Treatment of gram negative bacteraemia and shock with human antiserum to a mutant *Escherichia coli. New England Journal of Medicine,* **307,** 1225–1230

Part IV

Infection

Chapter 11

Prevention of postoperative sepsis

C. J. L. Strachan

Introduction

Despite the many advances in surgical technique, theatre asepsis, antibiotic potency, nutritional support and monitoring systems, sepsis after surgery continues to be a major cause of morbidity and mortality. In spite of an increasing interest of surgeons in the science of prevention, avoidable deaths from sepsis are still reported from intensive care units with embarrassing frequency. While most surgeons agree in principle, very few have unit or hospital antibiotic policies. Although they would always scrub before surgery and wear a mask, they rarely check that the appropriately prescribed antibiotic has been given. In 1977, a study of patients referred to a regional hyperbaric oxygen unit with gas gangrene found the majority had either no antibiotic prophylaxis or an antibiotic with the wrong spectrum given (Darke, King and Slack, 1977). In 1975, a broad survey of general surgeons performing colorectal surgery found either the wrong prophylactic antibiotic used or none at all (Condon *et al.*, 1979). In 1979, a Veterans Administration study showed 16% preoperative prophylaxis (Munster, Weiner and Gibson, 1979).

There are many deaths from sepsis which are associated with multiple organ failure following multiple injuries or faecal peritonitis, but there are still a few patients who die of septic complications following routine elective surgery. This cost, in life, is not the only price to be paid. The cost of postoperative infection has been analysed in terms of 'morbidity, mortality and money' (Watts, 1981).

The morbidity consists of pain, anxiety, loss of function and loss of confidence, in addition to the morbidity of unsightly scarring, contractures, persistent wound sinus, incisional and recurrent hernias. The morbidity includes further surgery to scars and the wounds to replace prostheses – the latter at enormous cost to health care systems. The cost of an infected hip prosthesis in the UK is currently around £8000.

The cost of infection is not merely prolonged bed stay, which can be 3–4 days post-appendicectomy or up to 15 days extra after cholecystectomy (Strachan *et al.*, 1977), or a month in an intensive care unit. A survivor from sepsis after intensive therapy cost $27 951 in 1976 in the USA (Cullen *et al.*, 1976) and $18 900 in Australia in 1980 (Watts, 1981). In a National Nosocomial Infections study, patients with infected surgical wounds spent an average of 7.4 extra days in hospital (Brachman *et al.*, 1980). Based on an economic analysis from the University of Virginia by Swartz in 1969, the total All American bill, then, for surgical infection, was 9.8 billion dollars (Altemeier, 1982). This was based on an average 23.87 extra days at $6700–9477 each – matched controls were not used however (Green and Wenzel, 1977).

Classification of operation according to risk factors

It can only be assumed that reduction in overall sepsis rates will lower the annual cost of post-surgical sepsis. There are no studies, which is strange at a time when cost-cutting exercises are rampant.

Operative classification

The only study which has tackled the long-term assessment of relationship of risk factors and subsequent sepsis is the Foothills Hospital, Calgary, Canada, long-term prospective surveillance programme. Set up in 1967, the 5- and 10-year results have been published (Cruse and Foord, 1973, 1980). Infection rates analysed according to the type of surgery performed on a total of 62 939 patients showed a reduction in clean infection rates from 1.8% to 1.5%; in clean-contaminated surgery, in which the gastrointestinal tract was entered electively with minimal spillage, from 8.1% to 7.7% and in contaminated (gross spillage) 18.4% to 15.2%. In the final, highest risk, 'dirty' group with pus or perforation in the second quinquennium, the sepsis rate remained around 40%. It will be interesting to read the third report from this group, which covers the period 1977–82. In this 5 years, short-term perioperative prophylactic antibiotics, effective against the bacterial flora of the organ system breached, have significantly reduced postoperative sepsis in many centres, but are usually compared with much higher control rates.

Microbiological classification

This method of classification is based on the number of swabs with pathogenic bacteria at the primary operation (Pollock, 1979), i.e. not the probable prospective but the actual retrospective contamination:

(1) Clean – both visceral and parietal swab on closing sterile.
(2) Potentially contaminated – visceral swab only contaminated.
(3) Lightly contaminated – single bacterial species from the parietal swab.
(4) Heavily contaminated – two or more species grown from the parietal swab.

This should provide similar rates of sepsis to the NRC categories, but wide variations will of course identify the presence or absence or surgical skill!

The incidence of wound infection is frequently reported at a higher rate in the UK than in the USA. This represents a confusion in the definition, particularly of wound infection. Here, based on Ljungquist's definition, we would include not only pus but inflammation associated with a fluid discharge colonized by pathogenic micro-organisms (Ljungquist and Lund, 1964; Geddes and Williams, 1981). The single stitch abscess or non-purulent wound discharge which does not require debridement might be omitted in the USA. Similarly, under-reporting of infection from private wards (Polk and Ehrenkrantz, 1982) may be politically expedient.

Surgical audit of sepsis and choice of antibiotic

As mentioned above, few surgeons and only a few hospitals have an antibiotic policy linked with the quarterly returns of preoperative isolates from all the operations in which organisms are encountered. Surgeons must audit their sepsis rates, decide whether an antibiotic is needed and then select according to the type of operation, bacteria encountered and their sensitivity. Both human nature and the seemingly bottomless advertising budget of the pharmaceutical industry are great obstacles to the published trials. The choice of antibiotic may be local as long as the extent of sepsis is assessed by internationally recognized criteria. The end points of a surgical infection trial should always include intra-abdominal or distant sepsis and septic death as well as the standard, ill-defined entity, wound infection. This is best classified as major if it has a systemic effect and prolongs hospital stay, or minor if it does not. The time of contamination can usually be determined from the number of postoperative days and the pathogen isolated into primary or secondary infection.

One of the recent difficulties in separating primary from secondary infection, is the growing realization that short-term perioperative prophylaxis is associated with delayed wound infection 1–2 weeks after discharge, despite a normal-looking wound prior to suture removal.

Few attempts have been made to assess the extent of sepsis with a therapeutic or prognostic index. In a study of 11 physiological variables, each patient was classified within a 'multidimensional physiological hyperspace' (Siegel *et al.*, 1979). The complex requirements deterred most clinicians. On more readily obtained bedside information, a system for grading sepsis has been proposed, but is difficult to apply in practice. This scoring gives a weighting to local signs and effects rather than secondary or laboratory abnormalities (Elebute and Stoner, 1983). Further refinements eventually may provide a clinical aid.

Prevention of infection in clean surgery

Two-thirds of all surgical procedures are 'clean'. In general surgery operations, e.g. breast, thyroid, varicose veins and hernia, there is no need for antibiotic prophylaxis unless the host defence is impaired or a condition such as psoriasis or diabetes cannot be improved further. One of the few indications is the performance of mastectomy shortly after needle or open biopsy (Beatty *et al.*, 1983), and probably any major surgery within a week of open biopsy at the same site should be covered.

The majority of clean operations should be attended by meticulous asepsis which should commence as soon as the patient is admitted for surgery. The preoperative day should concentrate on the elimination of exogenous organisms, particularly *Staphylococcus aureus* in the skin, by bathing or showering with chlorhexidine gluconate or povidone iodine (Seeberg and Bergman, 1980). Nasal antibacterial cream in the preoperative week may be indicated if there had been a previous staphylococcal infection, history of boils or hidradenitis. One-third of patients on admission and one-half of ward staff carry *S.aureus*.

Operations on the groin or perineum have an increased risk and, since routine on-table preparation of skin has insufficient contact time to kill all clostridial spores, a povidone iodine soak for 30–40 min is a valuable adjunct, particularly in vascular surgery. The elderly have an increased nasal carriage of staphylococci, due to the heavy contamination which can follow even minor degrees of incontinence and to much thicker groin skin folds (Selwyn and Chalmers, 1965).

The presence of hair at the incision can also be a risk factor. The shave should be as close to the time of operation as possible, but not in the theatre, since loose hair constitutes a bacterial particle risk. The blade should be discarded after each patient and the geometry of the razor must cut the hair above the root infundibulum to avoid epidermal wounding attracting bacteria (Edlich *et al.*, 1979).

The prevention of postoperative chest infection is a controversial topic. Any patient undergoing a general anaesthetic is at risk – many house surgeons would claim that the greatest risk factor is the anaesthetist himself and that certain operating lists produce more 48-hour pyrexial events than others. It is traditionally recognized that patients with chronic bronchitis, heavy smokers and the aged should have physiotherapy, at least, since antibiotics may confer no additional advantage (Litchfield *et al.*, 1979). Chest infection rates commonly vary with the quality of the ward physiotherapy staff. Somc authors claim not only a reduction in wound sepsis with preoperative antibiotic prophylaxis, but if the spectrum is sufficient for respiratory organisms reduction in pulmonary infection can also be achieved with, for example, cotrimoxazole (Morran and McArdle, 1980).

The evidence that nutritionally deficient patients might benefit from preoperative intravenous or enteral feeding is conflicting (*see also* Chapter 7B). Small studies have reported benefits to include reduction in sepsis after gastric cancer surgery (Heatley, Williams and Lewis 1979), but others have not found any benefit (Yeung *et al.*, 1979).

The operating theatre environment

The majority of clean surgical infections are exogenous – from ward bedding and surfaces, other patients, medical and nursing personnel, bed linen, trolleys and finally the theatre environment. Included in the environmental consideration is not only the ultimate architectural dream of the perfect layout, but the pattern of traffic through the suites of materials, personnel and patients. The two methods currently in vogue are the vestibule and the multi-entrance plans, involving air locks, filter systems and security problems (Laufman, 1982).

There is a great deal of unsubstantiated 'folklore' about some of the methods used to maintain 'outer world' to 'inner sanctum' sterility. Blue lines are violated, 'zoning' from protective to aseptic is an uncertain science (MRC Report, 1968), and there is no uniform policy on controlling the vector potential of the trolley (Howard, 1982).

Orthopaedic surgery

The airborne bacterial contamination of wounds during operations, particularly those involving total joint replacement, has been extensively studied in the past 5–10 years. The recent series of MRC reports on the effect of ultra-clean air in operating rooms, involving 8000 major joint replacements, has shown that, when conventionally ventilated operating rooms are compared with ultra-clean rooms, the majority of bacteria which contaminate the conventional group is derived from the air (Lidwell *et al.*, 1983). The reduction in numbers of bacteria found in washouts when operations were done in clean air paralleled the reduction in joint sepsis. The reduction in numbers of bacteria associated with the use of antibiotics is similar to the 4 : 1 reduction in the incidence of sepsis in the prophylactic antibiotic group, and body exhaust systems reduced infections by a factor of two (Lidwell *et al.*, 1982). Sepsis occurred in 34 out of 5831 cases given antibiotics, compared with 52 cases out of 2221 operations without antibiotic cover. This 4 : 1 ratio compares with a 2.6 : 1 ratio in a better controlled ultra-clean air trial of 3175 patients (Salvati *et al.*, 1982). It would appear that the Charnley (1979) figure of 0.4% sepsis may represent the best possible.

It is no longer assumed that deep infections during the first 4 postoperative years are seeded during operation – organisms identical to distant intercurrent infections, e.g. lobar pneumonia, dental sepsis, urinary infection, etc., can be found in an acute unheralded joint infection years later (Laurence, 1983). Surgeons must inform each patient of the potential risk of late haematogenous seeding, for example following trauma, dentistry, cystoscopy or pneumonia. The use of gentamicin-containing cement is also favoured in some centres. At Lund University, Sweden, in 1981, Josefsson, Lindberg and Wiklander found, in a trial with 1633 patients, comparing systemic antibiotic with gentamicin cement only, that there were 6% superficial and 1.6% deep infections in the systemic group compared with 8.6% and 0.4% in the cement group (Josefsson, Lindberg and Wiklander, 1981). The Lund group would therefore use ultra-clean air with antibiotic systemically and in cement.

Peripheral vascular surgery

Despite the correlations which can be drawn between orthopaedic and vascular surgery and the more lethal consequences of reoperation to remove or bypass an infected thrombosed graft, vascular surgeons have been slow to adopt or to assess the role of advanced sepsis (Dale and Kaiser, 1980). Infection of a vascular prosthesis is a catastrophe as it usually leads to amputation of one or both legs in up to 75% of patients (Bradham, Cordle and McIver, 1961). In the prospective Nashville, USA, study of four graft infections, two died and the other two had limb amputations (Kaiser *et al.*, 1978).

There are certain vascular operations on carotid, vertebral and subclavian vessels where infection is rare. Anatomically, the greater risk of sepsis is around the abdominal aorta. The ruptured aorta has a threefold rate of bacterial isolation from the wall, compared with elective aneurysms, and the subsequent graft infection is usually with the same organism. Dissection of the duodenum, ligation of the inferior mesenteric artery, subsigmoid or subcaecal tunnelling and intestinal transudate within intestinal bags can all produce infection of body or limbs of the graft with a bowel organism. In one series, coliform organisms were more frequently isolated from the body of a bifurcated graft than *Staphylococcus aureus* (Jamieson, De Weese and Rob, 1975).

The most statistically frequent site of graft infection is the groin – the importance of an aseptic skin surface has been discussed earlier. Primary graft infections in the groin may arise from a distant septic or gangrenous focus, or from haematoma from the harvest of the long saphenous vein. Mutilation of lymphatics may allow both primary seeding of the wound or secondary infection due to a chronic lymphatic fistula. Incisions involving the groin have been associated with infection rates around 20% in some series (Shaw, Doig and Douglas, 1973; Christienson and Eklof, 1977). Diabetics are more liable to develop wound problems, yet no specific immunological deficiency has been identified (Casey *et al.,* 1983). Hyperglycaemia is associated with defects in neutrophil chemotaxis and phagocytosis (Bagdade, Root and Bulger, 1974) and often diabetics have low serum albumin at operation. As in other nutritional studies, patients undergoing vascular surgery had significantly fewer wound problems if their serum transferrin levels were over 150 mg/dl (Casey *et al.*, 1983).

Almost all peripheral vascular surgeons use some form of antibiotic prophylaxis despite the paucity of prospective controlled studies. At one time ampicillin plus cloxacillin was the combination of choice in the UK and cephalothin or clindamycin in the USA. Now, most surgeons use a first- or second-generation cephalosporin such as cephradine, cephazolin, cefamandole or cefuroxime. There is some evidence that some of the new third-generation cephalosporins have less than adequate antistaphylococcal activity and would be less effective.

The first controlled prospective study of 565 patients from Nashville, USA, demonstrated a significant reduction in wound infection rates if antibiotics were commenced just before surgery, when compared with a placebo group (Kaiser *et al.*, 1978). Skin preparation was not standardized until the mid-point of the study, when wounds in skin treated with hexachlorophane plus ethanol had 10.3% infection compared with 2.8% infection in those painted with povidone iodine. All patients subsequently had povidone iodine, and no brachiocephalic procedures were included since the first 109 head and neck operations had no single infection. Another study, of 217 patients, showed that either systemic or topical cephradine could reduce sepsis (Pitt *et al.,* 1980). The merits of topical or intra-incisional antibiotics are discussed below.

Cardiovascular and thoracic surgery

Antibiotic prophylaxis is now considered routine for most cardiovascular operations (Myerowitz, 1980; Michaelis and Locicero, 1983). As in peripheral vascular surgery, protection includes coverage of multiple temporary catheters, balloons and pacing wires and this percutaneous assault should be covered by a systemic antibiotic prior to line insertion.

The dose should be repeated at least every 4–6 h or earlier if blood loss is heavy. The organisms encountered are staphylococci, streptococci and peptostreptococci, pneumococci and *Bacteroides* spp., and so the choice of antibiotic again should be broad spectrum. Cefamandole, cefuroxime and cefotaxime are commonly used. The result of failure is endocarditis, mycotic infection of valves and prostheses, mycotic aneurysm and the extreme morbidity of sternal wound infection – which was 21% in one series (Fong, Baker and McKee, 1979).

Even more important than perioperative cover for major surgery is the prevention of infection in patients with cardiac disease having surgery on another organ system. This has been divided into a *mandatory group*, with congenital or valvular disease, with a prosthesis of any kind, floppy mitral valve or documented bacterial endocarditis; and a *theoretical group*, where antibiotics are indicated but clinical proof of need is lacking (Michaelis and Locicero, 1983). In thoracic surgery, the opened bronchus must always be considered contaminated and appropriate antibiotic cover selected for Gram-negative organisms in particular (Cameron *et al.*, 1981).

Gastro-oesophageal surgery

The transected oesophagus spills organisms peculiar to that locus. Anaerobes increase in the presence of carcinoma from 80% to 96%, but the isolation rate of all species of aerobic and anaerobic bacteria was similar in both groups (Mannell, Plant and Frohlich, 1983). Organisms identified are often anaerobic peptostreptococci and *Bacteroides melaninogenicus* from the oropharynx. These and aerobes can be recovered from an empyema thoracis after oesophagectomy (Lau *et al.*, 1981), and the value of pre-resection lavage with metronidazole is being assessed by Lau and her group in Hong Kong. The coliforms and other aerobes can be covered by cefuroxime or cefamandole, but additional cover against streptococci can be achieved by mezlocillin or piperacillin.

The operative classification of all upper gastrointestinal tract surgery when a viscus is opened is clean-contaminated, thus gastric operations such as highly selective vagotomy should not need antibiotic cover. There is a close correlation between intragastric pH and total numbers of bacteria isolated (Gorbach, 1971). When the pH rises in gastric carcinoma, ulcer, previous resection or haemorrhage, gastric aspirates with $>10^6$ organisms/ml have been associated with a wound infection rate of over 90% (Gatehouse *et al.*, 1978). Preoperative identification both in stomach and duodenum for biliary flora is too costly and selective prophylactic antibiotic prescribing still produced a 10% sepsis rate in those with $<10^6$ organisms/ml. Thus, all gastroduodenal surgery should be covered by either a single dose cephalosporin or ureidopenicillin parenterally.

There is current controversy in the lower risk operations of upper gastrointestinal surgery as to whether intra-incisional antibiotics or antiseptics at the end of surgery, or preoperative wound infiltration, might be as effective as either parenteral route. Intra-incisional application fails to reach protective serum levels and only protects the wound (Greenall *et al.*, 1981).

The most relevant trial comparing intra-incisional prophylaxis with intravenous prophylaxis is in high risk gastric surgery (Hares *et al.*, 1981).

The protection afforded by a single intravenous dose of 1.5 mg cefuroxime at induction and that of the same dose placed in the incision at the end of surgery were compared with results from a third unrelated control group. The control group had an unacceptably high rate of sepsis: 35% wound infection; 19% abscess; 21% septicaemia. The wound sepsis rates among the intra-incisional and systemic groups were similar, 4% and 7%, respectively. The most important finding was that intra-abdominal abscess and septicaemia were absent in the systemic group, whereas 19% developed abscesses and 4% septicaemia in the intra-incisional group. The reasons for lack of systemic effect are apparent from the cefuroxime assays. The peak serum cefuroxime level after injection into the wound was only a little more than half the level achieved by intramuscular injection and was not reached until 1 h after injection.

There has been a great vogue to instil povidone iodine into the wound during closure. Despite the initial wave of enthusiasm following the trials of Gilmore's group (Gilmore, Martin and Fletcher, 1973; Gilmore and Sanderson, 1975), others have shown no benefit (Pollock and Evans, 1975; Rogers, Blouin and O'Leary, 1983). These variable reports of efficacy may be due to stronger than 1% solutions interfering with normal wound healing and paradoxically increasing the infection rate (Viljanto, 1980).

Of more interest and theoretically more value is the concept of pre-incisional intraparietal injection of antibiotics (Armstrong, Taylor and Reeves, 1982; Armstrong *et al.*, 1984). By intramuscular injection at the site of wounding, adequate serum levels are achieved but further controlled trials from other centres with long postoperative surveillance are needed.

Biliary surgery

Many biliary operations are potentially contaminated and 20–30% of patients have pathogenic bacteria in their bile. Sepsis rates are 40-fold greater in patients with bacteria and the jaundiced patient has a high risk of sepsis and septic death (Chetlin and Elliott, 1971). The use of percutaneous transhepatic drainage procedures is associated with increasing rates of cholangitis and liver abscess formation, the longer the drainage tubes remain. The Hammersmith, UK, study of major liver resection for cholangiocarcinoma found that 25% of patients undergoing hepatic resection following decompression died of an uncontrollable sepsis due to organisms acquired during drainage (Blumgart *et al.*, 1984). Indeed, any amelioration of the pathophysiological effects of jaundice seem entirely negated by increased septic morbidity.

Seven years ago, in elective cholecystectomy, a study of 214 patients showed that a single 1 g intramuscular injection of cephazolin significantly reduced wound infection from 16.9% to 3.2%. Those patients given a 5-day course had a 5.5% infection rate (Strachan *et al.*, 1977). A further study of 416 patients from our group again showed the efficacy of single dose prophylaxis without any evidence of the development of resistance (Hurlow *et al.*, 1981). It had been agreed until 1981 that only 'high risk' cases should have antibiotic prophylaxis (Watts, Roberts and Finlay-Jones,

1981), but accurate preoperative identification is impossible and intraoperative Gram staining of bile too late, costly and time consuming. It has taken 6 years since first proposed (Strachan, 1978) for universal agreement that all elective gall bladder procedures should have single dose prophylaxis (Keighley, 1982a; Stubbs, 1983; Gruber *et al.*, 1983).

Elderly jaundiced patients have a much higher risk of sepsis and septic death after duct exploration or bypass surgery. In a recent series of 118 obstructive jaundice patients from Birmingham, 3 septic deaths were recorded – 37% of the patients were diabetics and they had a significantly greater wound infection rate (20% *v.* 4%) following single dose cephazolin prophylaxis (Keighley, Razay and Fitzgerald, 1984). Diabetic infection was due mainly to *Staphylococcus aureus* and it would appear that more attention is needed both pre- and postoperatively in this doubly compromised group, with better Gram-positive cover. Anaerobes are also important when bowel is opened for bypass. Thus, any single agent used should be broad spectrum. In a prospective study of 45 patients undergoing bypass surgery for jaundice, we compared single dose cefoxitin with single dose cefotaxime. There were fewer diabetic patients in the study and no *S. aureus* infections. Only 3 patients developed sepsis and one of these died of bronchopneumonia following drainage of a bacteroides/coliform subphrenic abscess (Binu *et al.*, 1983).

Appendicectomy

Although appendicectomy is often the first operation which surgeons 'in embryo' are allowed to perform unaided, it can still be lethal. In 1982, in England and Wales, 154 patients died from appendicitis (Office of Population Census and Surveys, 1983), the majority either very young or very old. Infection should rarely follow the removal of a normal or acutely inflamed appendix. If the appendix is gangrenous or perforated, infection can be frequent and severe. The organisms are commonly a mixed aerobic/anaerobic combination of bacteroides (especially *B. fragilis*), *Escherichia coli* and faecal streptococci. The most common organism in early studies was *B. fragilis* (Veillon and Zuber, 1898), yet it is only in the last decade that we have been able to provide total cover against the anaerobes with metronidazole. This agent in suppository form is widely used preoperatively as the only prophylaxis when there is no clinical evidence of septicaemia or peritonitis.

When the appendix is found to be gangrenous or perforated at operation, then 'treatment' antibiotics to cover all possible aerobic organisms should be given. The duration of this 'treatment' has never been properly determined and depends greatly on the quality of the host defence, with age the greatest risk factor. From the hundreds of antibiotic trials in appendicectomy and work on experimental models (Weinstein *et al.*, 1975), it appears that early septic deaths are caused by Gram-negative aerobic bacteria and late abscess formation is due to anaerobes. Gentamicin reduced early mortality and is still widely used. Those who believe streptococcal organisms important used ampicillin as well.

More recent studies have tried to achieve the optimum effect with a single agent such as cefoxitin (Hoffman, McDonald and Watts, 1981), cefazolin (Morris, 1981), cefotaxime with and without metronidazole (Lau *et al.*, 1983) and cefotetan (Tanner, Thom and Strachan, 1985). In none of these studies did the single agent completely abolish anaerobic infection and metronidazole alone was inadequate. In the cefotetan study, it appears that the isolation of *Streptococcus milleri* at the time of operation represented an important risk factor for subsequent sepsis. It is present in the lumen of 50% of inflamed appendices (Poole and Wilson, 1977).

Of the 10 patients with *S. milleri* isolated there was a 40% wound sepsis rate despite antibiotic cover, and it was more prevalent in the group receiving gentamicin and timidazole. Some authors claim that antibiotic lavage of the peritoneal cavity is the best method, as it deals directly with contaminated peritoneal exudate. In the USA it is often supplemented by systemic prophylaxis and delayed closure (Sherman, Luck and Borger, 1976) and thus is difficult to evaluate. The benefits listed include earlier resolution of abdominal pain, pyrexia and tachycardia when tetracycline 1 g/l was used (Stewart, 1979). This gave a 15% total infection rate in perforated appendicitis (Stewart and Matheson, 1978). This same group has now produced a 5-year prospective study of 1504 abdominal operations under the care of a single surgeon. All potential or actual peritoneal contamination was treated by tetracycline lavage plus 500 mg tetracycline intravenously – in only 23 cases was metronidazole with or without other antibiotics used preoperatively. The incidence of wound (2.8%) and intraperitoneal (0.8%) infection is dramatically lower than world literature (Krukowski *et al.*, 1984). Very few surgeons use tetracycline lavage – there are no advertising or marketing pressures on them to do so. Is this the only reason? Haffner found doxycycline lavage no better than with ampicillin (Haffner *et al.*, 1976).

Another old chestnut is the debate on whether the heavily contaminated wound should be primarily closed or delayed until clean and granulating. It is not well accepted by nurses or patients and most of the literature in favour is retrospective. Indeed, one prospective study concluded 'delayed primary closure has an important place in the history of contaminated wound management not in the modern management of perforated or gangrenous appendicitis' (Pettigrew, 1981).

Colorectal surgery

As in appendicectomy studies, results vary widely as the variety of operations included range from right to left colectomies and resections for inflammatory bowel disease to perineal procedures for anal canal malignancy and colostomy. The incidence of sepsis can be reduced by adequate bowel preparation whether by whole bowel irrigation, mannitol or old-fashioned purgation with magnesium sulphate and low residue diet. Anastomotic dehiscence is more common if preparation is poor and is related to age and nutritional state (Irvin and Goligher, 1973). Surgical skill is vital in providing maximal blood supply to the cut edges and accurate apposition, now made simpler in low anterior resection of rectum by the use of the staple gun. It is more difficult to clear faeces from the obstructed bowel, and intraoperative irrigation of the colon may permit primary anastomosis (Dudley, Radcliffe and McGeehan, 1980).

There are several specific and general reviews worth reading (Dudley and Fielding, 1980; Keighley, 1982b). Whichever technique is used, the addition of antibiotics reduces postoperative sepsis rates. The debate on whether systemic prophylaxis is better than the oral route is still extant and well reviewed by Hunt's group (Guglielmo *et al.*, 1983). They conclude that oral neomycin and erythromycin (Condon *et al.*, 1979) or metronidazole are inexpensive and easy to administer in the elective case, but the supplement of a broad spectrum cephalosporin, aminoglyside or mezlocillin may be of value. In the Aberdeen, Scotland, paper on tetracycline lavage, the infection rate of 1.8% wound infection in elective colorectal operations and 6.7% in emergency procedures more than halves the previously best recorded figures on either side of the Atlantic (Krukowski *et al.*, 1984). No doubt lively debate on this and the many other colorectal studies will continue.

The quality of surgery and an almost obsessional regard to all the many risk factors including the timing and prescription of antibiotics will continue to produce the best results. Despite the many new antibiotics on the horizon, only marginal advantage will be possible with penems, thienamycins, monobactams or semi-synthetic quinolone derivatives.

The future

Much of the residual postoperative sepsis is found in the patient whose immune responses are suppressed. Perhaps when we learn enough about the natural mechanisms of host defences to maintain them, antibiotics and their abuse will decline in importance.

At present, the enhancement of non-specific host defence mechanisms is in its infancy. Reticulo-endothelial stimulators include *Corynebacterium parvum* (Calhoun *et al.*, 1980) or bacterial products such as phospholipid (Fauve and Hevin, 1974), cold insoluble globulin (fibronectin) and levamisole (Meakins *et al.*, 1979). Unfortunately, the low level of significance in reducing septic episodes achieved in the levamisole study was not reproduced elsewhere (Ausobsky, Evans and Pollock, 1982). Muramyl dipeptide from bacterial cell wall has provided enhancement against antibiotic resistant organisms and higher survival rates in experimental animals compared to those receiving antibiotics alone (Polk and Galland, 1982).

The ease with which leucocytes migrate into an area of potential infection correlates with subsequent infection (Meakins, 1979). This is adversely affected by distant sepsis, malnutrition and anoxia, whether preoperative or anaesthetic. Infusing phagocytes intraperitoneally in rats failed to prevent peritonitis by *Escherichia coli* (Flint *et al.*, 1981). Chemo-attractants attract granulocytes into a site of bacterial challenge (Hau and Simmons, 1980), and intraperitoneal stimulation by increasing local reticulo-endothelial activity by zymosan may be beneficial (Joyce *et al.*, 1978). Successful augmentation of the host defect in anergic patients now seems possible. Perhaps Shaw should have the last word:

> 'There is at bottom only one genuinely scientific treatment for all diseases, and that is to stimulate the phagocytes. Stimulate the phagocytes. Drugs are a delusion.'
>
> G. B. Shaw (1906), *The Doctor's Dilemma,* Act 1.

References

ALTEMEIER, W. A. (1982). Hospital acquired infections: a personal perspective. In *Infection and the Surgical Patient* (Polk, H. C. Jr., Ed.). London; Churchill Livingstone, pp. 207–211

ARMSTRONG, C. P., DIXON, U. M., DAVIES, G. C., DUFFY, S. R. and CHETTY, U. (1984). A prospective randomised trial of pre-incisional injection of cephamandole in wound infection prophylaxis. *Surgery, Gynecology and Obstetrics* (in press)

ARMSTRONG, C. P., TAYLOR, T. V. and REEVES, D. S. (1982). Pre-incisional intra-parietal injection of cephamandole: a new approach to wound infection prophylaxis. *British Journal of Surgery,* **69,** 459–460

AUSOBSKY, J. R., EVANS, M. and POLLOCK, A. V. (1982). Levamisole and postoperative complications: a controlled clinical trial. *British Journal of Surgery,* **69,** 447–448

BAGDADE, J. D., ROOT, R. K. and BULGER, R. J. (1974). Impaired leukocyte function in patients with poorly controlled diabetes. *Diabetes,* **23,** 9–14

BEATTY, J. D., ROBINSON, G. V., ZAIA, J. A., BENFIELD, J. R., KEMENY, M. M., MEGIND, M. M., RIIHIMAKI, D. U., TERZ, J. J. and LEMMELIN, M. E. (1983). Prospective analysis of nosocomial wound infection after mastectomy. *Archives of Surgery,* **118,** 1421–1424

BECK, W. C. (1981). Aseptic barriers in surgery. *Archives of Surgery,* **116,** 240

BINU, P. S., HARVEY, M., THOM, B. T. and STRACHAN, C. J. L. (1983). Prophylactic use of cefotaxime or cefoxitin in jaundiced patients. Proceedings of the 13th International Congress of Chemotherapy, Vienna (Spitzy, K. H. and Karter, K., Eds), SY.55–9/17

BLUMGART, L. H., BENJAMIN, I. S., HADJIS, N. S. and BEAZLEY, R. (1984). Surgical approaches to cholangiocarcinoma at the confluence of the hepatic ducts. *Lancet,* **1,** 66–70

BRACHMAN, P. S., DAN, B. B., HALEY, R. W., HOOTON, T. M., GARNER, J. S. and ALLEN, J. S. (1980). Nosocomial infections: incidence and cost. *Surgical Clinics of North America,* **60**(1), 15–26

BRADHAM, P. R., CORDLE, F. and MCIVER, F. A. (1961). Effect of bacteria on vascular prosthesis. *Annals of Surgery,* **154,** 187

CALHOUN, K., TRACHTENBERG, L., HART, K. and POLK, H. C. (1980). *Corynebacterium parvum:* immunomodulation in local bacterial infections. *Surgery,* **87,** 52–58

CAMERON, J. L., IMBEMBO, A., KIEFFER, R. F., SPRAY, S. and BAKER, R. R. (1981). Prospective clinical trial of antibiotics for pulmonary resections. *Surgery, Gynecology and Obstetrics,* **152,** 156–158

CASEY, J., FLINN, V., PAWLOWSKI, J. and BERGAN, J. J. (1983). Correlation of immune and nutritional status with wound complications in patients undergoing vascular operations. *Surgery,* **93,** 822–827

CHARNLEY, J. (1979). *Low Friction Arthroplasty of the Hip.* Berlin; Springer Verlag, p. 158

CHETLIN, S. H. and ELLIOTT, D. W. (1971). Biliary bacteraemia. *Archives of Surgery,* **102,** 303–307

CHRISTIENSON, J. and EKLOF, B. (1977). Synthetic arterial grafts: infection complications. *Scandinavian Journal of Thoracic and Cardiovascular Surgery,* **11,** 43–50

CONDON, R. E., BARTLETT, J. G., NICHOLS, R. L., SCHULTE, W. J., GORBACH, S. L. and OCHI, S. (1979). Preoperative cephalothin fails to control septic complications of colorectal operations; results of controlled clinical trial. A Veterans Administration cooperative study. *American Journal of Surgery,* **137,** 68–74

CRUSE, P. J. E. and FOORD, R. (1973). A five year prospective study of 23,648 wounds. *Archives of Surgery,* **107,** 206–210

CRUSE, P. J. E. and FOORD, R. (1980). The epidemiology of wound infection in surgical infections. *Surgical Clinics of North America,* **60,** 27–40

CULLEN, D. J., FERRARA, I. C., BRIGGS, B. A., WALKER, P. F. and GILBERT, J. (1976). Survival hospitalisation charges and follow-up results in critically ill patients. *New England Journal of Medicine,* **294,** 982–987

DALE, W. A. and KAISER, A. B. (1980). Prevention of infection in vascular surgery. In *Controversies in Surgical Sepsis* (Karran, S., Ed.). Eastbourne; Praeger, pp. 277–284

DARKE, S. G., KING, A. M. and SLACK, W. K. (1977). Gas gangrene and related infection: classification, clinical features and aetiology, management and mortality. A report of 88 cases. *British Journal of Surgery,* **64,** 104–112

DUDLEY, H. A. F. and FIELDING, L. P. (1980). Management of patients undergoing colorectal surgery with particular reference to sepsis. In *Controversies in Surgical Sepsis* (Karran, S., Ed.). Eastbourne; Praeger, pp. 303–310

DUDLEY, H. A. F., RADCLIFFE, A. G. and MCGEEHAN, D. (1980). Intra-operative irrigation of the colon to permit primary anastomosis. *British Journal of Surgery,* **67,** 80–81

EDLICH, R. F., RODEHEAVER, G., THACKER, J. G. and EDGERTON, M. T. (1979). Technical factors in wound management. In *Fundamentals of Wound Management* (Hunt, T. K. and Dunphy, J. E., Eds). New York; Appleton Century Crofts

ELEBUTE, E. A. and STONER, H. A. (1983). The grading of sepsis. *British Journal of Surgery,* **70,** 29–31

FAUVE, R. M. and HEVIN, B. (1974). Immunostimulation with bacterial phospholipid extracts. *Proceedings of the National Academy of Sciences, U.S.A.,* **71,** 573–577

FLINT, L. M., CALHOUN, J. H., ANDERSON, M. D. and RICHARDSON, J. D. (1981). Studies of peritoneal phagocytes as therapy for faecal peritonitis. *Journal of Surgical Research,* **30,** 154–158

FONG, I. W., BAKER, C. B. and MCKEE, D. C. (1979). The value of prophylactic antibiotics in aortocoronary by-pass operations. *Journal of Thoracic and Cardiovascular Surgery,* **78,** 908–910

GATEHOUSE, D., DYMOCK, F., BURDON, D. W., ALEXANDER-WILLIAMS, J. and KEIGHLEY, M. R. B. (1978). Prediction of wound sepsis following gastric operations. *British Journal of Surgery,* **65,** 551–554

GEDDES, A. M. and WILLIAMS, J. D. (1981). *Control of Hospital Infection* (Lowbury, E. J. L. and Ayliffe, G. A. J., Eds). London; Chapman and Hall

GILMORE, O. J., MARTIN, T. D. and FLETCHER, B. N. (1973). Prevention of wound infection after appendicectomy. *Lancet,* **1,** 220–222

GILMORE, O. J. and SANDERSON, P. J. (1975). Prophylactic interparietal povidone-iodine in abdominal surgery. *British Journal of Surgery,* **62,** 792–799

GORBACH, S. L. (1971). Intestinal microflora. *Gastroenterology,* **60,** 1110–1129

GREEN, J. W. and WENZEL, R. P. (1977). Postoperative wound infection: a controlled study of the increased duration of hospital stay and direct cost of hospitalisation. *Annals of Surgery,* **185,** 264–268

GREENALL, M. J., ATKINSON, J. E., EVANS, M. and POLLOCK, A. V. (1981). Single dose antibiotic prophylaxis of surgical wound sepsis: which route of administration is best? A controlled clinical trial of intra-incisional against intravenous cephaloridine. *Journal of Antimicrobial Chemotherapy,* **7,** 223–227

GRUBER, U. F., ELKE, R., WIDMER, M., TRIPPEL, M. and GERBER, H. (1983). Soll man in der Gallenwegchirurgie eine Antibiotika-Prophylaxe machen? (Antibiotic prophylaxis in gall bladder surgery?). *Schweizerische Medizinische Wochenschrift,* **113,** 558–559

GUGLIELMO, B. J., HOHN, D. C., KOO, P. J., HUNT, T. K., SWEET, R. L. and CONTE, J. E. (1983). Antibiotic prophylaxis in surgical procedures: a critical analysis of the literature. *Archives of Surgery,* **118,** 943–955

HAFFNER, J. W., ENG, J., LOTVEIT, T. and AUNE, S. (1976). Peritoneal lavage with doxycycline in acute diffuse peritonitis. *Annals Chirurgica Gynaecologica Fenn.,* **65,** 22–26

HARES, M. M., HEGARTY, M. A., WARLOW, J., MAKINS, D., YOUNGS, D., BENTLEY, S., BURDON, D. W. and KEIGHLEY, M. R. B. (1981). A controlled trial to compare systems and intra-incisional cefuroxime in high risk gastric surgery. *British Journal of Surgery,* **68,** 276–280

HAU, T. and SIMMONS, R. L. (1980). Chemotactic substances in the treatment of experimental intra-peritoneal infections. *Annals of Surgery,* **192,** 625–628

HEATLEY, R. V., WILLIAMS, R. H. and LEWIS, M. H. (1979). Preoperative intravenous feeding – a controlled trial. *Postgraduate Medical Journal,* **155,** 541–545

HOFFMAN, C. E. J., MCDONALD, P. J. and WATTS, J. MCK. (1981). Cefoxitin prophylaxis for non-perforated appendicitis. In *Infections in Surgery* (Watts, J. McK., McDonald, P. J., O'Brien, P. E., Marshall, V. R. and Finlay-Jones, J. J., Eds). Edinburgh; Churchill Livingstone, pp. 217–219

HOWARD, R. J. (1982). The environment. In *Infections and the Surgical Patient* (Polk, H. C., Ed.). London; Churchill Livingstone, pp. 30–42

HURLOW, R. A., STRACHAN, C. J. L., WISE, R., ELLIS, D., ERNST, D., GATEHOUSE, D., GRENILY, R. P., LITTLE, G., POWIS, S., STAMATAKIS, J. D. and SYNOTT, M. (1981). A comparative study of the efficacy of cefuroxime for preventing wound sepsis after cholecystectomy. In *Cefuroxime Update,* International Congress and Symposium No. 38. London; Royal Society of Medicine and Academic Press

IRVIN, T. T. and GOLIGHER, J. C. (1973). Aetiology of disruption of intestinal anastomoses. *British Journal of Surgery,* **60,** 461–464

JAMIESON, G. G., DE WEESE, J. A. and ROB, C. G. (1975). Infected arterial graft. *Annals of Surgery,* **90,** 427–435

JOFESSON, G., LINDBERG, L. and WIKLANDER, B. (1981). Systemic antibiotics and gentamicin-containing bone cement in the prophylaxis of postoperative infections in total hip replacement; multicenter investigation. *Clinical Orthopaedics,* **159,** 194

JOYCE, L. D., HAU, T., HOFFMAN, R., SIMMONS, R. L. and LILLEHEI, R. C. (1978). Evaluation of the mechanism of zymosan-induced resistance to experimental peritonitis. *Surgery,* **83,** 717–725

KAISER, A. B., CLAYSON, K. R., MULHEIM, J. L., ROACH, A. C., ALLEN, T. R., EDWARDS, W. H. and DALE, W. A. (1978). Antibiotics prophylaxis in vascular surgery. *Annals of Surgery,* **188,** 283–289

KEIGHLEY, M. R. B. (1982a). Infection and the biliary tree. In *The Biliary Tract* (Blumgart, L. H., Ed.). Edinburgh; Churchill Livingstone, pp. 219–235

KEIGHLEY, M. R. B. (1982b). Prevention and treatment of infection in colorectal surgery. *World Journal of Surgery,* **6,** 312–320

KEIGHLEY, M. R. B., RAZAY, G. and FITZGERALD, M. G. (1984). Influence of diabetes on mortality and morbidity following operations for obstructive jaundice. *Annals of the Royal College of Surgeons of England,* **66,** 49–51

KRUKOWSKI, Z. H., STEWART, M. P. M., ALSAYER, H. M. and MATHESON, N. A. (1984). Infection after abdominal surgery: five year prospective study. *British Medical Journal,* **60,** 461–464

LAU, W. F., FAN, S. T., YIU, T. F., POON, G. P. and WONG, S. H. (1983). Prophylaxis of post-appendicectomy sepsis by metronidazole and cefotaxime: a randomised prospective and double blind trial. *British Journal of Surgery,* **70,** 670–672

LAU, W. F., WONG, J., LAM, K. H. and ONG, G. B. (1981). Oesophageal microbial flora in carcinoma of oesophagus. In *Infection in Surgery* (Watts, J. McK., McDonald, P. J., O'Brien, P. E., Marshall, V. R. and Finlay-Jones, J. J., Eds). Edinburgh; Churchill Livingstone, pp. 177–180

LAUFMAN, H. (1982). Environmental aspects of infection. In *Surgical Infectious Diseases* (Simmons, R. L. and Howard, R. J., Eds). New York; Appleton Century Crofts

LAURENCE, M. (1983). Ultraclean air. *Journal of Bone and Joint Surgery,* **65-B,** 375–377

LIDWELL, O. M., LOWBURY, E. J. L., WHYTE, W., BLOWERS, R., STANLEY, S. J. and LOWE, D. (1982). The effect of ultraclean air in operating rooms on deep sepsis in the joint after total hip or knee replacement: a randomised study. *British Medical Journal,* **285,** 10–14

LIDWELL, O. M., LOWBURY, E. J. L., WHYTE, W., BLOWERS, R., STANLEY, S. J. and LOWE, D. (1983). Airborne contamination of wounds in joint replacement operations: the relationship to sepsis rates. *Journal of Hospital Infections,* **4,** 111–131

LITCHFIELD, J. C., KEIGHLEY, M. R. B., MYATT, I. W. and EDWARDS, M. C. (1979). Randomised controlled trial of cefuroxime for established postoperative respiratory infection. *British Journal of Surgery,* **66,** 188–190

LJUNGQUIST, U. and LUND, M. D. (1964). Wound sepsis after clean operations. *Lancet,* **1,** 1095–1097

MANNELL, A., PLANT, M. and FROHLICH, J. (1983). The microflora of the oesophagus. *Annals of the Royal College of Surgeons of England,* **65,** 152–154

MEAKINS, J. L. (1979). Host defence mechanisms, wound healing and infection. In *Fundamentals of Wound Management* (Hunt, T. K. and Dunphy, J. E., Eds). New York; Appleton Century Crofts

MEAKINS, J. L., CHRISTOU, N. V., SHIZGAL, H. M. and MACLEAN, L. D. (1979). Therapeutic approaches to allergy in surgical patients. Surgery and levamisole. *Annals of Surgery,* **190,** 286–296

MICHAELIS, L. L. (1981). Letter to all physicians, dentists and osteopathic physicians in metropolitan and suburban Chicago from the Cardiovascular Surgery Committee of the Chicago Heart Association

MICHAELIS, L. L. and LOCICERO, J. (1983). The use of prophylactic antibiotics in cardiovascular and thoracic surgery – symposium – perioperative prevention of infection with antibiotics. In Proceedings of 13th International Congress of Chemotherapy, Vienna (Spitzy, K. H. and Karter, K., Eds), SY.9., pp. 33–38

MORRAN, C. and MCARDLE, C. S. (1980). The reduction of postoperative chest infection by prophylactic co-trimoxazole. *British Journal of Surgery,* **67,** 464–466

MORRIS, W. T. (1981). Control of infection after appendicectomy: metronidazole and cefazolin. In *Infection in Surgery* (Watts, J. McK., McDonald, P. J., O'Brien, P. E., Marshall, V. R. and Finlay-Jones, J. J., Eds). Edinburgh; Churchill Livingstone, pp. 220–222

MRC REPORT (1968). Aseptic methods in the operating suite. *Lancet,* **1,** 705–763

MUNSTER, A. M., WEINER, J. and GIBSON, G. (1979). Prophylactic antibiotics in surgery: practices within surgical services of the Veterans Administration. *Journal of the American Medical Association,* **241,** 177–178

MYEROWITZ, D. L. (1980). Surgery of the chest. In *Antimicrobial Chemotherapy* (Kagan, B. M., Ed.). Philadelphia; Saunders, pp. 361–369

OFFICE OF POPULATION CENSUSES AND SURVEYS (1983). *Mortality Statistics – Cause.* Review of the Registrar General 1982. London; *Her Majesty's Stationery Office,* Series DH2, No. 9

PETTIGREW, R. A. (1981). Delayed primary wound closure in gangrenous and perforated appendicitis. *British Journal of Surgery,* **68,** 635–638

PITT, H. A., POSTIER, R. G., MACGOWAN, W. A. L., FRANK, L. W., SURMAK, A. J., SITZMAN, J. V. and BOUCHIER-HAYES, D. (1980). Prophylactic antibiotics in vascular surgery – topical, systemic or both? *Annals of Surgery,* **192,** 356–364

POLK, H. C. and EHRENKRANTZ, N. J. (1982). Hospital acquired infections: a personal perspective. In *Infection and the Surgical Patient* (Polk, H. C., Ed.). Edinburgh; Churchill Livingstone, p. 211

POLK, H. C. and GALLAND, R. B. (1982). Enhancement of non-specific host defence mechanisms. In *Infection and the Surgical Patient* (Polk, H. C., Ed.). Edinburgh; Churchill Livingstone, pp. 101–109

POLLOCK, A. V. (1979). Surgical wound sepsis. *Lancet,* **1,** 1283–1286

POLLOCK, A. V. and EVANS, M. (1975). Povidone iodine for the control of surgical wound infection: a controlled clinical study against topical cephaloridine. *British Journal of Surgery,* **62,** 292–294

POOLE, P. M. and WILSON, G. (1977). *Streptococcus milleri* in the appendix. *Journal of Clinical Pathology,* **30,** 937–942

ROGERS, D. M., BLOUIN, G. S. and O'LEARY, J. P. (1983). Povidone iodine wound irrigation and wound sepsis. *Surgery, Gynecology and Obstetrics,* **157,** 426–430

SALVATI, E. A., ROBINSON, R. P., ZENO, S. M., KOSTIN, B. L., BRAUSE, B. D. and WILSON, P. D. (1982). Infection rates after 3175 total hip and total knee replacements performed with and without a horizontal undirectional filtered air flow system. *Journal of Bone and Joint Surgery,* **64A,** 525–535

SEEBERG, S. and BERGMAN, B. R. (1980). Preoperative total body washing with chlorhexidine gluconate performed by patients undergoing orthopaedic surgery. In *Problems in the Control of Hospital Infections* (Newson, S. W. B. and Caldwell, A. D. S., Eds). London; Royal Society of Medicine and Academic Press

SELWYN, S. and CHALMERS, D. (1965). Disposal of bacteria from skin lesions: a hospital hazard. *British Journal of Dermatology,* **77,** 349–356

SHAW, D., DOIG, C. M. and DOUGLAS, D. (1973). Is airborne infection in operating theatres an important cause of wound infection in general surgery? *Lancet,* **1,** 17–19

SHERMAN, J. O., LUCK, S. R. and BORGER, J. O. (1976). Irrigation of the peritoneal cavity for appendicitis in children: a double blind study. *Journal of Paediatric Surgery,* **11,** 371–374

SIEGEL, J. H., CERRA, F. B., COLEMAN, B., GIOVANNI, I., SHETYE, M., BORDER, J. R. and MCMENEMY, R. H. (1979). Physiological and metabolic correlations in human sepsis. *Surgery,* **86,** 163–193

STEWART, D. J. (1979). Peritoneal lavage and the perforated appendix. In *Surgical Sepsis* (Strachan, C. J. L. and Wise, R., Eds). London/New York; Academic Press/Grune and Stratton, pp. 123–131

STEWART, D. J. and MATHESON, N. A. (1978). Peritoneal lavage in appendicular appendicitis. *British Journal of Surgery,* **65,** 54–56

STRACHAN, C. J. L. (1978). Antibiotics for biliary infections. Symposium on Biliary Tract Disorders. *Scottish Medical Journal,* **22,** 241–244

STRACHAN, C. J. L., BLACK, J., POWIS, S. J. A., WATERWORTH, T. A., WISE, R., WILKINSON, A. R., BURDON, D. W., SEVERN, M., MITRA, B. and NORCOTT, H. (1977). Prophylactic use of cephazolin against wound sepsis after cholecystectomy. *British Medical Journal,* **i,** 1254–1256

STUBBS, R. S. (1983). Wound infection after cholecystectomy: a case for routine prophylaxis. *Annals of the Royal College of Surgeons of England,* **65,** 30–31

TANNER, A. G., THOM, B. T. and STRACHAN, C. J. L. (1985). A comparative study of cefotetan versus gentamicin and tinidazole as prophylaxis in emergency abdominal surgery. *Journal of Hospital Infections* (in press)

VEILLON, A. and ZUBER, A. (1898). Recherches sur quelques microbes strictement anerobies et leur role en pathologie. *Archives de Médecin Experimentale at Anatomié pathologique,* **10,** 517

VILJANTO, J. (1980). Disinfection of surgical wounds without inhibition of normal wound healing. *Archives in Surgery,* **115,** 253–256

WATTS, J. MCK. (1981). The cost of infection. In *Infection in Surgery* (Watts, J. McK., McDonald, P. J., O'Brien, P. E., Marshall, U. R. and Finlay-Jones, J. J., Eds). Edinburgh; Churchill Livingstone, pp. 10–13

WATTS, J. MCK., ROBERTS, A. B. and FINLAY-JONES, J. J. (1981). Infection in biliary surgery, Flinders Medical Centre experience. In *Infection in Surgery* (Watts, J. McK., McDonald, P. J., O'Brien, P. E., Marshall, U. R. and Finlay-Jones, J. J., Eds). Edinburgh; Churchill Livingstone, pp. 187–193

WEINSTEIN, W. M., ONDERDONK, A. B., BARTLETT, J. G., LOUIE, T. J. and GORBACH, S. L. (1975). Antimicrobial therapy of experimental abdominal sepsis. *Journal of Infectious Diseases,* **132,** 282–286

YEUNG, C. K., YOUNG, G. A., HACKETT, A. F. and HILL, G. L. (1979). Fine needle catheter jejunostomy – an assessment of a new method of nutritional support after major gastrointestinal surgery. *British Journal of Surgery,* **66,** 727–732

Chapter 12

Changes in immunological parameters following surgery and other severe trauma

J. Watkins

Introduction

There is a widespread belief that a significant fall in host immunity follows surgery and that the extent of the fall relates to the severity of the surgical procedure. The consequences are considered to be severe postoperative infections, poor wound healing and possibly disorders of blood coagulation. With the cancer patient, an additional worry for the surgeon is the possible establishment of micrometastases in an environment of reduced immune surveillance. Unfortunately, there is no entirely satisfactory way of measuring immunity and clinical observations are of necessity largely subjective in the absence of a control situation.

It is established that as a result of operative trauma the patient in the perioperative period will exhibit marked but variable changes in his blood. The changes involve quantitative and qualitative variations in immunoglobulins and the humoral inflammatory systems, as well as in immunocompetent cell populations, the lymphocytes, macrophages and cells of the myeloid series. Such changes may disappear or become consolidated during the recovery phase. Similar changes in *clinical disease* states would be associated with a degree of immuno-incompetence (Oppenheim *et al.*, 1975) and a poor prognosis. It is reasonable therefore to ask whether or not in the postoperative patient they infer a similar degree of harmful immuno-incompetence. If so, can they be manipulated by selective anaesthetic and surgical procedures? At a different level, can the changes be seen as harbingers of future disaster and hence have prognostic value?

Although immunity cannot be measured directly, there are nevertheless numerous techniques available which measure such changes in the blood and are conventionally employed in immunology as 'measures of immunity'. The majority of these tests are concerned with cellular immunity, as indeed are the few *in vivo* procedures, whereas the humoral aspect generally receives scant attention. The fundamental purpose of this chapter is to survey the various techniques, their limitations and their interpretations.

Immunity

'Immunity' is used mostly in a very vague sense, even by immunologists! Immunity defines the ability of the animal to mount a satisfactory attack on an invasive organism and its toxic products, such that proliferation of that organism and consequent tissue damage to the host is kept to a minimum. In its simplest practical sense immunity is seen as active and directed phagocytosis of identified harmful material which has entered the body. However, only in the invertebrates is life so simple. Here, glycoprotein 'agglutinins' coat invading parasitic protozoans, presumably as a result of chemical affinity to their cell coats, making them succulent or more attractive to the host's wandering hungry phagocytes. Although this represents the beginnings of immunity, in the mammals and particularly man such a vague identification and phagocytosis system would be totally inadequate and the host would have succumbed to tissue damage and toxin poisoning long before the source of infection had been controlled.

Complex systems have been evolved to deal rapidly with any invasive situation, each system being designed to magnify or enhance the signal from the preceding one, generating both local and systemic response. It is useful to visualize five separate phases in the immunity process, although in truth the edges between these phases are continuous and blurred except in certain disease states. The overall concept is shown in *Figure 12.1*. The phases are as follows:

(1) *Identification* of the invader as foreign or otherwise, involving the interplay of T and B lymphocytes and macrophages.
(2) The *immune response and antibody formation* if the invader is considered to be harmful.
(3) The extremely important (and usually misunderstood) formation of the *antigen–antibody complex* which has both critical size and concentration in normal health (probably genetically defined).
(4) The activation by the complex of the *inflammatory systems* (particularly complement) which actively direct and regulate the final phase.
(5) *Phagocytosis* of the immune complex.

Although this framework effectively defines the process of human immunity, and more specifically Types II and III 'mechanisms' of the Gell and Coombs classification of disease defence, we can graft on two special loops (*Figure 12.1*, heavy lines) operating with different speed of response and combining two or more phases of the basic immunity processes, to end up with the same objective – phagocytosis of the invader.

The first of these is the extremely rapid mechanism of immediate hypersensitivity (Type I) which replaces the separate formation of immune complex and subsequent triggering of inflammatory response by causing the antigen to combine with a specific antibody, a reagin usually of the IgE immunoglobulins class. The latter has particularly strong affinity for the surface membranes of mast cells and basophils. Once a critical concentration of these antibodies has built up on the cells, further exposure to antigen produces a complex *on* the cell surface. The physical change in the antibody molecule is then transferred directly through the cell

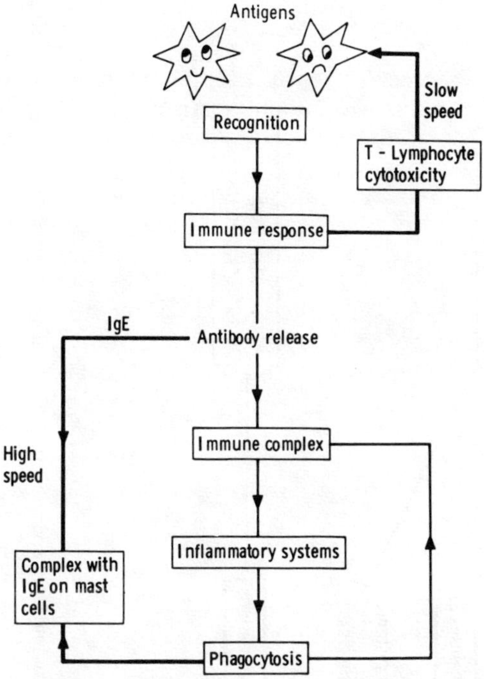

Figure 12.1. The biological processes which give rise to immunity in man. The central pathway equates with the Types II and III disease defence mechanisms of Gell and Coombs. The 'loops' (heavy lines) represent the specialized defence or reaction mechanisms, Types I and IV (From Watkins, 1984, by permission of the publishers)

microtubule system, leading to degranulation and the rapid release of vasoactive chemicals such as histamine and serotonin, as well as biologically active peptides *without* the intermediate involvement of complement activation and anaphylatoxin release. Reagin–antibody response has genetic implications and since some 10% of the population exhibit an appreciable degree of allergy it should imply some evolutionary benefit to the host. As with most enhancement mechanisms, the ease with which inappropriate activation can occur makes the possession of this trait most undesirable.

The second loop is concerned directly with cellular immunity, the Type IV mechanism. Here, having primed the immunocompetent cells to recognize a foreign cellular antigen, an excessive production of T-lymphocytes results in action against the target, effected not through antibody synthesis but through lymphokines released from the T-lymphocytes. The inflammatory response is brought about by the secretion products of the attacking lymphocyte but other cells, such as eosinophils, are also involved. Debris is again cleared by phagocytosis. Although classic involvement of this mechanism is in the rejection of tissue and organ grafts, as well as in contact dermatitis, all hardly beneficial to the host, some other aspects of T-lymphocyte activity, such as natural killer (NK) cell activity may be of considerable importance for their cytotoxic action on escaping cancer cells during surgery.

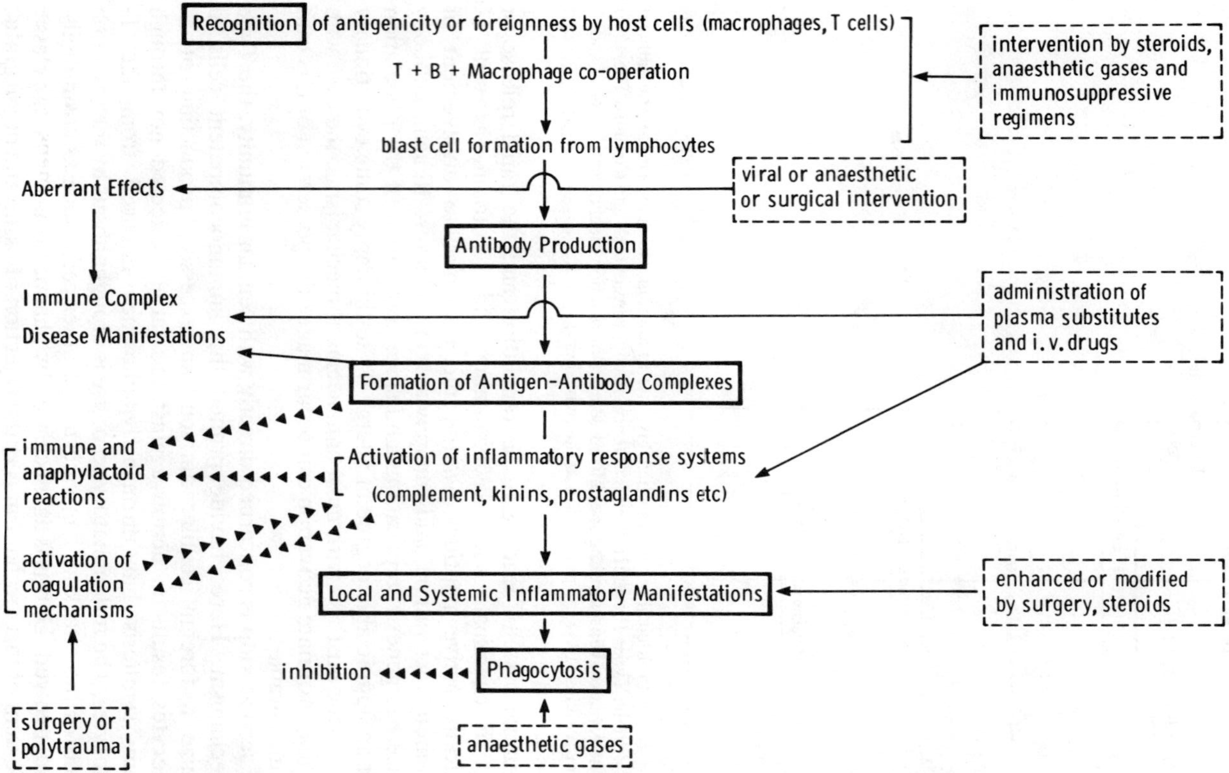

Figure 12.2. Interference with the biological processes of immunity by virus infections and predominantly by the intervention of anaesthesia and surgery

Penalties of sophistication

The very complexity of the systems comprising human immunity are both the strength and weakness of the overall system, since this provides endless opportunity for inappropriate activation (*Figure 12.2*).

Natural interference

Viral infections modify antibody synthesis producing antibodies specific to invading antigens but with poor *avidity* (adherence) to the antigen. The consequence is the production of faulty immune complexes which fail to trigger the inflammatory processes and hence phagocytosis – such that they are not cleared from the circulation and may precipitate in various organs around the body. The best known example is the near 100% incidence of rashes in patients with infectious mononucleosis who are treated with ampicillin. More tragic immune complex mediated effects of viral infection are encountered in neurological disease such as subacute sclerosing panencephalitis, a disease attributed to persistent infection by measles virus. Genetic features resulting in inadequate complexes are considered to be the cause of human immune complex disease such as systemic lupus erythematosus, while in some families who are abnormally sensitive to Epstein–Barr virus there is a progressive infection of the B-lymphocytes which terminates in hypogammaglobulinaemia.

Surgical and anaesthetic interference

The systems of immunity evolved tens of thousands of years prior to the advent of anaesthetics and surgery and are poorly equipped to deal with their onslaught. Modern surgery places high demands on anaesthesia and this has led to a considerable degree of polypharmacy with several drugs, both intravenously administered and gaseous, necessary to maintain the patient. The intravenous route of drug administration places the patient at immediate risk since, in a way, the process of evolution is reversed. Instead of an orderly presentation of antigens to the host's processing system through mucous membranes, there is direct entry to his own internal sea, the blood system. Here, a number of systems may be fired, particularly direct vasoactive substance release (such as histamine) as a result of the high chemical energy of the intravenous drug bolus, or alternatively there may be activation of the inflammatory systems such as complement. The use of plasma substitutes may generate convincing (to the host) immune complexes or aggregates and produce either local or systemic effects. Cardiopulmonary bypass procedures and dialysis may activate complement as a result of surface phenomenon. Although considered as 'immediate reactions', the consequences of such response not infrequently manifest in the perioperative recovery period, particularly with 'short' surgical procedures.

The trend of anaesthesia towards total intravenous regimens, particularly when these are used for prolonged sedation in patients requiring mechanical ventilation over several days or even weeks, can only increase the incidence of delayed reactions, particularly of the serum sickness type. Evidence of this is already occurring in the literature (Lawler, McHutchon and Bamber, 1983).

The interplay of the biological systems involving wound healing and immunity is often overlooked. Of necessity, these systems have evolved in parallel, since there would be little point in mounting a sophisticated attack on an invading organism if steps were not also taken to close up the point of entry into the body. The complement system in particular shares function with coagulation and fibrinolytic pathways with several 'common' inhibitor and activator enzymes. Thus, excessive activation of C3 will lead to platelet aggregation and if compounded by surgery, in terms of cut collagen fibres, may lead in *some* individuals to disseminated intravascular coagulation (DIC) postoperatively. Multiple trauma, such as encountered in road traffic accidents, may give rise to leuco-emboli in the patient's lungs producing the symptoms of shock lung and adult respiratory distress syndrome (ARDS). The latter is thought to occur by action of Factor XII upon complement C5 which then releases a potent polymorph clumping agent (C5a anaphylatoxin) systemically. The clumped cells are pumped into the capillaries of the lung, which they block, causing an inflammatory response (Hammerschmidt *et al.,* 1980).

Several effects of anaesthesia and surgery with major sequelae postoperatively can be seen to represent little more than interference with the delicately balanced enzyme systems rather than 'immunosuppression'. Before this brief survey is concluded, the effect of pre-existing disease in the patient should be considered, other than that necessitating surgery. Such disease may be totally unexpected by the clinician. Thus, the appearance of cytomegalovirus in renal transplant patients may be due as much to the stimulation of latent virus by a chronic graft versus host immune stimulation as to the deliberate immunosuppressive regimen. Finally, the patient with underlying chronic disease may be at high risk postoperatively simply because his immune systems are finite and are probably working near full capacity. The extra requirements to cope with new demands created by the surgical wound may indeed be the last straw and these demands may prove too much. No complex immunosuppressive theory applied to anaesthesia and surgery is required to explain the postoperative complications of these unfortunates.

Tests of immunity

In vivo *tests*

Since immunity is seen as a whole body function, any assessment should ideally be made on this basis. As immunity cannot be quantitated absolutely, assessments can only be made on the basis of *change* between pre- and postoperative measurements. *In vivo* tests provide a measure of delayed hypersensitivity, the prototype reaction being the lesion produced by the intradermal injection of tuberculin PPD, although other antigenic substances (e.g. mumps, Candida) may be employed in this manner. Unlike *immediate* antibody mediated reactions, cell mediated responses cannot be observed macroscopically until several hours after exposure to the antigen (hence, *delayed*). Reactions may thus be assessed at 24 h and 48 h. At its peak the lesion is characterized macroscopically by induration and erythema and microscopically by the large infiltrate of lymphocytes and macrophages. The skin responses – good, bad or indifferent – classify the patient as normal or anergic (Meakins *et al.*, 1977). Whether or not these tests provide useful information regarding the development of postoperative infection in any particular patient is open to debate (Pietsch, Meakins and Maclean, 1977; Brown *et al.*, 1982). The incidence of infection in most studies appears to be related more to the severity of the operation and the nature of the disease rather than to immune factors.

A version of such testing, anergy testing with dinitrochlorobenzene (DNCB), makes use of the fact that most individuals develop allergic cutaneous reactions following sensitization by repeated exposure to this simple but highly reactive chemical. The basis of the test is that DNCB becomes covalently linked to skin proteins which the body then no longer recognizes as 'self'. Following this latent sensitization, further exposure to the chemical (known as a hapten or incomplete antigen) results in the delayed hypersensitivity lesion. This test has been found useful in the selection of cancer patients for surgical resection of their tumours. In a study of 83 patients with malignant disease, Eilber and Morton (1970) showed that almost all those who reacted positively to DNCB had resectable tumours and were disease free at six months, in marked contrast to those who were DNCB negative.

An interesting corollary to both 'tuberculin PPD' and DNCB testing is that these parameters of immunity, and hence the systemic immunological features to which they are linked, are not significantly modified by anaesthesia and surgery.

In vitro *tests*

These tests measure the changes in peripheral blood in one or more of the parameters indicated in *Figure 12.1*. Despite the intrinsically unsatisfactory nature of such measurements, based on single function rather than a whole body function assessment of immunity, their non-invasive nature makes their use an attractive proposition. Indeed, such measurements present a perfectly respectable approach to immunity in *classic* immunology, concerned as this subject is with basic measurements in small animals such as mice, rats and guinea pigs. Here, quite large groups of littermates may be employed, with individual groups of these sacrificed for measurements on blood, spleen and lymph nodes at appropriate intervals, i.e. single function tests are made on organs representative of the body's system of immunity. In man, things are very different as there are no related control subjects and, except under conditions of accidental trauma requiring for example removal of the spleen, measurements are confined to the most ephemeral of organs, the peripheral blood circulation. Peripheral blood shows very marked and rapid changes following surgical trauma as a result both of endocrine stimulation altering leucocyte movements between compartment pools and of changes in the compartments themselves. Pre- and post-surgery observations on blood are not directly comparable and care must be taken in the interpretation of experimental observations.

The tests themselves fall into two categories: relatively non-specific *quantitations* and the measurements of *antigen specific recognition* by leucocytes. The former are easy to do and should not be dismissed as 'too obvious' in favour of more sophisticated (usually meaning complicated) techniques. The quantitation tests (Watkins and Salo, 1982) are as follows:

(1) Measurement of immunoglobulin levels (giving a simple assessment of humoral competence).
(2) Measurements of changes in inflammatory systems, albumin, and most particularly changes in levels and *function* of the various complement components.
(3) Simple measurements of changes in levels and types (IgG, IgA and IgM) of circulating immune complexes; various techniques have been recommended (Creighton, Lambert and Meischer, 1973; Theofilopoulos, 1982).
(4) Changes in plasma histamine levels (Lorenz *et al.*, 1981).
(5) Measurement of total white cell count, its differential, T- and B-lymphocyte proportions and T-helper cell and T-suppressor cell ratios. The latter may be measured most conveniently with commercially available monoclonal antisera. Overall, these assays give a surprisingly good assessment of cellular immunity.
(6) *In vitro* assessment of phagocytic function (Jarstrand, Lahnborg and Palmblad, 1978).

It is desirable that a full 'routine' haematological profile is obtained for each sample, irrespective of the chosen parameter of immunity, in order to correct for any fluid changes arising from compartment changes, blood loss and from the administration of exogenous fluids. Further, marked platelet aggregation in any sample indicates mishandling of that sample and should cast doubt on the validity of any leucocyte function tests made upon that sample.

Tests involving antigen specific recognition by blood leucocytes (Watkins and Salo, 1982) may be subdivided as follows:

(a) Tests in which the recognition of a specific antigen is reflected in some physical property change in the cells present in the test culture. These changes might be in the mixed lymphocyte culture (MLC), in cell migration inhibition (factor) tests (MIF) or the very interesting and relative newcomer to the immunologist's armoury, leucocyte adherence inhibition (LAI) which is considered below in more detail. Natural killer cell function falls into this group as a very specialized test; NK cells, a type of T-lymphocyte, are involved in cytotoxicity without previous sensitization to their target cells. The function of these cells is of considerable interest and importance to the cancer patient where resection of his tumour may liberate myriads of malignant cells. Its assay in the laboratory makes use of commercially available tumour cell lines, e.g. Raji cells, as target cells labelled with ^{51}Cr.
(b) Tests measuring immunoglobulin production. The original Jerne haemolytic plaque assay, which involves the lysis of sheep red blood cells incorporated into an agar plate together with guinea-pig complement by stimulated lymphocytes, has been extended to human peripheral blood samples (Bird and Britton, 1979). Not only can the number of antibody-forming cells be evaluated by counting plaques

(PFC technique), but radioimmunoassay can be used to evaluate the quantity and immunoglobulin class of the antibody secreted into the medium. The human lymphocytes may be stimulated to specific antigenic response (Fauci and Pratt, 1976) or simply activated in the presence of *polyclonal b-cell mitogens*.

(c) Tests in which are measured the proportion of lymphocytes capable of transforming into immunocompetent blast cells. As in (b) above, the degree of response of lymphocytes directly to specific antigens could be measured, but almost universal practice is to use mitogenic stimulation of lymphocyte cultures with plant, bacterial and viral extracts. In both cases, the technique essentially consists of incubating a known number of lymphocytes harvested from the peripheral circulation with tritiated thymidine and the appropriate antigen or mitogen. The cells are then harvested, washed and the level of radioactivity incorporated measured, thus providing a measure of synthesis of nuclear content.

While most mitogens act as polyclonal B-cell activators (PBA) some produce T-lymphocyte transformation and some both, presumably expressing the heterogeneity of the mitogen preparations. The most widely used PBA mitogens in general immunological practice are phytohaemagglutinin (PHA), pokeweed mitogen (PWM) and concanavalin A (Con A). These all nevertheless show a degree of T-cell dependence, and although under 'normal' conditions this may be unimportant, in the rapid changes of blood leucocyte populations encountered following anaesthetic and surgical trauma marked changes may be observed and erroneously ascribed to reduced B-cell activity and hence compromised host immunity.

The use of mitogens rather than specific antigens poses considerable practical experimental advantage, since rather than a narrow clone of cells being activated specifically, with relatively low radioactive incorporation, the 'polyclonal' function of mitogens increases the total incorporation of radioactivity with a subsequent increase in accuracy of measurement. Nevertheless, mitogen activation is not theoretically equivalent to the activation of lymphocytes by antigens and it is therefore rather reassuring to note that Jubert *et al.* (1973), studying the effects of anaesthesia, surgery and intraoperative blood loss on immunocompetence, used both mitogens and specific bacterial antigens in lymphocyte transformation experiments and obtained substantially similar results from both.

The lymphocyte preparation itself provides the major stumbling block to all such investigations of immunity. Whereas humoral factors like proteins and even individual blood cells can be identified and quantified, the lymphocyte preparation is of necessity a heterogeneous collection of various types of lymphocytes, and will also contain polymorphs and other cells of the myeloid series, as well as small numbers of red blood cells. The preparations themselves range from whole blood, through crude leucocyte suspensions to fractionated, enriched, lymphocyte preparations. Indeed, the crudity of the preparation is often essential to the immunological technique; for example, blood polymorphs are essential 'marker cells' in both the MIF and LAI tests. The variability of the preparations becomes 'normalized by experience' within each laboratory but gives rise to considerable inter-laboratory variation in reporting, although general patterns of response are reasonably reproducible. Transformation tests, particularly with mitogens, are particularly sensitive to the *source* of the mitogen (reflecting its heterogeneous nature) and this should always be stated in any reports.

Profiles of immunity

General observations

Since lymphocyte transformation tests, particularly to PHA, are those most frequently encountered in the literature, the profiles of such tests pre-, per- and post-surgery provide a good starting point for these discussions.

Figure 12.3 illustrates a profile typical of that encountered in patients following anaesthesia and surgery. There is inevitably a rapid fall (50–75%) from the preoperative value of this immunity 'index', following the onset of trauma, and a much slower recovery to the preoperative value, usually over 7 days. The response is non-specific in that it simply represents changes associated with the body's stress response to trauma, predominantly surgical trauma. The illustration herc is particularly interesting since it is adapted from Doenicke's experiments (Doenicke *et al.*, 1981) in which

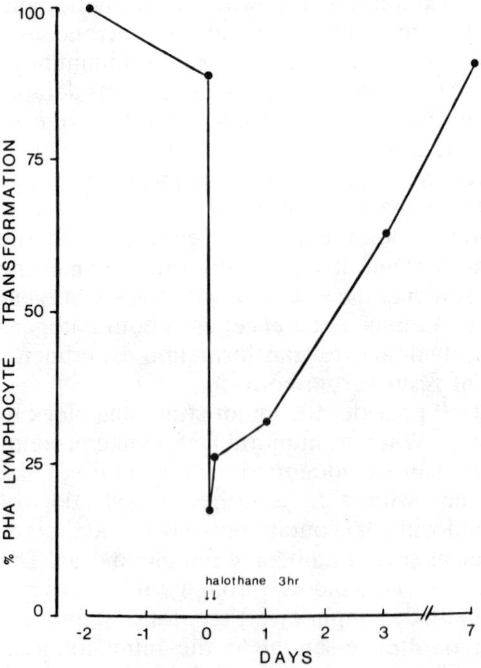

Figure 12.3. PHA transformation curve for peripheral blood lymphocytes taken pre-, peri- and postoperatively, exhibiting the body's typical stress response to trauma (After Doenicke *et al.*, 1981)

informed volunteers were exposed to halothane anaesthesia for 3 h without surgical intervention. Here, the stress response is to prolonged anaesthetic trauma alone and in this parameter is quite indistinguishable from that encountered in minor surgical procedures. While few workers would consider that the percentage fall in transforming cells correlates directly with a proportionate loss of host immunity, it is nevertheless frequently quoted as evidence of a *harmful* fall in immunity, to be avoided whenever possible by the use of appropriate anaesthetic techniques, e.g. stress-free anaesthesia.

However, an alternative explanation is that immunity evolved long before anaesthesia and surgery came upon the scene and there are no provisions to cope with wounding on the scale encountered in modern surgery. Without modern drugs and the skill of the anaesthetist, the patient would simply die. All that the body can do, in fact, is to reduce immune surveillance to prevent a further possibility of autoimmune stimulation to the unusual cell products released by surgery if the host should indeed survive the surgical assault – a beneficial effect! In any case preformed antibodies against most common pathogens persist in the body even when 'production' is reduced. IgG antibodies, the major immunoglobulin class, have a biological half-life of 25–28 days.

Although the fall–rise curve is typical of the body's stress response curve, and is reflected in immunoglobulin levels as well as cellular functions, it is a resultant profile and its components may not always be obvious or indeed identical. Thus, in *Figure 12.3* the dramatic fall observed within a few minutes of the commencement of anaesthesia represents not a loss of immunoresponsiveness by the cells but simply the fact that the cells suffered a change in physiological functioning, i.e. they went to 'sleep', not surprisingly, as a result of the anaesthesia. Their *apparent* behaviour is not much different from that encountered in the cells 24 h later when another mechanism must be involved.

The severely burned patient

A much more important example of the hidden consequences of immunity profiles is encountered in the plasma immunoglobulin (IgG) levels of severely burned children. In *Figure 12.4* are illustrated the fall–rise curves for serum gamma globulin (early nomenclature, predominantly IgG), during the first week after burn injury, with the lowest levels between the third and fifth days, in two age groups, 0–4 years and 4.1–12 years (Kefalides *et al.*, 1964). The early fall in level does to some extent represent fluid and protein loss from the burn area and, of course, haemadilution following fluid replacement. Despite the similarities in the IgG curves in terms of shape and protein concentrations, fatal septicaemia is prevalent only in the younger age group, despite similar therapy. This observation indicates that something is wrong with the *quality* of the immunoglobulin, not its quantity, in the under-4 age group, leading to the formation of inadequate immune complexes to the burn-associated bacteria and their toxins. This probably correlates with the immaturity of the immune systems in very young children who are thus less able to cope with their system's stress response to the burn trauma than older children.

Realization of this type of immunological problem in the burn patient triggered a number of trials to boost the burn patients' (particularly children) flagging immunity either by exogenous immunoglobulin preparations or by vaccination with vaccine made from the surface antigens of burn bacteria (Jones, Roe and Gupta, 1979), additional to the usual antibiotic regimen. Appreciable benefits have been claimed by some groups (Jones, Roe and Gupta, 1979) and at worst no significant difference between control and treated groups (Stone *et al.*, 1965). In Sheffield, investigations have been made into the use of exogenous immunoglobulin which has been enzymatically modified to make it non-antigenic to the recipient. Such a product is Gamma-Veinine (Behringwerke A.G., Marburg).

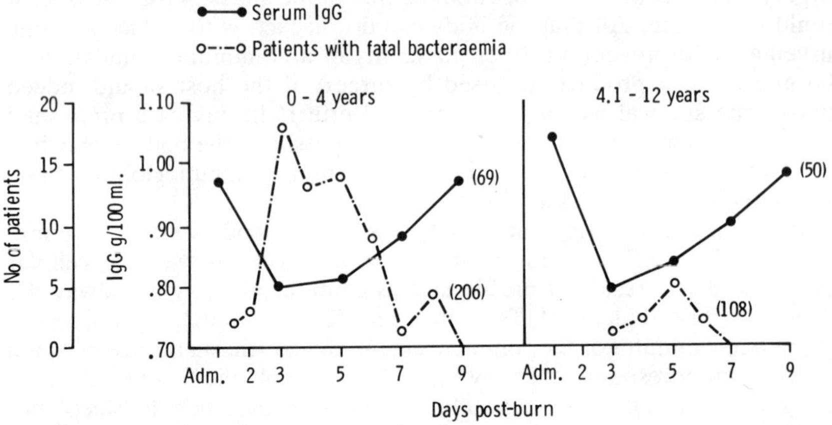

Figure 12.4. Serum gamma globulin levels and day of onset of fatal septicaemia in two groups of severely burned children, ages 4 months to 4 years and 4.1–12 years, respectively. Figures in parentheses refer to the number of patients studied. There were 64 fatal septicaemias among 206 children in the younger group, and 10 among 108 children in the older age group (From Kefalides *et al.*, 1964, by permission of the publishers)

Unlike intact antibodies, which function by producing immune complexes, Gamma-Veinine probably functions simply by neutralizing toxins. Its small size compared with the untreated molecule enables it to penetrate rapidly into deeply infected tissues. This is theoretically desirable in the deep burn victim. Only one case report involving such therapy occurs in the literature (Noesberger, 1974), but we have ourselves recently used Gamma-Veinine therapy to treat severe burns in a 5-year-old girl presenting with 22% surface burns and who, despite conventional burn therapy involving antibiotics, developed septicaemia on the twelfth day post-burn (Watkins and Appleyard, in preparation).

The decision to use Gamma-Veinine was based on the patient's clinical deterioration and also her plasma protein profile which showed a rather low IgG, low albumin and a raised IgM (*Table 12.1*). The inference was that although IgM antibodies were being produced they were in too low a concentration, or too large in size, or both, to cope with deep-seated infection. Moreover, although the smaller IgG immunoglobulin was undoubtedly being synthesized, it was probably being lost through the burn

Table 12.1. Burn patient – female (age 5 years, weight 22 kg)

Day post-burn	*Gamma-Veinine*	*Plasma proteins* (g/l) IgG	IgA	IgM	Albumin
13	no	6.0	1.5	4.4	30.2
14	yes	–	–	–	–
15	yes	8.6	1.5	2.0	33.6
16	yes	9.6	1.7	1.8	36.0
17	no	–	–	–	–
18	no	10.1	1.8	2.7	42.9
19	no	14.0	2.3	2.9	49.9

area. It seemed reasonable that infusion of Gamma-Veinine might 'break' the vicious cycle of events and enable normal immune control to be regained. Following infusion of 5% Gamma-Veinine solution, there was a marked improvement of the patient's clinical condition within the first 24 h, her temperature returned to normal and the total white cell count recovered near 'normal' levels (*Figure 12.5*). Her plasma IgG immunoglobulin and albumin levels increased markedly during therapy and continued to do so after completion of therapy (*Table 12.1*). Her general clinical condition continued to improve and she was finally discharged to the plastic surgical unit for grafting on the twenty-fourth day.

The role of Gamma-Veinine and similar related modified immunoglobulins is of current interest in the treatment of the surgical septicaemic patient as well as for treatment of bacterial infections in patients with antibody deficiency syndromes, either primary or resulting from 'therapy'. It should be used in addition to antibiotic therapy and other general measures, and not as a replacement for these. Monitoring of its effectiveness, as distinct

```
T. GENTAMICIN------------------------
E. WBC.
M 24.9 19.7  17.9  16.0  11.2  12.7
P.
40C   .     .     .     .     .     .
 .   *.     .     .     .     .     .
 .    .     .     .     .     .     .
39  * .   * .     .     .     .     .
 .    .*    .*   *.     .     .     .
 . *  .    *.     .     .     .     .
38    .     .   * .*    .     .     .
 .    .     .     .     .     .*    .
 .    . *   .     . *   *   * .  *  .*
37* . . . . . . . . . . . . . . . .*.
 .    .     .     .  *  .     .     .
 .    .     .     .     .  *  .     .
36C   .     .     .     .     .     .
 .    .     . GV  . GV  . GV  .     .
DAY12....13....14....15....16....17
```

Figure 12.5. Intensive care ward computer print-out for the young burn patient (see text). This shows body temperature and total white blood cell count (WBC) pre-, per- and post-Gamma-Veinine (GV) therapy. Antibiotic therapy (gentamicin) was maintained throughout from assessment of general clinical improvement, lies mainly in simple day-to-day laboratory monitoring of immunoglobulin levels, albumin (as in *Table 12.1*) and leucocyte counts.

There is considerable literature involving preliminary studies with Gamma-Veinine, well abstracted by Hoechst Pharmaceutical Ltd (1979) in their three-part publication 'Gamma-Veinine, polyvalent immunoglobulin for intravenous use'. All these studies carry the message that Gamma-Veinine must be used as early as possible following the onset of the disease. A recent multicentre international trial of Gamma-Veinine has investigated its usefulness in the treatment of the septicaemic surgical patient. Although most centres, including Sheffield, had anecdotal cases of critically ill patients responding dramatically to this immunoglobulin therapy, the overall findings were equivocal as to whether or not immunoglobulin therapy provided any additional advantage in clinical recovery. This outcome may have been biased by the imprecise protocol for admitting patients to the trial.

Comment

Thus it is clear that simple measurements of immunoglobulin and albumin levels in plasma give rise to an understanding of a mechanism of fatal septicaemia in young children. This, in turn, has generated an interest in immunotherapy which has extended beyond the original situation to encompass surgical septicaemia and immuno-incompetent situations in general. The response to such therapy may now be monitored in the laboratory by measuring the changes in the immunoglobulin levels, particularly IgG (see review by Pirofsky, 1984).

Continuing the theme of simplicity in immunological tests, attention is turned to a 'new technique' which is widely acclaimed as providing a valid measure of cellular immunity – leucocyte adherence inhibition (LAI).

Leucocyte adherence inhibition

This technique evolved as a result of attempts to improve upon macrophage migration inhibition, which uses capillary tubes as the 'focus' for migration. Halliday and Miller (1972) tested the ability of murine peritoneal cells to adhere to glass and exhibit antigen induced adherence inhibition during a 1 h incubation. The only satisfactory glass surface fortunately turned out to be haemocytometer slides! The grids etched upon these glass slides permitted cells to be counted before and after washing of the slide, to determine the degree of adherence. This particular technique is still considered to be the most sensitive form of LAI assay, although two other experimental variations – the microplate assay and the tube assay – have been developed which not only have technical advantage but also appear to exploit different immunological phenomena.

Appropriately enough, the term 'leucocyte adherence inhibition' was chosen with care. It was appreciated that leucocytes of all types adhered to the glass surface and that inhibition of this adherence occurred in a non-cell specific manner in the presence of antigen to which some of these cells were sensitized. The mechanism of LAI is still not fully resolved, but it is most likely that a T-lymphocyte subset (suppressor cells) liberate lymphokines (in response to the antigen) which then inhibit adherence by other types of leucocytes.

Clinical role

From being an obscure phenomenon associated with murine tumours, LAI has evolved as a practical clinical tool with both diagnostic and prognostic capabilities (Thomson, 1982). It was inevitable that, with its antigen related specificity, much of the interest should be in its predictive role in human cancer, but it has also attracted attention in non-malignant situations involving microbial antigens and autoimmune disease (rheumatoid arthritis) as well as a general measure of cellular immunity. Thus, Tannenbaum (1982) reported LAI studies which appeared to identify a subgroup of RA patients who were destined to have a more aggressive illness than others who initially presented with the same clinical symptoms.

In the *early diagnosis* of cancer, the LAI assay appears to compare favourably with established clinical procedures in terms of both specificity and sensitivity for colorectal cancer (Ayeni *et al.*, 1981), prostatic carcinoma (Bhatti, Ablin and Guinan, 1982) and to a lesser extent breast and lung cancer. Early detection of these cancers obviously increases the possibility of successful treatment and less radical methods, in turn reducing postoperative trauma. If the LAI techniques can be developed accurately enough to detect malignancy in its early stages and provided as a simple *routine test kit*, then this will indeed represent a breakthrough of immunological testing. A particular virtue of the antigen responsive LAI tests is that they are more sensitive to early rather than later stages of cancer. Essentially this is because in advanced cancer the patient's sensitive leucocytes are already coated maximally with tumour specific antigens (or complexes of these) so that they are in fact paralysed to further challenge *in vitro*.

Following radical surgery on the cancer patient there is a profound depressive effect on patients' LAI reactivity, similar to that encountered with other cellular techniques, e.g. PHA responsiveness, this index falling to about 50% of its preoperative value. The depressive effect has been encountered following radical prostatectomy (Bhatti, Ablin and Guinan, 1982), in patients with melanoma, and following mastectomy. These observations in large part are due to the body's non-specific stress response to severe surgical trauma, rather than to the nature of the disease.

A *prognostic role* for LAI following cancer surgery is proposed by Lopez *et al.* (1978). Briefly, as has been seen following surgery, all patients' positive assay results are lost and remain so for about 2 weeks. After this time, the positive LAI response returns, remains for 3–5 months and disappears again unless the patient has residual tumour sufficient in size to act as a stimulus to maintain immune reactivity. In patients harbouring micrometastases, the LAI positive response again disappears after 3–5 months, only to reappear again when the cancer reaches a specific size. Positive LAI assays may precede clinical observations by a year.

There are exciting possibilities here, but inevitably pitfalls exist. Not all patients show positive results, even with advanced cancer. Concomitant immunosuppressive therapy, irradiation or chemotherapy can adversely affect the LAI response, as does steroid and anti-inflammatory drug therapy. Results, as with other laboratory tests, should be interpreted in the light of clinical experience to add weight to an otherwise uncertain decision rather than creating the decision.

Unusual profiles, histamine and immune complexes

Despite the fact that trauma is considered to release histamine in a variety of species, and that many drugs administered in the postoperative period are quite clearly capable of releasing substantial plasma histamine, few studies have been made of histamine changes following surgery (Roher *et al.,* 1982; Lorenz *et al.,* 1984). Although the role of histamine in 'immediate hypersensitivity' reactions is well appreciated, its pathophysiological role in surgery is less clear. Major surgery, particularly abdominal, generates plasma histamine release at pathological levels (>1 ng/ml) postoperatively, and it is suggested that the release is involved in postoperative problems associated with blood coagulation, respiration and cardiac output (Lorenz *et al.,* 1984). This is clearly an area requiring further investigation and clinical trials before guidelines can be established for the usefulness of histamine assays in predicting postoperative complications. Nevertheless, surgeons should be aware of this further potential complication of surgical trauma.

As already discussed, the importance of changes in levels of circulating immune complexes is less theoretical, although generally these refer to viral effects, perhaps stimulated by operative trauma.

Direct effects of surgery itself may only be significant in the cancer patient. Here, the removal of the bulk of the tumour may enable further lymphocytes to mature without 'tumour tolerance' induced by high concentrations of anti-tumour immune complexes usually present in these patients. These new lymphocytes may well regulate residual tumour cells and metastases, contributing to a long, symptom-free period of normal life for the patient. The case for immune complexes in cancer has been the subject of a review by Theofilopoulos (1982). He concluded that non-specific measurement of immune complexes was a useful tool in monitoring the treatment and relapse of some forms of cancer.

In an interesting non-malignant situation, the deliberate formation of *controlled* immune complexes to dextran in patients' plasma has proved advantageous. Dextran has been widely used in the prevention of postoperative thromboembolic complications. Unfortunately, it has also precipitated a number of life-threatening anaphylactoid reactions. Noting that many individuals have naturally occurring antibodies which cross-react to dextran, Messmer *et al.* (1980) decided that reactions would occur from immediate precipitation of these antibodies by administered dextran (aggregate anaphylaxis). They reasoned that administering a small quantity of a low molecular weight dextran prior to the 'clinical' dextran would result in the formation of a small soluble complex which would be harmless and effectively remove all the patient's dextran-reactive antibodies, after which the clinical dextran could be safely administered. The initial studies of this hapten therapy on some 35 000 patients were impressive and justified the belief that immune complexes were certainly involved in some dextran reactions.

Changes in inflammatory systems

The stress response to trauma may be divided into two major components. The first is concerned with maintaining blood flow and energy supplies to vital organs and is mediated by changes in levels of catecholamines, ADH, renin and aldosterone. The second component provides the enormous metabolic stimulation necessary to supply energy for 'flight or fight' and later to supply energy for recovery and repair. From the immunological point of view, the first of these is the more important since studies of changes in the blood provide early warning of postoperative problems and the possibility of controlling these problems. The problems of the patient entering negative nitrogen balance are better monitored by metabolic techniques than immunological measurements.

Problems of blood coagulation

Changes in the blood occur soon after surgery commences, leading to an increased tendency to coagulation. The mechanism by which platelets become more 'sticky' is rather uncertain, but they respond to the catecholamine increase and to the release of tissue thromboplastins from endothelial cells as a result of any local (e.g. surgery) or generalized (multiple trauma, e.g. road traffic accident victims) tissue damage. Indeed, thromboplastins will be liberated as a result of various trauma including burns, hypoxia and acidosis. While the ability of increased haemostasis is clearly valuable to the patient during the initial surgery, in excess it can result in pulmonary microembolization and postoperatively to venous occlusion and pulmonary embolism.

While bacterial infections, particularly Gram-negative septicaemia, are probably the most important cause of disseminated intravascular coagulation (Cash, 1977), the initiation of disseminated intravascular coagulation (DIC) is by the release of tissue thromboplastins. This may be aided by complement (C3) activation in certain surgical procedures, e.g. cardiopulmonary bypass. In contrast to elective surgery, multiple trauma such as that encountered in road traffic accidents may give rise to the symptoms of shock lung and ARDS. While ARDS may result from complement (C5a anaphylatoxin) mediated clumping of polymorphs leading to leucoemboli in the capillaries of the lung (and subsequent tissue damage by superoxide release; McCord, English and Petrone, 1980), it may also arise from vasoconstriction of these capillaries. It would seem useful to have some distinguishing test for these two possibilities rather than a 'blanket' treatment with high doses of steroids for all multiple trauma patients arriving at hospital. Unfortunately, there are no *established* tests as yet for predicting all patients at risk to ARDS and not entirely satisfactory ones for DIC, although certain clinical conditions, such as dissecting aneurisms of the aorta (*Table 12.2*), are known to place patients at high risk. In the absence of predictive tests, anticoagulation therapy, steroid therapy and possibly superoxide dismutase therapy (for ARDS) are sensible practical procedures.

Table 12.2. Haematological complications in intensive care unit patients (from Watkins and Thornton, 1982, by permission of the publishers)

Patient	*'Trauma'*	*Haematological complication*	*C3 involved*	*C5 involved*	*Outcome*
BC	Colostomy	ARDS	Trace	Yes	Death
GB	Leukaemia (+ septicaemia)	ARDS	Yes	Yes	'Recovery'
RK	Colonic replacement oesophagus	ARDS	No	Yes	Recovery
LP	RTA*	ARDS	No	Yes	Recovery
EH	RTA	ARDS	No	Yes	Recovery
JW	RTA	ARDS	No	Yes	Recovery
AW	Lap/ischaemic colitis	DIC	Yes	No	Death
PJ	RTA	?DIC	Yes (limited)	No	Recovery
FS	Aortic aneurism	DIC	Yes	No	Death
JH	Perf. gut postop.	DIC	Yes	No	Death
Control subjects					
4 patients	Various, RTA, etc.	None	No	No	Recovery
SD	Leg amputation	None	Yes	Yes	Death
DF	RTA head injury → diabetes mel.	None	No	No	Death

* RTA = road traffic accident.

Predictive tests of coagulopathies

Generally, the concentration responses of the acute phase proteins, such as complement components and albumin, are too slow to be of clinical value in the early diagnosis of septicaemia or of blood coagulation problems. However, the measurement of the highly sensitive *activation* of complement systems is another matter. Several laboratories, including the Sheffield unit, are investigating the involvement of non-immune complement activation in DIC and ARDS.

The experimental techniques for the most part are relatively simple. Conversion of the complement components C3 and C5 is a measure of how much of the 'native components' are converted to inactive proteins as a result of the release of the biologically active entities, the C3a and C5a anaphylatoxins. In simple terms, the degree of conversion defines the likely clinical effects of the activation (Watkins, 1981). It is necessary to take serial blood samples from the patients (into EDTA), at least at daily intervals, and analyse these both quantitatively for the appropriate C3 or C5 levels (watch for haemadilution in the patient as a result of his therapy) using radial immunodiffusion techniques against the appropriate 'commercial' antiserum, and functionally by assessing the degree of conversion in single dimension immunoelectrophoresis (Watkins, 1982). It is necessary to demonstrate that other complement components (particularly C4) are not involved, since this would simply imply 'immune' response. Some laboratories prefer to measure more specific breakdown products of C3 and C5 directly, namely C3d and C5a (anaphylatoxin). These pose considerable technical problems and pitfalls for those without immunochemical expertise.

Retrospective studies on patients who had developed DIC or ARDS showed a remarkably clear division between the involvement of the non-immune mediated activation of the C3 and the C5 pathways, respectively, in these diseases (*Table 12.2*). This stimulated the possibility of screening patients' plasma prospectively for early indication of these coagulopathies.

Preliminary prospective studies were made on plasma samples supplied 'blind' from intensive care units and subjected to the simple immunochemical procedures outlined above, radial immunodiffusion for quantitation and immunoelectrophoresis for measurement of complement C3 and C5 component conversion. The results were impressive (*Table 12.3*). There

Table 12.3. Patients developing coagulopathies: comparison of positive immunological tests with haematological and clinical data

No. patients	*Suspected coagulopathy*	*Positive by:* Immunology	Haematology	*Clinically proven*
23	ARDS	18	not done	18/23
42	DIC	35	40	24/42

are no routine haematological tests for ARDS, but here the immunological involvement of C5 correctly identified impending clinical disease in 18 out of 23 patients suspected of developing this disease. In the early interpretation of DIC, C3 involvement was not significantly less sensitive than the various parameters of coagulation measured by the Sheffield Blood Coagulation Unit (Preston, 1979), although admittedly it was slower technically. Interpretation of ARDS by this method appears to give an advantage of 24 h over the appearance of the clinical manifestations. Whether or not this is sufficient time for practical treatment of the patient, only a proper clinical trial can evaluate.

Modification of immunity by anaesthetic techniques

Although the surgeon can do little to minimize the degree of surgical trauma other than by operating in early diagnosed disease states, the anaesthetist is in a unique position to intervene in the stress response with an ever increasing armoury of drugs and a choice of anaesthetic technique. The choice includes general anaesthesia involving volatile anaesthetic substances and various gases, or total intravenous anaesthesia, or analgesia, or regional anaesthesia. It is appropriate to end this chapter with some of the controversies and some prospects for immunological improvement in patient care provided by this approach. Interest effectively centres upon 'stress-free' analgesic anaesthesia and total intravenous anaesthesia. Regarding the former, it may be that blocking of any physiological function such as the stress response is not always a good thing. It is, after all, an important biological defence mechanism and only the seriously ill patient is likely to be at risk by its activation. Nevertheless, anaesthetic agents and anaesthetic techniques can play a major role in the modification of the stress response at afferent, central and efferent sites of the reflex arc. Several studies have indicated that patients are better clinically in the postoperative period if reflex responses to surgery are reduced by the administration of analgesic drugs, typically pethidine, morphine and morphine-like drugs such as fentanyl and alfentanyl (Dundee, Brown and Hamilton, 1969; Henderson and Parbrook, 1976).

Analgesic anaesthesia ranges from neuroleptanalgesia alone (useful for short but painful procedures where there is advantage in keeping the patient awake but free from pain) to the addition of the drug(s) to otherwise conventional anaesthesia. The use of analgesic drugs provides a high degree of cardiovascular stability, of particular advantage for cardiovascular and neurological surgery and for anaesthesia in the elderly and the poor risk patient. Neurolept techniques and the use of high dose fentanyl and morphine regimens in conventional anaesthesia abolish the cortisol stress response as well as changes in growth hormone and adrenocorticotrophic hormone (ACTH) levels (Brandt *et al.*, 1978; Ellis and Humphrey, 1982). Salo and his collaborators (Eskola *et al.*, 1984) have recently reported immunological studies on two groups of patients undergoing open heart surgery. One group was operated on under conventional balanced anaesthesia including fentanyl (17±3 μg/kg body weight), the other by the high dose fentanyl technique (72±22 μg/kg) and their pre- and postoperative immunity assessed in lymphocyte transformation and PFC immunoglobulin synthesis experiments. Despite the highly significant difference in cortisol secretion between the two groups, their immunological parameters were indistinguishable, although both cell-mediated immunity and humoral immunity were decreased, as expected, postoperatively. Thus, highly significant changes in the endocrine stress response do not automatically have identifiable immunological consequences.

For general surgery, high dose fentanyl and morphine regimens create practical recovery room problems (*see* Chapter 1 and Blunnie *et al.*, 1983) and epidural blocks may prove more satisfactory to ablate the stress response for lower abdominal surgery. However, for upper abdominal and thoracic surgery the picture is less satisfactory, since the cortisol responses are not abolished (Blunnie *et al.*, 1983).

Total intravenous anaesthesia has much to recommend itself to the anaesthetist (Wright and Dundee, 1982) and to the immunologist. Not only is there scope for controlled administration of the hypnotic drug, but the absence of noxious anaesthetic gases, particularly nitrous oxide and halothane, further reduces damage to the patient's system of cellular immunity (Sturrock and Nunn, 1976). The general effects of volatile anaesthetic agents upon host cellular immunity are far more important than commonly believed and completely outweigh the quite rare cases of delayed hypersensitivity associated with halothane (Walton, 1981).

The technique is dependent upon the rapid metabolism of the hypnotic drug and for this reason 'newer' drugs like Althesin and etomidate are preferable to the barbiturates. These drugs may be combined with fentanyl to provide 'stress-free' anaesthesia, as before.

It has recently been demonstrated (Griffith *et al.*, 1983) that patients with malignant disease undergoing surgery with total intravenous anaesthesia exhibit a rise in NK cell activity. This rise is not observed in patients with similar malignant disease operated upon with conventional inhalational anaesthesia. This observation suggests that the choice of anaesthetic technique may be of particular importance in the surgical cancer patient in maintaining cytotoxic mechanisms to circulating tumour emboli liberated by surgery and thus preventing tumour metastases.

Conclusions

'Immunity' and 'impaired immunity' are terms frequently quoted by anaesthetist and surgeon to explain their patients' postoperative or post-trauma condition, despite the fact that there is no totally acceptable method of measuring these functions. This chapter has provided a critical view of the various immunological tests at present available, each of which measures one or more of the biological systems which together constitute host immunity.

Most of the changes encountered are not specific and represent the body's endocrine mediated stress response, essentially to surgical trauma. The very young 'burn victim' is an exception to this, appears genuinely immunosuppressed and immune stimulation or replacement of some type seems essential for the patient's survival.

Tests which appear to have particular virtue, such as LAI and early diagnostic tests for impending blood coagulopathies in the postoperative period, have been particularly emphasized. The more popular tests such as 'PHA response' and beliefs associated with such tests have been put into perspective to aid the reader about to embark upon research to a more critical appraisal of the situation.

References

AYENI, R. O., THOMSON, D. M. P., MACFARLANE, J. K. and DALY, D. (1981). A comparison of tube leucocyte adherence inhibition assay and standard physical methods for diagnosing colorectal cancer. *Cancer,* **48,** 1855–1862

BHATTI, R. A., ABLIN, R. J. and GUINAN, P. D. (1982). Evaluation of leucocyte adherence inhibition in prostate cancer. In *Assessment of Immune Status by the Leucocyte Adherence Inhibition Test* (Thomson, D. M. P., Ed.). New York; Academic Press, pp. 185–206

BIRD, A. G. and BRITTON, S. (1979). A new approach to the study of human B lymphocyte function using an indirect plaque assay and a direct B cell activator. *Immunological Reviews,* **45,** 41–67

BLUNNIE, W. P., MCILROY, P. D. A., MERRETT, J. D. and DUNDEE, J. W. (1983). Cardiovascular and biochemical evidence of stress during major surgery associated with different techniques of anaesthesia. *British Journal of Anaesthesia,* **55,** 611–618

BRANDT, M. R., KORSHIN, J., HANSEN, A. P., HUMMER, L., NISTRUP-MADSEN, S., RUGG, I. and KEHLET, H. (1978). Influence of morphine anaesthesia on the endocrine–metabolic response to open heart surgery. *Acta Anaesthesiologica Scandinavica,* **22,** 400–412

BROWN, R., BANCEWICZ, J., HAMID, J., TILLOTSON, G., WARD, C. and IRVING, M. (1982). Failure of delayed hypersensitivity skin testing to predict post-operative sepsis and mortality. *British Medical Journal,* **284,** 851–853

CASH, J. D. (1977). *Recent Advances in Blood Coagulation,* No. 2 (Poller, L., Ed.). Edinburgh; Churchill Livingstone, p. 293

CREIGHTON, W. D., LAMBERT, P. H. and MEISCHER, P. A. (1973). Detection of antibodies and soluble antigen–antibody complexes by precipitation with polyethylene glycol. *Journal of Immunology,* **3,** 1219–1227

DOENICKE, A., GROTE, B., SUTTMAN, H., GRAF, K. J., SPRECHT, U. V., OTT, H., SARAFOFF,, B. and BRETZ, C. (1981). Effects of halothane on the immunological system in healthy volunteers. *Clinical Research Reviews,* **1,** 23–25

DUNDEE, J. W., BROWN, S. S., HAMILTON, R. C. and MCDOWELL, S. A. (1969). Analgesic supplementation of light general anaesthesia. A study of its advantages using sequential analysis. *Anaesthesia,* **24,** 52–61

EILBER, F. R. and MORTON, D. L. (1970). Impaired immunological reactivity and recurrence following cancer surgery. *Cancer,* **35,** 362–367

ELLIS, F. R. and HUMPHREY, D. E. (1982). Clinical aspects of endocrine and metabolic changes relating to anaesthesia and surgery. In *Trauma, Stress and Immunity in Anaesthesia and Surgery* (Watkins, J. and Salo, M., Eds). London; Butterworths, pp. 189–208

ESKOLA, J., SALO, M., VILJANEN, M. J. and RUUSKANEN, O. (1984). Impaired B lymphocyte function during open heart surgery. Effects of anaesthesia and surgery. *British Journal of Anaesthesia,* **56,** 333–338

FAUCI, A. S. and PRATT, K. R. (1976). Polyclonal activation of bone marrow derived lymphocytes from human peripheral blood measured by a direct plaque-forming cell assay. *Proceedings of the National Academy of Sciences, USA,* **73,** 3676–3679

GRIFFITH, C. D. M., REES, R. C., PLATTS, A., LAURENCE, A. S. and RODGERS, J. (1983). Enhanced natural killer cell activity in patients with malignant disease during intravenous anaesthesia. *Journal for Experimental and Clinical Cancer Research,* **1,** 399–402

HALLIDAY, W. J. and MILLER, S. (1972). Leucocyte adherence inhibition: a simple test for cell mediated immunity and serum blocking factors. *International Journal of Cancer,* **9,** 477–483

HAMMERSCHMIDT, D. E., WEAVER, L. J., HUDSON, L. D., CRADDOCK, P. R. and JACOB, H. S. (1980). Association of complement activation and elevated plasma C5a with adult respiratory distress syndrome. *Lancet,* **i,** 947–949

HENDERSON, J. J. and PARBROOK, G. D. (1976). Influence of anaesthetic technique on post-operative pain. *British Journal of Anaesthesia,* **48,** 587–592

HOECHST PHARMACEUTICAL LTD (1979). Gamma-Veinine, polyvalent immunoglobulin for intravenous use, Parts 1, 2, 3. Frankfurt

JARSTRAND, C., LAHNBORG, G. and PALMBLAD, J. (1978). Phagocyte function in various situations in surgery. *Acta Chirurgica Scandinavica,* (Stockholm), Supplement 482, 79–82

JONES, R. J., ROE, E. A. and GUPTA, J. L. (1979). Controlled trials of a polyvalent pseudomonas vaccine in burns. *Lancet,* **ii,** 977–983

JUBERT, A. V., LEE, E. T., HERSH, E. M. and MCBRIDE, C. M. (1973). Effects of surgery, anaesthesia and intraoperative blood loss on immunocompetence. *Journal of Surgical Research,* **15,** 399–403

KEFALIDES, N. A., ARANA, J. A., BAZAN, A., VELARDE, N. and ROSENTHAL, S. M. (1964). Evaluation of antibiotic prophylaxis and gammaglobulin, plasma, albumin and saline solution therapy in severe burns. *Annals of Surgery,* **159,** 496–506

LAWLER, P. G. P., MCHUTCHON, A. and BAMBER, P. A. (1983). Potential hazards of prolonged steroid anaesthesia. *Lancet,* **i,** 1270–1271

LOPEZ, M. J., O'CONNER, R., MACFARLANE, J. K. and THOMSON, D. M. P. (1978). The natural history of antitumour immunity in human breast cancer assayed by tube leucocyte adherence inhibition. *British Journal of Cancer,* **38,** 660–673

LORENZ, W., DOENICKE, A., SCHÖNING, B. and NEUGEBAUER, E. (1981). The role of histamine in adverse reactions to intravenous agents. In *Adverse Reactions of Anaesthetic Drugs* (Thornton, J. A., Ed.). Amsterdam; Elsevier/North-Holland, pp. 169–238

LORENZ, W., ROHER, H. D., DOENICKE, A., LENNARTZ, H., FISCHER, M., THERMANN, M., LARGIADER, F., NEUGEBAUER, E. and WATKINS, J. (1984). Systemic and local changes of histamine concentrations in plasma and wound exudates in the post-operative period. In *Clinical Research Reviews* (Janssen Research Foundation), Vol. 4, p. 151. Proceedings of a Symposium 'Care of the Postoperative Patient', Edinburgh, 1983

MCCORD, J. M., ENGLISH, D. K. and PETRONE, W. F. (1980). Role of superoxide in granulocyte mediated inflammation. In *Biological and Clinical Aspects of Superoxide Dismutase. Developments in Biochemistry,* Vol. 11B (Bannister, W. H. and Bannister, J. V., Eds). New York; Elsevier, pp. 154–159

MEAKINS, J. L., PIETSCH, J. B., BUBENICK, O., KELLY, R., RODE, H., GORDON, J. and MACLEAN, L. D. (1977). Delayed hypersensitivity: indicator of acquired failure of host defences in sepsis and trauma. *Annals of Surgery,* **186,** 241–250

MESSMER, K., LJUNGSTRÖM, K. G., GRUBER, U. F., RICHTER, W. and HEDIN, H. (1980). Prevention of dextran-induced anaphylactoid reactions by hapten inhibition. *Lancet,* **i,** 975

NOESBERGER, B. (1974). Immunoglobulin – Therapie bei gramnegativer Sepsis nach Verbrennungen. *Die Gelben,* **XIV,** 97–103

OPPENHEIM, J. J., DOUGHERTY, S., CHAN, S. P. and BAKER, J. (1975). Use of lymphocyte transformation to assess clinical disorders. In *Laboratory Diagnosis of Immunological Disorders* (Vyas, G. N., Stites, D. P. and Brecher, G., Eds). New York; Grune and Stratton, pp. 87–109

PIETSCH, J. B., MEAKINS, J. L. and MACLEAN, L. D. (1977). The delayed hypersensitivity response: application in clinical surgery. *Surgery,* **82,** 349–355

PIROFSKY, B. (1984). Intravenous immune globulin therapy in hypogammaglobulinaemia. *The American Journal of Medicine,* **76** (3A), 53–60

PRESTON, F. E. (1979). Haematological problems associated with shock. *British Journal of Hospital Medicine,* **21,** 232–245

ROHER, H. D., LORENZ, W., LENNARTZ, H., KUSCHE, J., DIETZ, W., GERDES, G. and PARKIN, J. V. (1982). Plasma histamine levels in patients in the course of several standard operations. Influence of anaesthesia, surgical trauma and blood transfusion. *Klinische Wochenschrift,* **60,** 926–934

STONE, H. H., GRABER, C. D., MARTIN, J. D. and KOLB, L. (1965). Evaluation of gammaglobulin for prophylaxis against burn sepsis. *Surgery,* **58,** 810–814

STURROCK, J. E. and NUNN, J. F. (1976). Synergism between halothane and nitrous oxide in the productions of nuclear abnormalities in the dividing fibroblast. *Anesthesiology,* **44,** 461–471

TANNEBAUM, H. (1982). The leucocyte adherence inhibition assay in human and experimental rheumatic diseases. In *Assessment of Immune Status by the Leucocyte Adherence Inhibition Test* (Thomson, D. M. P., Ed.). New York; Academic Press, pp. 207–231

THEOFILOPOULOS, A. N. (1982). Immune complexes in cancer. *The New England Journal of Medicine,* **307,** 1208–1209

THOMSON, D. M. P., Ed. (1982). *Assessment of Immune Status by the Leucocyte Adherence Inhibition Test.* New York; Academic Press, p. 380

WALTON, B. (1981). Immunological aspects of adverse reactions to inhalational anaesthetic agents. In *Adverse Reactions of Anaesthetic Drugs* (Thornton, J. A., Ed.). Amsterdam; Elsevier/North-Holland, pp. 239–277

WATKINS, J. (1981). Mechanisms and factors predisposing towards adverse response to intravenous anaesthetic substances. In *Adverse Reactions of Anaesthetic Drugs* (Thornton, J. A., Ed.). Amsterdam; Elsevier/North-Holland, pp. 137–167

WATKINS, J. (1982). Evaluation pratique de l'implication du complément au cours des réaction anaphylactoides. *Annales Françaises d'Anaesthesia et de Réanimation,* **1,** 279–284

WATKINS, J. (1984). Immunological effects of anaesthetic drugs. *Clinics in Anaesthesiology,* **2,** 463–483

WATKINS, J. and SALO, M., Eds (1982). *Trauma, Stress and Immunity in Anaesthesia and Surgery.* London; Butterworths, p. 378

WATKINS, J. and THORNTON, J. A. (1982). Immunological and non-immunological mechanisms involved in adverse reactions to drugs. *Klinische Wochenschrift,* **60,** 958–964

WRIGHT, P. J. and DUNDEE, J. W. (1982). Attitudes to intravenous infusion anaesthesia. *Anaesthesia,* **37,** 1209–1211

Chapter 13

Problems of the immunosuppressed patient

G. R. D. Catto and N. Velasco

Introduction

During the past 20 years, the increasing use of immunosuppressive drugs has resulted in a large number of patients who have impaired immunological defences and who are, therefore, at risk of developing opportunistic infections. Many patients with malignant disease, organ transplants and collagen vascular diseases among others, no longer die rapidly of their primary disease but survive on immunosuppressive therapy and are able to return to a relatively normal way of life. As they are now encountered in all branches of medical practice, it is important to appreciate that for many of these patients infection, not their original illness, has become the major cause of mortality (Brunner *et al.,* 1979).

In order to explain the high incidence of severe, often fatal, opportunistic infections in homosexuals and haemophiliacs, the acquired immuno-deficiency syndrome (AIDS) has been postulated. The pattern of morbidity in these groups resembles that of patients on immunosuppressive therapy as they have impaired cell mediated immunity with preservation of humoral immunity (Gottlieb *et al.,* 1981; Hymes *et al.,* 1981; Masur *et al.,* 1981; Pinching, 1984).

This chapter will concentrate on the particular problems which may be experienced by the immunosuppressed renal transplant recipient. With the exception of metabolic bone disease discussed later in the chapter, these problems are, to a greater or lesser extent, common to all patients who require immunosuppressive drugs. Indeed, it has long been accepted that many of the complications of transplantation are related to the immunosuppressive therapy rather than to the procedure itself.

Immunosuppressive therapy

Non-specific immunosuppression

Azathioprine and corticosteroids, although used in clinical practice for more than 20 years, remain the drugs most commonly prescribed to suppress the almost inevitable immunological response mounted by the host against an allograft. The recently developed fungal metabolite, cyclosporin A, which causes depression of both cellular and humoral immunity, is likely to become widely used in future (Calne *et al.,* 1981), while other measures such as antilymphocyte globulin (Bach *et al.,* 1973;

Turcotte *et al.*, 1973) and radiotherapy to the host or graft (Morris, 1979a) have been investigated previously. All these therapeutic approaches, however, have the major disadvantage that they are non-specific and result in a general depression of the recipient's immune system with a concomitant increased risk of opportunistic infections (Salaman, 1979).

Corticosteroids

Corticosteroids are potent immunosuppressive agents which act on both cell mediated and humoral immunity in ways which are at present not well understood. When given in high dosage over prolonged periods of time, they unfortunately produce a large number of potentially serious side effects including increased susceptibility to infection, growth retardation, osteoporosis and myopathy, diabetes mellitus, gastrointestinal haemorrhage and hypertension.

In renal transplantation, corticosteroids are administered for two principal reasons: (a) the prophylaxis of allograft rejection, and (b) in increased dosage as treatment for episodes of rejection. Until recently, the total dosage of corticosteroid administered to an individual patient was often enormous. One accepted regimen advocated methylprednisolone 20 mg/kg/d for 3 days, then prednisolone 2 mg/kg/d decreasing to 0.5 mg/kg/d in the first month after transplantation (Simmons *et al.*, 1977). With this schedule, the total dosage of prednisolone given in the first postoperative month as maintenance or prophylactic therapy was approximately 7 g. In 1977, McGeown and colleagues from Belfast published a paper which not only presented successful transplant results, but also revealed that they had been giving very much smaller doses of corticosteroids to their patients (McGeown *et al.*, 1977). Their regimen of hydrocortisone 200 mg i.v., q.i.d., for the first 24 h after surgery, followed by prednisolone 20 mg orally for 6 months, gave only prednisolone 0.6 g during the first postoperative month. The difference in total steroid dose between these high and low dose schedules is thus considerable. Those transplant centres which have adopted the low dose regimen have detected no decrease in graft survival, but have reported decreased patient morbidity mainly from a reduced incidence of gastrointestinal haemorrhage and opportunistic infections (Morris *et al.*, 1982).

Following those studies on the advantages of low dose steroid therapy in the prophylaxis of rejection, the increased steroid dosages required in the treatment of established rejection have also been investigated. Ten years ago, rejection was commonly treated by giving the patient methylprednisolone 1 g i.v. daily for several days. This form of rejection therapy added considerably to the already large doses of corticosteroids administered as maintenance therapy. At the present time, one of the following two regimens is commonly used and is seldom repeated on more than two occasions during the first three months after transplantation:

(1) Patients may be given methylprednisolone 1 g intravenously on three occasions at intervals of 12 or 24 h (Bell *et al.*, 1971). Recent studies have indicated that smaller doses of methylprednisolone (0.5 g or 0.25 g) may be equally effective.

(2) The dosage of oral prednisolone may be increased to 200 mg for 3 days and then gradually reduced to maintenance levels (McGeown *et al.*, 1977).

There is no evidence that any particular form of treatment for rejection is more effective than another. It therefore seems reasonable to select a regimen with the lowest effective dosage of corticosteroids.

Azathioprine

Azathioprine, an imidazole derivative, is rapidly converted in the liver to 6-mercaptopurine and effectively depresses both cellular and humoral arms of the immune response. The usual dose is 1.5–3.0 mg/kg/d, but tolerance of individual patients to the drug varies widely. Rapidly absorbed from the gastrointestinal tract, azathioprine is metabolized into inactive products which are secreted in the urine. Because of this, the dosage need not, in theory, be reduced in renal failure (Bach and Dardenne, 1971); such a reduction in dose is, however, commonly recommended (Monaco, 1979; McGeown, 1981). Bone marrow depression with leucopenia and thrombocytopenia is the most frequent and important side effect, but hepatitis and jaundice may also occur. Clinically, it is important to remember that the dosage of azathioprine should be reduced when allopurinol is administered. Allopurinol slows the degradation of azathioprine, and thus increases the risk of toxicity and opportunistic infections.

Cyclosporin A

Cyclosporin A has been shown in animal and clinical studies to suppress allogeneic rejection by inhibiting differentiation of T-lymphocytes. In effect, it is the first partially selective immunosuppressive drug to be developed and is likely to become widely used in the future (Calne *et al.*, 1981). However, despite its proven value in increasing graft survival rates, problems of renal and hepatic damage are not inconsiderable, while severe infections and occasional lymphomas have been reported in patients treated with cyclosporin A (Calne *et al.*, 1979).

Antilymphocyte globulin

Prepared by immunizing a horse or other animal with human lymphocytes, antilymphocyte globulin has potent immunosuppressive properties which are aimed principally at recipient T-lymphocytes. The value of this preparation in preventing or treating transplant rejection remains controversial, but an increase in viral and mycotic infections has been reported in patients given antilymphocyte globulin.

Radiotherapy

Radiation to the recipient caused considerable morbidity and mortality, while radiation restricted to the graft has not been shown to be of value in preventing rejection (Morris, 1979a). For these reasons radiotherapy is no longer routinely used in renal transplantation, but remains part of the standard therapy in bone marrow transplantation.

Within the past five years, however, it has been shown that the technique of total lymphoid irradiation, developed for the treatment of Hodgkin's disease, can produce donor specific immune unresponsiveness (Kaplan, 1981). In animal transplant models, total lymphoid irradiation of recipient animals pre-transplant caused improved graft survival rates, while preliminary results from clinical studies are apparently encouraging (Najarian, 1981).

Specific immunosuppression

The disadvantages and side effects of non-specific immunosuppression will be evident from the previous section. The necessity for reliable and safe immunosuppression has been recognized for many years; the ideal has been to produce immunosuppression only of that part of the recipient's immune system responsible for rejection of the specific graft (Morris, 1979b). Such an approach has proved possible in animal transplant models but, with the possible exception of the beneficial blood transfusion effect on allograft survival rates, has not been applicable clinically (MacLeod *et al.*, 1982). Several investigators have speculated that the survival of a fetus, despite the presence of maternal antibodies directed to paternal antigens expressed on the fetal tissue, may depend upon a type of specific immunosuppression (Gill, 1983; Power *et al.*, 1983). Further information on the factors involved in protecting the fetus may be of value in the quest for donor-specific immunosuppression.

Gastrointestinal haemorrhage

Gastrointestinal haemorrhage is a not infrequent complication of renal transplantation and has a mortality of up to 50%. The incidence, shown to be related to the total steroid dosage administered, was 18% in a transplant unit using conventional, relatively high dose corticosteroid therapy (Jones *et al.*, 1978), but only 7% in a unit which had adopted the low dosage regimen (Doherty *et al.*, 1977). Although H2 antagonist drugs such as cimetidine have also been shown to decrease the incidence of gastrointestinal haemorrhage following renal transplantation, it would seem more logical to reduce the total steroid dose than to add additional prophylactic drug therapy (Doherty, 1978).

Metabolic bone disease

At present, disabling metabolic bone disease affects 14% of successful renal transplant recipients after five years (Brynger *et al.*, 1980). However, as recently as 1968 avascular necrosis of bone, commonly affecting the femoral head, was reported in as many as 30% of transplant recipients (Cruess *et al.*, 1968). The gradual reduction in the prevalence of this disabling condition has been achieved by decreasing the total steroid dosage given after transplantation and by improvements in the pretransplant treatment of the metabolic bone diseases associated with chronic renal failure – a complex mixture of osteitis fibrosa, osteomalacia and osteoporosis. The most effective treatment at present is a combination of (a) vitamin D as 1α-hydroxycholecalciferol (alfacalcidol) or 1,25-dihydroxycholecalciferol (calcitriol) in a dose of 0.5–1.0 μg/d; (b) oral calcium carbonate supplements to provide a total of 1–1.5 g elemental calcium per day; and (c) the maintenance of normal serum phosphate concentrations (Catto and MacLeod, 1976). Parathyroidectomy may be indicated for intractable hypercalcaemia. Careful control of metabolic bone disease before transplantation should decrease the prevalence of bone disease after transplantation when such additional factors as continuing hypophosphataemia may cause osteomalacia and corticosteroid therapy may predispose to osteoporosis. For those unfortunate patients who do develop avascular necrosis of the femoral head, total hip replacement is the treatment of choice.

Malignant disease

It has been appreciated for several years that cancer may be transplanted with the donor kidney. For this reason, patients with malignant diseases are not suitable as potential kidney donors. However, following the investigations of Penn and Starzl (1972), renal transplant recipients have been suspected of having an increased prevalence of neoplasms arising *de novo*. It has been reported that the prevalence increased from 0.2% pre-transplant to 1.3% post-transplant for recipients of cadaver allografts, whereas there was no comparable increase in the frequency of malignant disease among recipients of living-related grafts (Brynger *et al.*, 1980). As the former group receive large amounts of immunosuppressive drugs, this observation was thought to provide indirect evidence for the reactivation of oncogenic viruses. There was, moreover, an increased risk of only certain types of malignancy. Malignant lymphoma was reportedly more common in transplant recipients than in normal individuals, while there was also an increase in carcinoma of the cervix and in both squamous and basal cell carcinoma of the skin. More recently, an increased incidence of cancer was reported in patients with chronic renal failure treated by maintenance haemodialysis (Lindner, Farewell and Sherrard, 1981).

These reports, however, emanated from relatively small series. Data from larger surveys and from the Registry of the European Dialysis and Transplant Association have not wholly supported the initial observations (Wing, Jacobs and Selwood, 1982). Only by analysis of combined data for different ages, sexes, countries and cancers will this important issue be resolved (Wing *et al.*, 1983).

Infectious diseases

Bacterial infections

Contrary to widespread belief, infections occurring during the first month after renal transplantation are not commonly caused by exotic or unusual pathogens, but by conventional bacteria. Exceptions to this general rule are due to exacerbations of unrecognized pre-existing infections when immunosuppressive therapy is started; this probably explains the rare but reported examples of miliary tuberculosis, invasive aspergillosis and Legionnaire's disease occurring in the early post-transplant period. In general, however, the major causes of infection in the recent transplant recipient are the same as in any post-surgical patient and include wound sepsis, pneumonia and urinary tract infection.

Perhaps surprisingly, the incidence of wound infection, despite the preceding period of chronic uraemia, is no different from that reported for clean surgical procedures in non-immunized patients – approximately 2%. The incidence, of course, is increased in the presence of urinary leaks, wound haematomata and re-exploration of the wound. The organisms involved in these infections and the arguments for and against the use of prophylactic antibiotics do not differ in this situation from any operative procedure. The only significant difference is that immunosuppressive therapy, especially corticosteroid therapy, may mask the usual signs of infection – fever, inflammation and tenderness. Therefore, as the usual diagnostic signs may be absent, any patient in whom a wound infection is suspected should have an abdominal ultrasound examination and, when necessary, needle aspiration of the wound and adequate broad spectrum antibiotic treatment.

The incidence of postoperative pneumonia is not increased after transplantation and such infections as do occur are produced by common bacterial pathogens. Ureteric and bladder catheters, now removed as soon after operation as practicable, predispose to an increase in urinary tract infections after transplantation. The organisms responsible are once again the recognized bacterial pathogens such as *Escherichia coli* and *Streptococcus faecalis*. More unusual organisms are usually found only after prolonged periods of catheterization or following antibiotic therapy.

Viral infections

Cytomegalovirus infection

After the immediate postoperative period, infection with more uncommon pathogens – viruses, fungi and protozoa, predisposing to superinfections with increasingly resistant bacteria and fungi – becomes a significant cause of morbidity. Infection with cytomegalovirus (CMV) is widely encountered among transplant recipients (Craighead, 1969; Armstrong *et al.*, 1976; Ho *et al.*, 1976; Balfour *et al.*, 1977; Betts *et al.*, 1977). Activation of the latent virus in the immunosuppressed patients is the most common cause, as more than half of transplant recipients have detectable amounts of CMV antibody present in their sera before transplantation (Craighead, 1969; Armstrong *et al.*, 1976; Naragi *et al.*, 1977). In patients who have not previously been exposed to CMV, blood transfusions (Paloheimo *et al.*, 1968; Bayer and Tegtmeier, 1976) or the transplanted kidney (Betts *et al.*, 1975; Ho *et al.*, 1975; Betts *et al.*, 1977) itself may transmit the infection. Primary infection with CMV may be prevented if only kidneys from CMV-negative donors are given to negative recipients and CMV-negative blood is used for blood transfusions (Betts *et al.,* 1975; Ho *et al.,* 1975). Several recent studies have indicated that the incidence of symptomatic CMV infection in transplant recipients can be decreased when a low dose steroid regimen is adopted (Morris *et al.,* 1982; Velasco *et al.,* 1984).

Infection with CMV remains by far the most common cause of unexplained fever in the early months after transplantation. Clinically, the symptoms are extremely variable. An insidious onset with anorexia, fever and malaise may be the only features, while other patients may become extremely ill with pneumonia, prolonged fever, deranged liver function tests and such haematological abnormalities as leucopenia and thrombocytopenia. These last features predispose to a bleeding diathesis and to superinfection with bacteria and other pathogens such as *Pneumocystis carinii* and *Clostridium difficile* (Rubin *et al.,* 1977).

The gastrointestinal bleeding in CMV infections has been ascribed to direct viral involvement, particularly in the caecum (Sutherland *et al.,* 1979), to the concomitant thrombocytopaenia or, more recently, to superinfection with *Clostridium difficile*. Another factor which facilitates superinfection is a direct effect of the CMV virus on the immune system as shown by abnormalities of the cell mediated response, skin test recall and lymphocyte stimulation tests (Linnemann *et al.,* 1978; Rytel *et al.,* 1978; Rinaldo *et al.,* 1980).

Renal impairment may also be produced by infection with CMV (Richardson *et al.,* 1981; Schooley *et al.,* 1983). The combination of fever and an increasing serum creatinine concentration caused by CMV is often incorrectly interpreted as evidence of a rejection episode. In this situation, prolonged courses of high doses of corticosteroids may cause exacerbation of the infection and indeed may rarely result in the death of patient. CMV infections may cause graft dysfunction by stimulating the production of IgM lymphocytotoxins (Baldwin *et al.,* 1983). Finally, chorioretinitis may occur as a late complication of CMV infection (Fiala *et al.,* 1977; Murray *et al.,* 1977).

Management of the transplanted patient with CMV infection may be difficult. A decrease in immunosuppressive therapy, which might strengthen host defences and help control the infection, might also predispose to graft rejection. Conversely, an increase in steroid therapy might predispose to a fatal illness. At present no specific drug therapy has been shown to be of value in treatment of CMV infection, but considerable efforts have been made to develop effective (a) active immunization with attenuated live vaccines, and (b) passive immunization with hyperimmune globulin. Preliminary data suggest that the latter approach may be of value for seriously ill patients (Brown *et al.,* 1983).

Other viral infections

Although CMV is the most frequently identified viral infection after transplantation, other members of the herpesvirus group (Epstein–Barr virus, herpes simplex virus and varicella zoster virus), the hepatitis viruses and more rarely both the adenoviruses and papovaviruses may all be excreted to excess after transplantation. The presence of an excess of herpesviruses in malignant cells from patients receiving long-term immunosuppression has caused speculation about their role in carcinogenesis since, as already discussed, renal transplant recipients may have an increased incidence of malignancy (Matas, Simmons and Najarian, 1975). Although all the mentioned viruses may cause recognizable illnesses, a definitive clinical diagnosis is seldom possible and laboratory investigations may identify the pathogen only after the acute clinical problem has been resolved. The value of such antiviral agents as acyclovir in established or suspected viral infection, although promising (Balfour *et al.*, 1983), remains to be further assessed. For the future, therapy with interferon may benefit many transplanted patients who subsequently develop severe viral infections (Hirsch *et al.*, 1983).

Fungal infections

Fungal infections in transplant recipients are more commonly suspected than proved. Once again, they may be due to reactivation of a latent infection or to acquisition of an opportunistic infection post-transplant. In the former, more uncommon category are such infections as histoplasmosis, coccidioidomycosis and blastomycosis; all of these fungal infection, which usually present with respiratory symptoms, are rare in the UK. Opportunistic infections, however, with *Aspergillus fumigatus, Candida albicans* and *Cryptococcus neoformans* are less uncommon, may cause metastatic infection and should be suspected in a febrile transplant recipient. Treatment, when started early with amphotericin B, 5-fluocystosine, miconazole or ketoconazole, is usually effective. Fortunately, it seems likely that the incidence of these opportunistic fungal infections will decline as more transplant units adopt the low dosage steroid regimen.

Pneumocystis carinii

Pneumocystis carinii is a ubiquitous parasite which may cause a pneumonitis in immunosuppressed hosts. Clinically, the most frequently noted features of infection are dyspnoea, fever and cough; the latter, however, is seldom productive and only rarely associated with haemoptysis. Radiological features of diffuse bilateral infiltrate are relatively non-specific and pneumocysts are seldom identifiable in sputum – possibly because the cysts are anchored to alveolar walls by filopodia. Definite diagnosis depends upon histological identification of pneumocysts in biopsy samples of lung tissue. Until recently, treatment depended upon the toxic agent pentamidine. Fortunately, it has been shown that treatment with cotrimoxazole in a dosage three times greater than that usually recommended for the treatment of bacterial infection in adults is an effective and less toxic form of therapy. The efficacy and simplicity of this treatment has caused many transplant units to initiate therapy when *Pneumocystis carinii* infection is suspected and without obtaining a definite diagnosis using potentially dangerous lung biopsy. Although this approach is acceptable when the patient's clinical condition improves, it may cause major diagnostic difficulties when the condition continues to deteriorate despite adequate cotrimoxazole treatment. It is important to remember that CMV infection and superadded bacterial infection may be present at the same time as *Pneumocystis carinii*.

A prophylactic treatment regimen has been successfully introduced for patients who require bone marrow transplantation and who are, thus, immunosuppressed to a greater extent than patients undergoing renal transplantation. The regimen consists of antiviral, antifungal and antiprotozoal agents – acyclovir, ketoconazole or amphotericin and cotrimoxazole. However, the very nature of bone marrow transplantation implies specific problems not present in other immunosuppressed patients.

Conclusions

The chapter has outlined some of the problems that may be associated with immunosuppression in the renal transplant recipient. The morbidity associated with transplantation is caused not by the surgical procedure itself, but is directly related to the amount of immunosuppressive therapy administered. Patient morbidity has been shown to decrease in those transplant centres which have adopted a low corticosteroid dosage regimen.

References

ARMSTRONG, J. A., EVANS, A. S., RAO, N. and HO, M. (1976). Viral infections in renal transplant recipients. *Infection and Immunology,* **14,** 970–975

BACH, J. F. and DARDENNE, M. (1971). The metabolism of azathioprine in renal failure. *Transplantation,* **12,** 253–259

BACH, M. C., SAHYOUN, A., ADLER, J. C., SCHLESINGER, R. M., BREMAN, J., MADRAS, P., PENG FANG-KU AND MONACO, A. P. (1973). Influence of rejection therapy in fungal and nocardial infections in renal transplant recipients. *Lancet,* **i,** 180–184

BALDWIN, W. M. III, CLAAS, F. H. J., VAN ES, A., WESTEDT, W. L., VAN GEMERT, G., DAHA, M. R. and VAN ES, L. A. (1983). Renal graft dysfunction during infection with cytomegalovirus: association with IgM lymphocytotoxins and HLA DR 3 and DR 7. *British Medical Journal,* **287,** 1332–1334

BALFOUR, H. H., BEAN, B., LASKIN, O. L., AMBINDER, R. F., MEYERS, J. D., WADE, J. C., ZAIA, J. A., AEPPLI, D., KIRK, L. E., SEGRETI, A. C. and KEENEY, R. E. (1983). Acyclovir halts progression of herpes zoster in immunocompromised patients. *New England Journal of Medicine,* **308,** 1448–1453

BALFOUR, H. H., SLADE, M. S., KALIS, J. M., HOWARD, R. J., SIMMONS, R. L. and NAJARIAN, J. S. (1977). Viral infections in renal transplant donors and their recipients: a prospective study. *Surgery,* **81,** 487–492

BAYER, W. L. and TEGTMEIER, G. E. (1976). The blood donor: detection and magnitude of cytomegalovirus carrier states and the prevalence of cytomegalovirus antibody. *Yale Journal of Biology,* **49,** 4–12

BELL, P. R. F., CALMAN, K. C., WOOD, R. F., BRIGGS, J. D., PATON, A. M., MCPHERSON, S. G. and KYLE, K. (1971). Reversal of acute clinical and experimental organ rejection using large doses of intravenous prednisolone. *Lancet,* **i,** 876–880

BETTS, R. F., FREEMAN, R. B., DOUGLAS, R. G. and TALLEY, T. E. (1977). Clinical manifestations of renal allograft derived primary cytomegalovirus infection. *American Journal of Diseases of Childhood,* **131,** 759–763

BETTS, R. F., FREEMAN, R. B., DOUGLAS, R. G., TALLEY, T. E. and RUNDELL, B. (1975). Transmission of cytomegalovirus infection with renal allograft. *Kidney International,* **8,** 385–392

BROWN, C. B., NICHOLLS, A. J., EDWARD, N., CUTHBERTSON, B., YAP, P. L. and MCLELLAND, D. B. C. (1983). Hyperimmune immunoglobulin therapy for cytomegalovirus infections in renal transplant patients. *Proceedings of the European Dialysis and Transplant Association,* **20,** 271–279

BRUNNER, F. P., BRYNGER, H., CHANTLER, C., DONCKERWOLCKE, R. A., HATHWAY, R. A., JACOBS, C., SELWOOD, N. H. and WING, A. J. (1979). Combined report on regular dialysis and transplantation in Europe, IX, 1978. *Proceedings of the European Dialysis and Transplant Association,* **16,** 2–73

BRYNGER, H., BRUNNER, F. P., CHANTLER, C., DONCKERWOLCKE, R. A., HATHWAY, R. A., JACOBS, C., KRAMER, P., SELWOOD, N. H. and WING, A. J. (1980). Combined report on regular dialysis and transplantation in Europe, X, 1979. *Proceedings of the European Dialysis and Transplant Association,* **17,** 2–86

CALNE, R. Y., ROLLES, K., WHITE, D. J. G., THIRA, S., EVANS, D. B., MCMASTER, P., DUNN, D. C., CRADDOCK, G. N., HENDERSON, R. G., AZIZ, S. and LEWIS, P. (1979). Cyclosporin A initially as the only immunosuppressant in 34 recipients of cadaveric organs: 32 kidneys, 2 pancreases and 2 livers. *Lancet,* **ii,** 1033–1036

CALNE, R. Y., WHITE, D. J. G., EVANS, D. B., THIRU, S., HENDERSON, R. G., HAMILTON, D. V., ROLLES, K., MCMASTER, P., DUFFY, T. J., MACDOUGALL, B. R. D. and WILLIAMS, R. (1981). Cyclosporin A in cadaveric organ transplantation. *British Medical Journal,* **282,** 934–936

CATTO, G. R. D. and MACLEOD, M. (1976). The investigation and treatment of renal bone disease. *American Journal of Medicine,* **61,** 64–73

CRAIGHEAD, J. E. (1969). Immunological response to cytomegalovirus infection in renal allograft recipients. *American Journal of Epidemiology,* **90,** 506–513

CRUESS, R. L., BLENNERHASSETT, J., MACDONALD, R., MACLEAN, L. D. and DOSSETOR, J. (1968). Aseptic necrosis following renal transplantation. *Journal of Bone and Joint Surgery,* **50A,** 1577–1589

DOHERTY, C. C. (1978). Cimetidine prophylaxis of the renal transplantation. *British Medical Journal,* **1,** 717

DOHERTY, C. C., O'CONNOR, F. A., BUCHANAN, K. D., SLOAN, J. M., DOUGLAS, J. F. and MCGEOWN, M. G. (1977). Treatment of peptic ulcer in renal failure. *Proceedings of the European Dialysis and Transplant Association,* **14,** 386–395

FIALA, M., CHATTERJEE, S. N., CARSON, S., POOLSAWAT, S., HEINER, D. C., SAXON, A. and GUZE, L. B. (1977). Cytomegalovirus retinitis secondary to chronic viraemia in phagocytic leukocytes. *American Journal of Ophthalmology,* **84,** 567–573

GILL, T. J. (1983). Immunogenetics of spontaneous abortion in humans. *Transplantation,* **35,** 1–6

GOTTLIEB, M. S., SCHROFF, R., SCHANKER, H. M., WEISMAN, J. D., PENG THIM FAN, D. O., WOLF, R. A. and SAXON, A. (1981). *Pneumocystis carinii* pneumonia and mucosal candidiasis in previously healthy homosexual men. Evidence of a new acquired cellular immunodeficiency. *New England Journal of Medicine,* **305,** 1425–1431

HIRSCH, M. S., SCHOOLEY, R. T., COSIMI, A. B., RUSSELL, P. S., DELMONICO, F. L., TOLKOFF-RUBIN, N. E., HERRIN, J. T., CANTELL, K., FARRELL, M. L., ROTA, T. R. and RUBIN, R. H. (1983). Effects of interferon-alpha on cytomegalovirus reactivation syndromes in renal transplant recipients. *New England Journal of Medicine,* **308,** 1489–1493

HO, M., DOWLING, J. N., ARMSTRONG, J. A., SUWANSIRIKUL, S., WU, B., YOUNGBLOOD, L. A. and SASLOW, A. (1976). Factors contributing to the risk of cytomegalovirus infection in patients receiving renal transplants. *Yale Journal of Biology and Medicine,* **49,** 17–26

HO, M., SUWANSIRIKUL, S., DOWLING, J. N., YOUNGBLOOD, L. A. and ARMSTRONG, J. A. (1975). The transplanted kidney as a source of cytomegalovirus infection. *New England Journal of Medicine,* **293,** 1109–1112

HYMES, K. B., CHEUNG, T., GREENE, J. B., PROSE, N. S., MARCUS, A., BALLARD, H., WILLIAM, D. C. and LAUBENSTEIN, L. J. (1981). Kaposi's sarcoma in homosexual men. A report of eight cases. *Lancet,* **2,** 598–600

JONES, R. H., RUDGE, C. J., BEWICK, M., PARSONS, V. and WESTON, M. J. (1978). Cimetidine: prophylaxis against upper gastrointestinal haemorrhage after renal transplantation. *British Medical Journal,* **1,** 398–400

KAPLAN, H. (1981). Selective effects of total lymphoid irradiation (TLT) on the immune response. *Transplantation Proceedings,* **13,** 425–428

LINDNER, A., FAREWELL, V. T. and SHERRARD, D. J. (1981). High incidence of neoplasia in uremic patients receiving long-term dialysis. Cancer and long-term dialysis. *Nephron,* **27,** 292–296

LINNEMANN, C. C., KAUFFMAN, C. A., FIRST, M. R., SCHIFF, G. M. and PHAIR, J. P. (1978). Cellular immune response to cytomegalovirus infection after renal transplantation. *Infection and Immunology,* **22,** 176–180

MACLEOD, A. M., POWER, D. A., MASON, R. J., STEWART, K. N., SHEWAN, W. G., EDWARD, N. and CATTO, G. R. D. (1982). Possible mechanisms of action of transfusion effect in renal transplantation. *Lancet,* **ii,** 468–470

MASUR, H., MICHELIS, M. A., GREENE, J. B., ONORATO, I., STOUWE, R. A. V., HOLZMAN, R. S., WORMSER, G., BRETTMAN, L., LANGE, M., MURRAY, H. W. and CUNNINGHAM-RUNDLES, S. (1981). An outbreak of community-acquired pneumocystis pneumonia – initial manifestation of cellular immune dysfunction. *New England Journal of Medicine,* **305,** 1431–1438

MATAS, A. J., SIMMONS, R. L. and NAJARIAN, J. S. (1975). Chronic antigenic stimulation, herpesvirus infection, and cancer in transplant recipients. *Lancet,* **1,** 1277–1279

MCGEOWN, M. G. (1981). Clinical renal transplantation and immunosuppression. In *Immunosuppressive Therapy* (Salaman, J. R., Ed.). London; MTP Press, pp. 143–176

MCGEOWN, M. G., KENNEDY, J. A., LOUGHBRIDGE, W. G. G., DOUGLAS, J., ALEXANDER, J. A., CLARKE, S. D., MCEVOY, J. and HEWITT, J. C. (1977). One hundred kidney transplants in the Belfast City Hospital. *Lancet,* **ii,** 648–651

MONACO, A. P. (1979). Transplantation. In Strauss and Welt's *Diseases of the Kidney* (Earley, L. E. and Gottschalk, E. W., Eds), ch. 13. Boston; Little, Brown and Co., pp. 463–515

MORRIS, P. J. (1979a). Renal transplantation. In *Renal Disease* (Black, D. A. K. and Jones, N. F., Eds), ch. 18. London; Blackwell Scientific Publications, pp. 549–587

MORRIS, P. J. (1979b). Specific suppression of rejection in renal transplantation. *Proceedings of the European Dialysis and Transplant Association,* **16,** 310–315

MORRIS, P. J., CHAN, L., FRENCH, M. E. and TING, A. (1982). Low dose oral prednisolone in renal transplantation. *Lancet,* **i,** 525–527

MURRAY, H. W., KNOX, D. L., GREEN, W. R. and SUSE, R. M. (1977). Cytomegalovirus retinitis in adults: a manifestation of disseminated viral infection. *American Journal of Medicine,* **63,** 574–584

NAJARIAN, J. S. (1981). Total lymphoid irradiation. *Transplantation Proceedings,* **13,** 417–424

NARAGI, S., JACKSON, G. G., JONASSON, O. and YAMASHIROYA, H. M. (1977). Prospective study of prevalence, incidence and source of herpesvirus infections in patients with renal allografts. *Journal of Infectious Diseases,* **136,** 531–540

PALOHEIMO, J. A., VON ESSEN, R., KLEMOLA, E., KÄÄRIÄINEN, L. and SILTANEN, P. (1968). Subclinical cytomegalovirus infections and cytomegalovirus mononucleosis after open heart surgery. *American Journal of Cardiology,* **22,** 624–630

PENN, I. and STARZL, T. E. (1972). Malignant tumours arising de novo in immunosuppressed organ transplant recipients. *Transplantation,* **14,** 407–417

PINCHING, A. J. (1984). Acquired immune deficiency syndrome. *Clinical and Experimental Immunology,* **56,** 1–13

POWER, D. A., CATTO, G. R. D., MASON, R. J., MACLEOD, A. M., STEWART, G. M., STEWART, K. N. and SHEWAN, W. G. (1983). The fetus as an allograft: evidence for protective antibodies to HLA-linked paternal antigens. *Lancet,* **ii,** 701–704

RICHARDSON, W. P., COLVIN, R. B., CHEESEMAN, S. H., TOLKOFF-RUBIN, N. E., HERRIN, J. T., COSIMI, A. B., COLLINS, A. B., HIRSCH, M. S., MCCLUSKEY, R. T., RUSSELL, P. S. and RUBIN, R. H. (1981). Glomerulopathy associated with cytomegalovirus vivaemia in renal allografts. *New England Journal of Medicine,* **305,** 57–63

RINALDO, C. R., CARNEY, W. P., RICHTER, B. S., BLACK, P. H. and HIRSCH, M. S. (1980). Mechanisms of immunosuppression in cytomegaloviral mononucleosis. *Journal of Infectious Diseases,* **141,** 488–495

RUBIN, R. R., COSIMI, A. B., TOLKOFF-RUBIN, N. E., RUSSELL, P. S. and HIRSCH, M. S. (1977). Infectious disease syndromes attributable to cytomegalovirus and their significance among renal transplant recipients. *Transplantation,* **24,** 458–464

RYTEL, M. W., AGUILAR-TORRES, F. G., BALAY, J. and HEIM, L. R. (1978). Assessment of the status of cell mediated immunity in cytomegalovirus-infected renal allograft recipients. *Cellular Immunology,* **37,** 31–40

SALAMAN, J. R. (1979). Non-specific immunosuppression. In *Kidney Transplantation, Principle and Practice* (Morris, P. J., Ed.). London; Academic Press, pp. 161–182

SCHOOLEY, R. T., HIRSCH, M. S., COLVIN, R. B., TOLKOFF-RUBIN, N. E., MCCLUSKEY, R. T., BURTON, R. C., RUSSELL, P. S., HERRIN, J. T., DELMONICO, F. L., GIORGI, J. V., HENLE, W. and RUBIN, R. H. (1983). Association of herpes virus infections with T-lymphocyte-subset alterations, glomerulopathy and opportunistic infections after renal transplantation. *New England Journal of Medicine,* **308,** 307–313

SIMMONS, R. L., HOOK, E. J. VAN, YUNIS, E. J., NOREEN, H., KJELLSTRAND, C. M., CONDIE, R. M., MAUER, M., BUSELMEIER, T. J. and NAJARIAN, J. S. (1977). 100 Sibling kidney transplants followed 2 to 7½ years. A multifactorial analysis. *Annals of Surgery,* **185,** 196–204

SUTHERLAND, D. E. R., CHAN, F. Y., FOUCAR, E., SIMMONS, R. L., HOWARD, R. J. and NAJARIAN, J. S. (1979). The bleeding cecal ulcer in transplant patients. *Surgery,* **86,** 386–398

TURCOTTE, J. G., FEDUSKA, N. J., HAINES, R. F., FREIER, D. T., GIKAS, P. W., MCDONALD, F. D., JOHNSON, A. G., MORRELL, R. M., THOMPSON, N. W. and ARBOR, R. (1973). Antithymocyte globulin in renal transplant recipients, a clinical trial. *Archives of Surgery,* **106,** 484–488

VELASCO, N., CATTO, G. R. D., EDWARD, N., ENGESET, J. and MOFFATT, M. A. J. (1984). The effect of the dosage of steroids on the incidence of CMV infection in renal transplant recipients. *Journal of Infection,* **9,** 69–78

WING, A. J., BROYER, M., BRUNNER, F. P., BRYNGER, H., CHALLAH, S., DONCKERWOLCKE, R. A., JACOBS, C., KRAMER, P. and SELWOOD, N. H. (1983). Combined report on regular dialysis and transplantation in Europe, XIII, 1982. *Proceedings of the European Dialysis and Transplant Association,* **20,** 5–78

WING, A. J., JACOBS, C. and SELWOOD, N. H. (1982). Cancer and patients with end-stage renal failure. *British Medical Journal,* **284,** 504

Part V

Special situations

Chapter 14

The poor risk patient

F. R. Ellis and K. H. Simpson

Surgical risk has been defined as the probability of morbidity or mortality resulting from preoperative preparation anaesthesia, operation and convalescence (Feigal and Blaisdell, 1979). The concept of risk involves prediction of a wide variety of outcomes and should not be confused with prognosis, which refers to the natural history of a particular disease process and its modification by treatment.

The risk factor has always been of concern to anaesthetists and surgeons and is one of the determinants for a chosen type and timing of treatment. The risk of a surgical procedure can only be estimated in the light of previous experience and will change with time as the causes are elucidated and eliminated. Thus, risk can only be a relative term, and to designate a patient to be a 'poor risk' infers some form of categorization.

Methods of categorization of risk

American Society of Anesthesiologists (ASA) classification

There have been several attempts to grade patients for surgical procedures, this being the first and perhaps best known. In 1941, Saklad, Rovenstine and Taylor, acting as a committee for the American Society of Anesthetists, Inc., devised a system for the collection and tabulation of statistical data in anaesthesia (Saklad, 1941). Operative risk was a factor under consideration and it was realized that this could not be quantified, as it was dependent upon so many variables. The ASA system was devised to categorize the physical status of the patient and not as a measure of operative risk. The original classification had six groups of patients, a seventh group being added later to include the moribund patient who was expected to die within 24 h, with or without surgical intervention.

In 1962, the House of Delegates of the American Society of Anesthesiologists, Inc. (1963) simplified the original classification of physical status as follows:

Class 1: a normal healthy patient. No organic pathology, or patients in whom the pathological process is localized, e.g. fractures, congenital abnormalities, localized infections, bony deformities, hernias.

Class 2: a patient with a mild systemic disease. A moderate but definite systemic disturbance caused either by the condition that is to be treated by surgery, or by other existing pathological processes, e.g. mild diabetes, moderate anaemia, acute pharyngitis, chronic sinusitis, minor infection causing systemic disturbance, mild thyrotoxicosis.

Class 3: a patient with a severe systemic disturbance that limits activity, but is not incapacitating and includes severe systemic disease from any cause, e.g. combinations of cardiac and respiratory disease, complete intestinal obstruction causing serious physiological disturbance, debilitating long illness with weakness of several systems, severe trauma resulting in shock.

Class 4: a patient with an incapacitating systemic disease that is a constant threat to life and includes an extreme systemic disorder which has already become a threat to life regardless of treatment.

Class 5: a moribund patient not expected to survive 24 h, with or without an operation.

Emergency cases are designated by adding E to the classification number.

Physical status and outcome

The next logical step in the assessment of operative mortality was to ascertain whether classification of preoperative physical status correlated with outcome. Anaesthetic experience was surveyed during a 10-year period from 1947 to 1957 (Dripps, Lamont and Eckenhoff, 1961). General and spinal anaesthesia was performed in 120 000 patients with 1285 deaths within 30 days of surgery, producing a gross mortality rate of 1.1%. When this mortality was examined in terms of physical status, there were no deaths in patients in ASA class 1 and the death rate increased steadily as the physical status of the patients worsened.

Keats (1978), reviewing the use and value of the ASA classification, found good correlation with surgical mortality. Examining the data of Vacanti, Van Houten and Hill (1970) and Marx, Mateo and Orkin (1973), it was shown that mortality increased with each grade of the classification (*Table 14.1*). The difference in the mortality rates in the two studies is in

Table 14.1. Percentage surgical mortality and ASA physical status

ASA status	*Surgical mortality* (%) Vacanti *et al.* (1970) (68 388 patients)	Marx *et al.* (1973) 34 145 patients)
1	0.08	0.06
2	0.27	0.47
3	1.8	4.4
4	7.8	23.5
5	9.4	50.8

part due to the difference in patient populations. Vacanti's patients were from US naval hospitals and 74% of them were ASA class 1, whereas Marx's patients were from a large general hospital and only 54% of them were ASA class 1. This may also account for the different perceptions of 'sickness'. The definition of ASA class 5 states that patients are not expected to survive 24 h, yet only 9.4% of Vacanti's ASA class 5 patients died, suggesting that others might have placed these patients in lower classes.

Owens, Felts and Spitznagel (1978) investigated the consistency of ASA grading by asking 304 anaesthetists to assess 10 hypothetical patients using questionnaires. They concluded that the majority of American anaesthetists used the system and found it helpful. Overall, there was a good correlation between anaesthetists in assessing the cases, although factors such as obesity, hepatitis and a history of myocardial infarction led to variation in response.

Although ASA classification was designed purely to grade physical status, it obviously is a useful predictor in the assessment of operative risk. It is, however, used less by surgeons and anaesthetists in the UK than in the USA.

Cardiac Risk Index (CRI)

Goldman *et al.* (1977) examined 1001 patients, over 40 years of age, having major non-cardiac surgery, in a prospective study to determine preoperative factors which could predict postoperative cardiac problems. Using multivariate discriminative analysis, they were able to identify nine independent factors, which seemed to indicate the potential for development of life-threatening and fatal cardiac complications in the postoperative phase. A cardiac risk index was determined from this data by a scoring system for each of the nine discriminant factors, as follows:

Preoperative factor	*Points*
History:	
(a) Age over 70 years	5
(b) Myocardial infarct in previous six months	10
Examination:	
(a) Third heart sound, jugular venous distension	11
(b) Significant aortic stenosis	3
ECG:	
(a) Rhythm other than sinus, premature atrial contractions	7
(b) Five or more premature ventricular contractions per minute	7
General status: *	
PaO_2 <8 kPa, $PaCO_2$ >6.6 kPa	
potassium <3 mmol/l	
bicarbonate <20 mmol/l	
raised blood urea or creatinine	
elevated transaminases	
signs of chronic liver disease	
bedridden from a non-cardiac cause	3
Operation:	
(a) Intraperitoneal, intrathoracic or aortic surgery	3
(b) Emergency procedure	4

*PaO_2, partial pressure of oxygen in arterial blood; kPa, kiloPascal (1 mm Hg = 0.133 kPa; $PaCO_2$, partial pressure of carbon dioxide in arterial blood.

From the score each patient could be allotted to one of four risk categories, as follows:

Risk class	*Points*
I	0–5
II	6–12
III	13–25
IV	>26

The results of Goldman and co-workers' study are shown in *Table 14.2.* It can be seen that 10 of the 19 postoperative deaths were in class IV which contained only 18 patients, a mortality rate of 56%, whereas the death rate in group I was only 0.2%.

Table 14.2. Number of postoperative complications or cardiac deaths in Goldman's risk classes I–IV

Class (*N*)	*No. minor complications* (*N* = 943)	*Life-threatening complications* (*N* = 39)	*Cardiac deaths* (*N* = 19)
I (537)	532	4	1
II (316)	295	16	5
III (130)	112	15	3
IV (18)	4	4	10

Jeffrey *et al.* (1983) prospectively studied 99 patients undergoing elective abdominal aortic surgery, independently to validate the CRI. Life-threatening or lethal complications were seen in 11 of these patients, with an increased incidence in risk classes I, II and III. In making a comparison with Goldman's results, Jeffrey concluded that the CRI underestimated the complications in class I patients. *Table 14.3* shows a comparison of the results of the two independent studies to correlate the CRI with postoperative cardiac complications. It must be remembered that the two studies are taken from different patient populations; Goldman's study included both elective and emergency surgery involving a wide variety of procedures, whereas Jeffrey's patients were all undergoing the same elective operation. This may account for the difference in absolute values in the two studies.

Table 14.3. Comparison of two studies of cardiac complications in Goldman's risk classes I–III

Class	*No. patients*	*Patients with cardiac complications* (%)	*Source*
I	56	7	
II	35	11	Jeffrey *et al.* (1983)
III	8	38	
I	537	1	
II	316	1	Goldman *et al.* (1977)
III	130	14	

There is no doubt that the CRI is a useful objective method of classification of patients into groups, which will allow comparison of data within and between centres. The CRI seems to have a better predictive ability than the simple ASA classification.

Pulmonary risk factors

All patients undergoing anaesthesia and surgery are at risk of developing pulmonary complications, which are a common cause of morbidity and mortality. Dripps and Deming (1946) showed that good preoperative preparation of high risk patients can decrease morbidity by approximately 50%. Preoperative assessment of patients recognizes certain important factors including chronic pulmonary disease, smoking, age greater than 60 years, obesity, abnormal preoperative lung function tests, upper abdominal or thoracic surgery and anaesthesia lasting more than 3 h.

Milledge and Nunn (1975), studying criteria for fitness in 12 patients with chronic obstructive airways disease undergoing a variety of surgical procedures, were able to distinguish the following three groups of patients:

Group 1: Low FEV 1*, normal $PaCO_2$, PaO_2 >7.3 kPa, in which no pulmonary problems were seen following routine anaesthetic and postoperative management.

Group 2: Low FEV 1, normal $PaCO_2$, PaO_2 <7.3 kPa, in which patients required postoperative oxygen by facemask as a supplement to routine management.

Group 3: Greatly reduced FEV 1, $PaCO_2$ >5.9 kPa, PaO_2 reduced by more than 2 standard deviations below normal, in which patients needed ventilatory support in the postoperative period.

They concluded from the study that a reduction of FEV 1, in the presence of normal blood gases, was not a contraindication to routine surgery. Values of FEV 1 less than 50% of predicted are compatible with normal recovery, but adequate monitoring and perhaps admission to intensive care was advisable. Patients with hypoxaemia, but a normal $PaCO_2$, should likewise be considered for routine surgery with attention to the blood gases and oxygen therapy where necessary. Hypercapnia seems to be the most important indicator that the patient may be at high risk of needing ventilatory support after surgery. Other workers have studied patients having thoracic surgery in order to distinguish predictors of postoperative moribidity and mortality. Useful factors include abnormal exercise tests, abnormal electrocardiogram, maximum breathing capacity of less than 50% predicted and preoperative hypercapnia.

Rigg and Jones (1978) summarized the management of patients with reduced cardiopulmonary (CP) reserve in functional terms, as follows:

(1) Normal CP reserve, in which patients were managed routinely and given postoperative oxygen and physiotherapy.

*FEV 1, forced expiratory volume in 1s.

(2) Reduced CP reserve VC* and/or FEV 1 <50% predicted, $PaCO_2$ normal, PaO_2 >9.3 kPa, Q_s/Q_t† <10%. Elderly or obese patients for thoracic or abdominal surgery were considered for epidural blockade to control wound pain and permit effective physiotherapy.
(3) Severely reduced CP reserve, VC and/or FEV 1 25–50% predicted, $PaCO_2$ normal, PaO_2 <9.3 kPa, Q_s/Q_t >10%, exercise capacity <75% of normal. Patients were managed with local or regional technique if possible, and if general anaesthesia was indicated, positive pressure ventilation was used.
(4) No CP reserve, pre-anaesthetic cardiac and/or respiratory failure, VC and/or FEV 1 <25% predicted, $PaCO_2$ >6.4 kPa, PaO_2 <6.7 kPa, Q_s/Q_t >25%. In these patients again, local or regional techniques were preferred, but general anaesthesia with controlled ventilation, oxygen therapy and epidural blockade was used if necessary

It can be seen from these studies that preoperative categorization of patients can aid planning and encourages thoroughness in patient assessment.

Hepatic risk factors

A number of schemes have been proposed to estimate hepatic reserve prior to surgery in patients with chronic liver disease. In 1964, Child and Turcotte (*see* Strunin, 1978) described a multifactorial analysis of three clinical observations and two laboratory tests to give an indication of the risks of surgery and long-term prognosis. These are shown in *Table 14.4*. Pugh, Murray-Lyon and Dawson (1973) modified this system to include other tests and allocated points for abnormalities present (*Table 14.5*). Using this classification, operative risk can be graded as follows:

Operative risk	*Points*
Grade A (good)	5–6
Grade B (moderate)	7–9
Grade C (poor)	10–15

It is recommended that only patients in grade A should usually be considered 'fit for anaesthesia' and that in others measures should be taken to improve the preoperative state.

Rating schemes and clinical practice

When considering the application of preoperative rating schemes to clinical practice, it is doubtful if any classification will improve significantly the practice of experienced anaesthetists and surgeons, whose clinical assessment of the patient will, in all probability, correlate highly with these indices. It has been demonstrated that subjective preoperative assessment of patients by experienced anaesthetists shows good agreement with observed mortality rates (Urzua *et al.*, 1981).

*VC, vital capacity.
†Q_s/Q_t, flow of blood through shunt divided by cardiac output.

Table 14.4. Multifactorial risk index for surgery in patients with hepatic disease (from Child and Turcotte, 1964, in Strunin, 1978, by permission of the publishers)

	Group A	*Group B*	*Group C*
Serum bilirubin (μmol/l)	<40	40–50	>50
Serum albumin (g/dl)	>35	30–35	<30
Ascites	none	easily controlled	poorly controlled
Neurological disorder	none	minimal	advanced
Nutrition	excellent	good	poor
Operative risk	*good*	*moderate*	*poor*

Table 14.5. Multifactorial risk index for surgery in patients with hepatic disease (from Pugh, Murray-Lyon and Dawson, 1973, by permission of the publishers)

Clinical and biochemical measurements	*Points scored for increasing abnormalities* 1	2	3
Encephalopathy	none	grade 1 or 2	grade 3 or 4
Bilirubin (μmol/l)	<25	25–40	>40
Albumin (g/dl)	>35	28–35	<28
Prothrombin time (seconds prolonged)	1–4	4–6	>6

As an aid to teaching, these classifications encourage the trainee to focus on important aspects of preoperative evaluation, which otherwise might be neglected. The use of rating scales also encourages a thorough approach to anaesthetic assessment and generates interest. If monitoring equipment is limited it should perhaps be preferentially used for patients at high risk, and there may be justification for admission of such patients to an intensive care unit electively.

The original remit put to Saklad and his colleagues was to devise a format for collection and tabulation of data to facilitate common understanding and communication. The use of classifications such as those discussed may help to fulfil this ideal.

Mortality and anaesthesia

So far, poor risk patients have been considered prospectively in terms of preoperative assessment. An alternative evaluation could be a retrospective assessment in terms of post-anaesthetic mortality. The first anaesthetic mortality was recorded in 1848, with the death of Hannah Greener under light chloroform anaesthesia. Since then, several prospective and retrospective studies have been undertaken to try to elucidate the causes of deaths due to anaesthesia and provide guidelines to improve clinical practice.

Beecher and Todd (1954) performed a large survey of deaths associated with anaesthesia and surgery. They implicated neuromuscular blocking drugs in a sixfold increase in mortality, suggesting an inherent drug toxicity. It has since become apparent that this increase in death rate reflected inexperience in the use of these drugs, in that the patients had been inadequately ventilated. The inappropriate management of the paralysed patient remains a cause of death today. In 1949, the Council of the Association of Anaesthetists of Great Britain and Ireland appointed a committee to investigate anaesthetic deaths. During the next 5 years details of 1000 deaths following anaesthesia were analysed. In its publication it concluded that anaesthesia contributed to 59% of the deaths (Edwards *et al.*, 1956). The commonest aetiological factors were hypovolaemia, pulmonary aspiration of gastric contents and overdose of barbiturates.

Harrison (1978) published a 10-year survey of anaesthetic mortality at Groote Schurr in Capetown during the period 1967–76, and a comparison was made with the data collected during the previous decade 1956–66 (*Table 14.6*). Anaesthetic deaths were defined as those occurring within 24 h of surgery, although it was acknowledged that this would invariably lead to the omission of some cases. Anaesthesia was thought to be a contributory factor in the deaths of 53 patients during the period 1967–76 and assessment of the circumstances was made. Four factors were identified in two-thirds of the cases, namely, problems with intubation, hypovolaemia, respiratory inadequacy following the use of neuromuscular blockers and inadequate postoperative care.

Table 14.6. Ten-year survey of anaesthetic mortality 1967–76, compared with data collected for the previous decade (from Harrison, 1978, by permission of the publishers)

	Deaths 1956–66 (177 928 anaesthetics)	*Deaths 1967–76* (240 483 anaesthetics)
Total surgical deaths	2026 (11.38/1000)	2442 (10.15/1000)
Deaths associated with anaesthesia	414 (2.33/1000)	531 (2.20/1000)
Deaths to which anaesthesia contributed	58 (0.33/1000)	53 (0.22/1000)
Deaths due to other causes	261 (1.43/1000)	343 (1.42/1000)
Inevitable deaths	95 (0.53/1000)	135 (0.56/1000)

In 1982, a series of papers from Cardiff analysed epidemiology in anaesthesia. One of the studies evaluated mortality following anaesthesia and surgery (Farrow *et al.*, 1982). In the latter study, 2391 deaths occurred during or following the 108 878 anaesthetics, producing a crude death rate of 2.2%. Of these deaths, 102 occurred in theatre, 27 in the recovery room and 2262 on the wards. No attempt was made to assign the cause of death to anaesthesia or surgery. It was reiterated that the death rate increased with both age and poor preoperative condition. It was also shown that mortality was 3.5 times greater in emergency cases; and the finding that as the duration of anaesthesia increased so did the mortality, confirmed earlier work (Vandam, 1965).

In the Cardiff study, the surgical mortality was analysed in terms of the presence of common preoperative conditions (Fowkes *et al.*, 1982). The relative mortality rate was calculated from this data; it was defined as the mortality with a specified preoperative condition divided by the mortality without the preoperative condition. It was used to estimate the increase in mortality associated with each condition separately (*Table 14.7*). From these results it can be estimated that, for example, a patient with heart failure is approximately 30 times more likely to die from an emergency operation than a patient who was fit preoperatively. It was found that the

Table 14.7. Relative mortality rate with different preoperative conditions (from Farrow *et al.*, 1982, by permission of the publishers)

Preoperative condition	*Relative mortality rate* Emergency	Elective
Impairment of health by surgical diagnosis	10.6	10.5
Ischaemic heart disease	18.0	11.8
Chronic lower respiratory tract infection	13.2	8.5
Heart failure	31.1	25.0
Obesity	6.6	3.3
Impaired renal function	23.0	15.3
Diabetes mellitus	12.7	10.8

mortality rate increased with age although the relative mortality rate decreased. This suggested that, in older age groups, the presence of preoperative conditions is a less important determinant of mortality than in the younger age groups. Thus, the relative mortality rate can help to give an indication of risk.

Lunn and Mushin (1982) published a report on mortality associated with anaesthesia, based on documentation of patients dying within 6 days of surgery in 5 areas in England, Scotland and Wales. The anaesthetist was asked to complete a report if either the surgeon or anaesthetist considered anaesthesia to have contributed to a patient's death. The study included over 1.1 million operations and 6060 deaths within the first 6 postoperative days. As there was only a 61% response to requests for information, it was not possible to draw conclusions from a statistical analysis of the data. However, the authors found that only 1 in 10 000 patients undergoing surgery die totally as a result of anaesthesia, which represents 280 cases a year in the UK.

Anaesthesia may have played some role in a further 1800 deaths per annum reported by Lunn and Mushin. Many of these deaths were probably avoidable and the factors cited as contributing to mortality have remained depressingly similar over the past three decades, namely, inhalation of gastric contents, hypotension and relative drug overdose in ill patients. The report emphasizes the importance of preoperative assessment and consultation between anaesthetists and surgeons as to the timing of surgery and management. The importance of good monitoring of patients and detailed documentation of events was stressed and the provision of recovery room facilities was shown to be an area where considerable improvement could be made. The results of this report show clearly that anaesthesia may contribute to deaths occurring much later than the traditional 24 h postoperatively.

Mortality in obstetric patients

The triennial reports on maternal mortality show that general anaesthesia remains a constant cause of death during childbirth. The number of deaths associated with anaesthesia for Caesarian section has remained fairly constant over the years, despite an improvement in the total maternal mortality figures (*Table 14.8*). Thus, anaesthesia itself has become of

Table 14.8. Maternal deaths in England and Wales 1961–78

	1961–63	*1964–66*	*1967–69*	*1970–72*	*1973–75*	*1976–78*
Deaths due to pregnancy and childbirth (including abortions)	692	579	455	355	235	227
Rate/million maternities	274.6	222.7	185.2	154.5	122.3	129.8
Deaths associated with general anaesthesia for Caesarian section 1961–78	19	20	35	19	17	20

greater relative importance (Cloake, 1982). The latest triennial report shows that, apart from 'other causes', anaesthesia was the most important cause of maternal death and avoidable factors were considered to be present in all cases (HMSO, 1982). Thirty deaths were directly due to anaesthesia, and in a further 10 cases it was a contributory factor. The recurring problems of difficulty in intubation with resultant hypoxia and inhalation of gastric contents were present in many cases. Morgan (1980) suggested that the preferential use of regional blockade for operative intervention would reduce maternal mortality. It should, however, be noted that the last triennial report described four deaths in association with epidural anaesthesia. Carefully controlled epidural blockade would no doubt avoid some of the difficulties associated with general anaesthesia, but it is not feasible if fetal distress or haemorrhage are present. The emphasis should be on adequate training and supervision of junior anaesthetists in all forms of obstetric anaesthesia and the provision of trained assistance in the anaesthetic room, if the present situation is to be improved (Corall, 1982).

Conclusions

The mortality reports discussed are concerned with all categories of patient and not just the 'poor risk' group, but they serve to highlight factors which lead to deaths in all patients, including inadequacies in anaesthetic technique. It is obvious that these factors summate with poor preoperative status, to result in an increased mortality in high risk patients. It is important to apply the highest standards of preoperative preparation, anaesthesia, surgery and postoperative care to the patients at greatest risk, but the problem remains as to the best way to identify these patients preoperatively. Further careful prospective studies of surgical and anaesthetic outcome are required; a combined approach is necessary for the most meaningful results.

References

BEECHER, H. K. and TODD, D. P. (1954). A study of the deaths associated with anaesthesia and surgery; based on a study of 599 548 anaesthetics in ten institutions 1948–1952, inclusive. *Annals of Surgery,* **140,** 2–34

CLOAKE, E. (1982). Maternal deaths in England and Wales, 1976–78. *Health Trends,* **14,** 106–109

CORALL, I. (1982). Editorial. *Anaesthesia,* **37,** 711–713

DRIPPS, R. D. and DEMING, M. V. N. (1946). Postoperative atelecetasis and pneumonia: diagnosis, etiology and management based upon 1240 cases of upper abdominal surgery. *Annals of Surgery,* **124,** 94–110

DRIPPS, R. D., LAMONT, A. and ECKENHOFF, J. E. (1961). The role of anesthesia in surgical mortality. *The Journal of the American Medical Association,* **178**(3), 261–266

EDWARDS, G., MORTON, H. J. V., PASK, E. A. and WYLIE, W. D. (1956). Deaths associated with anaesthesia; a report on 1000 cases. *Anaesthesia,* **11**(3), 194–220

FARROW, S. C., FOWKES, F. G. R., LUNN, J. N., ROBERTSON, I. B. and SAMUEL, P. (1982). Epidemiology in anaesthesia II: factors affecting mortality in hospital. *British Journal of Anaesthesia,* **54,** 811–816

FEIGAL, D. W. and BLAISDELL, F. W. (1979). The estimation of surgical risk. *The Medical Clinics of North America,* **63**(6), 1131–1143

FOWKES, F. G. R., LUNN, J. N., FARROW, S. C., ROBERTSON, I. B. and SAMUEL, P. (1982). Epidemiology in anaesthesia III: mortality risk in patients with coexisting physical disease. *British Journal of Anaesthesia,* **54,** 819–824

GOLDMAN, L., CALDERA, D. L., NUSSBAUM, S. R., SOUTHWICK, F. S., KROGSTAD, D., MURRAY, B., BURKE, D. S., O'MALLEY, T. A., GOROLL, A. H., CAPLAN, C. H., NOLAN, J., CARABELLO, B. and SLATER, E. E. (1977). Multifactorial index of cardiac risk in noncardiac surgical procedures. *The New England Journal of Medicine,* **297**(16), 845–850

HARRISON, G. C. (1978). Deaths attributable to anaesthesia: a ten year survey (1967–1976). *British Journal of Anaesthesia,* **50,** 1041–1046

HMSO (1982). Report on confidential enquiries into maternal deaths in England and Wales, 1976–1978 (DHSS). *Reports on Health and Social Subjects,* No. 26. London; HMSO

HOUSE OF DELEGATES OF THE AMERICAN SOCIETY OF ANESTHESIOLOGISTS, INC. (1963). New classification of physical status. *Anesthesiology,* **24**(1), 111

JEFFREY, C. C., KUNSMAN, J. K., CULLEN, J. and BREWSTER, D. C. (1983). A prospective evaluation of cardiac risk index. *Anesthesiology,* **58**(5), 462–464

KEATS, A. S. (1978). The ASA classification of physical status – a recapitulation. *Anesthesiology,* **49**(4), 233–236

LUNN, J. N. and MUSHIN, W. W. (1982). *Mortality Associated With Anaesthesia.* London; Nuffield Provincial Hospitals Trust

MARX, G. F., MATEO, C. V. and ORKIN, L. R. (1973). Computer analysis of post anesthetic death. *Anesthesiology,* **39,** 54–58

MILLEDGE, J. S. and NUNN, J. F. (1975). Criteria of fitness for anaesthesia in patients with chronic obstructive lung disease. *British Medical Journal,* **3,** 670–673

MORGAN, B. M. (1980). Maternal death: a review of maternal deaths at one hospital from 1958 to 1978. *Anaesthesia,* **35,** 334–338

OWENS, W. D., FELTS, J. A. and SPITZNAGEL, E. L. (1978). ASA physical status classifications: a study of consistency of ratings. *Anesthesiology,* **49**(4), 239–243

PUGH, R. N. H., MURRAY-LYON, I. M. and DAWSON, J. L. (1973). Transection of the oesophagus for bleeding varices. *British Journal of Surgery,* **60,** 646–649

RIGG, J. R. A. and JONES, N. L. (1978). Clinical assessment of respiratory function. *British Journal of Anaesthesia,* **50**(3), 3–12

SAKLAD, M. (1941). Grading of patients for surgical procedures. *Anesthesiology,* **2**(3), 281–284

STRUNIN, L. (1978). Preoperative assessment of the patient with liver dysfunction. *British Journal of Anaesthesia,* **50,** 25–31

URZUA, J., DOMINGUEZ, P., QUIROGA, M., MORAN, S., IRARRAZAVAL, M., MATURANA, G. and DUBERNET, J. (1981). Preoperative estimation of risk in cardiac surgery. *Anesthesia and Analgesia,* **60**(9), 625–628

VACANTI, C. J., VAN HOUTEN, R. J. and HILL, R. C. (1970). A statistical analysis of the relationship of physical status to postoperative mortality in 68 388 cases. *Anesthesia and Analgesia,* **49,** 564–566

VANDAM, L. D. (1965). The unfavourable effects of prolonged anaesthesia. *The Canadian Anaesthetists' Society Journal,* **12,** 107–120

Chapter 15

Postoperative care in hazardous environments

J. Nelson Norman

Introduction

The earlier chapters have underlined recent advances in the technology available for the care of the complex postoperative patient. The modern hospital is indeed a sophisticated place, salvaging and offering the chance of survival to those suffering from the most desperate of postoperative complications. There is, however, no intensive care unit available if, for example, the appendix stump ruptures during the postoperative period when that takes place on an Antarctic station a few hundred miles from the South pole. Equally, an acid–base disturbance is difficult to control when the patient is a diver undergoing his postoperative phase in a pressure chamber on an offshore installation. It thus seems appropriate at this time to consider the problems of the postoperative period, when that phase takes place in a hazardous environment.

In recent years, the problem of providing high grade health care for those who become acutely ill in remote places with hostile environmental conditions has been addressed in Aberdeen (Norman, 1981). The subject of remote and exploration medicine has still to undergo considerable development, but it is making progress as more and more people are required to live and work in distant places in the continuing search for further sources of food and energy. Comments in this chapter are based on those areas with which the author has been associated, which are the development of medical systems for personnel working in the Antarctic on the one hand and for saturation divers on the other.

Health care for the polar worker

Antarctic stations vary in size, but those in the British sector usually employ between 10 and 20 personnel in winter time. There are also smaller units which are manned for varying periods of time. Most activity obviously takes place during the summer months. During winter, the group is on its own and thousands of miles from the nearest hospital. Surgical illness takes on a new magnitude of risk under these circumstances and the first big problem for the postoperative phase is the distance which may separate the patient – and his often junior medical adviser – from the facilities of a hospital.

The main immediate hazard is remoteness and isolation, yet much thought must be given to the consequences of attempting to reduce the distance between patient and hospital during the post-traumatic period. The journey may take several weeks at sea, and although a state of relative calm is likely while the ship is in ice, this will readily give way to considerable violent movement when it enters the stormy waters of the Forties and Fifties of latitude. Seasickness in both patients and attendants can be a serious complicating factor and continuing violent movements can result in much pain and risk of further trauma in the postoperative patient.

The range of surgical conditions which have presented during the past 25 years at one polar station is set out in *Table 15.1.* It can be seen that orthopaedic problems figure prominently. The doctor in charge has also to double as radiographer, radiologist, anaesthetist and surgeon. In the case of a spiral fracture of the tibia managed at one polar base last year, the range of problems in the postoperative period was novel and varied and included: (a) difficulties in taking and interpreting X-rays; (b) using all the plaster of Paris available and, consequently, leaving the final one on for too long for fear that more would be required; (c) lack of physiotherapy and the problems of combating the resulting oedema and ankle stiffness, together with fear for the Achilles tendon; and (d) the problem of mobilization of the post-fracture patient on ice!

Table 15.1. The spectrum of serious illness or injury developed during 25 years on a single polar station, involving a total of 555 subjects

Major fractures	9
Minor fractures	13
Dislocations	5
Head injuries	8
Appendicitis	3
Non-surgical abdomens	11

We have recognized that the problem of providing high grade health care for people who become ill in remote and isolated places is fundamentally one of the distance and the time which separates the patient from the hospital facilities which he requires. We have thus endeavoured to overcome this problem by elaborating a series of training courses for the personnel who work in these remote sites. Each course is designed for particular environmental conditions. Fundamentally, the courses advise the personnel of the action which should be taken in a variety of circumstances immediately, and also instruct them in the technique of communicating the nature of the problem to a medical authority at a distance in terms which will allow him to make a diagnosis. The first part of the training procedure is designed to allow a diagnosis to be made and the second part provides training in practical manoeuvres and techniques which are undertaken on the authority of the doctor at a distance. The doctor thus takes the authority for, and uses his judgement on, the action which should be taken. The second important priority in this system is the provision of a sophisticated and clear system of communication.

Considerable work has been done recently by the Department of Continuing Medical Education at the Memorial University of Newfoundland in the development of communication techniques such as slow-scan television and satellite systems, together with tele-conferencing facilities. This has resulted, together with adequate training programmes, in the development of high grade health care for the remote communities of Newfoundland and Labrador (Roberts, House and McNamara, 1977).

Health care for the offshore oil worker

The distance which separates the offshore oil industry installations in the North Sea from hospital facilities ashore is different from the polar situation in terms of time and distance. The populations are also very much larger. The offshore oil industry is a heavy industry which is required to function in difficult and hazardous environmental conditions and the facilities made available for emergency care have to be somewhat specialized. There are, for example, highly equipped emergency rescue vessels patrolling close to the installations and maintaining a wide range of specialist equipment and resources. The ships often have additional functions and they may also need to act in the fire-fighting mode. When this happens there may be a conflict of interest if a serious post-traumatic casualty needs to be transported to hospital ashore, as this would interfere with the other functions of such a vessel.

In developing medical systems for the offshore industry in eastern Canada, the presence of icebergs and fog which prevents a helicopter from landing on an offshore structure for more than 100 days per year are complicating factors which make it necessary to provide even higher standards of training and communications, in order to provide the same degree of care for acute illness as is currently found in the North Sea. No matter how sophisticated the facilities are, however, there is still the same problem of immediate care before specialist advice and action can be brought to bear. Highly trained groups of specialists can be transported to emergency vessels by helicopter to undertake continuing care of the traumatized patient or even the patient who has already been subjected to an operation, but there is still an inevitable time delay before such facilities can be brought into contact with the patient. There is thus still a requirement for pretraining, backed by high quality communication systems, if the best care is to be provided for such patients.

Health care for the saturation diver

The most inaccessible of all isolated workers is the saturation diver. When a surgical illness is developed in a diver in the saturation mode in an offshore pressure chamber, it may be several days or even weeks before the diver can be decompressed. When the surgical team eventually arrives offshore it will be met with a wall of steel which separates it from its patient. A series of priorities was thus developed some years ago for the

Table 15.2. Priorities for the management of sick or injured divers in an offshore pressure chamber. The items are listed in order of priority

1	Training of divers in first aid
2	Clear and precise communications
3	Trained doctors willing to go offshore
4	Mobile intensive care unit
5	Transfer under pressure facility

management of a serious surgical illness, when it occurred in such a situation, and these priorities are shown in order of importance in *Table 15.2*.

A decision which has to be taken following the diagnosis of a surgical illness in an offshore pressure chamber is where that illness should be managed. If an acute life-threatening condition has developed it seems clear that a surgical team must attend offshore with its equipment. The specialists may be compressed and should be prepared to undertake some form of intervention in the offshore pressure chamber, if necessary. An alternative would be to transfer the patient, in a capsule at the same pressure as the offshore chamber, to a large operating chamber onshore within which the surgical team had already set up its equipment. It is important to stress that this latter system can only be used when the patient is in a stable condition and not likely to develop a sudden, severe deterioration, since the transfer capsule is so small that urgent action could not be taken under these circumstances. When the operation has been completed, the saturation diver may still have to face a number of complications, some of which are directly associated with the hyperbaric environment. Consideration must be given to such questions as: (a) infection; (b) the action of drugs at increased atmospheric pressure; (c) the function of ventilators in pressure chambers; (d) the problems inherent in decompressing underperfused tissue; and (e) the diagnosis of chest infection in pressure vessels. These questions are considered below.

Infection in pressure chambers

Hyperbaric oxygen chambers have been used for surgical purposes for the past 20 years and have reached an advanced state of sophistication in Japan and the USA. An example of such an operating chamber is shown in *Figure 15.1*. The chambers function at atmospheric pressures in the region of 300 or 400 kPa (3 or 4 atm), at absolute maximum, and are normally compressed with air while only the patient breathes the appropriate pressure of oxygen through a mask or endotracheal tube. Since the atmosphere is constantly replaced by the continuing action of the compressors, the environment remains bacteriologically clean. Indeed, it is an ideal place to nurse the post-traumatic patient who has some degree of damage to his immune system or other cause of susceptibility to infection.

The saturation pressure chamber, however, normally functions greatly in excess of 500 kPa (5 atm) absolute and indeed may well function

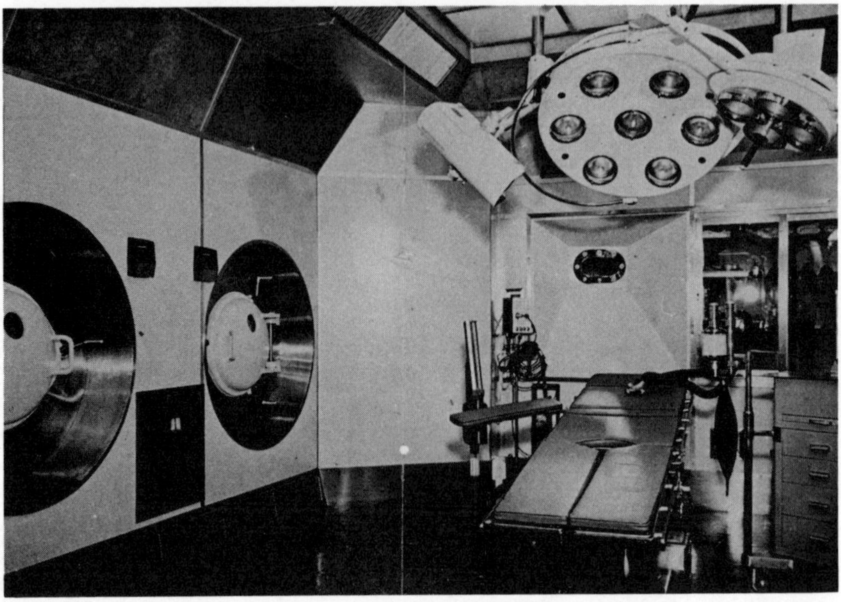

Figure 15.1. Hyperbaric operating theatre in a Japanese teaching hospital

somewhere in the region of 10 MPa (100 atm) absolute. The carrier gas used is helium. Since it is so expensive it is normally recirculated, by removing carbon dioxide and other noxious gases and adjusting the oxygen input with care. After some time, bacterial growth becomes established. Such a chamber is therefore a difficult environment in which to undertake any surgical procedure or within which to nurse a patient in the postoperative phase. A saturation chamber is normally run at a temperature of 33 or 34°C and it is somewhat difficult to maintain a low humidity due to the diving work with which it is associated. The normal Gram-positive flora which covers the skin under normal circumstances does not function well in such an environment and tends to die out, to become replaced by Gram-negative organisms which relish such environmental conditions. *Pseudomonas* spp. are particularly happy in these circumstances and indeed rather enjoy sea water! The whole bacteriological flora is, therefore, much more pathogenic than the normal and from the point of view of the postoperative patient the bacteriological environment becomes more and more hazardous with time. There has been so little experience of postoperative care in saturation chambers that the extent to which this would become a problem cannot be defined. *Pseudomonas pyocyanea* has caused the most trouble so far by being responsible for serious infections in the external auditory meatus of divers under these circumstances (Alcock, 1979).

Effect of increased atmospheric pressure on drugs

A very considerable increase in hydrostatic pressure is known to cause marked effects on the pharmacological action of certain drugs. The phenomenon of pressure reversal of anaesthetic agents has been known and widely investigated for many years (Lever *et al.*, 1971). The pressure required for such an occurrence is very much greater than that to which man is currently being exposed in underwater work-sites. Nevertheless, it is important to point out that certain drugs may act differently at increased atmospheric pressure, and analgesics and anaesthetics come into this category. In general, the work done so far suggests that an increased dosage of both analgesics and anaesthetics is required to produce the same effect, although precise dose–response curves have not been made for more than a few intravenous agents (Bailey *et al.*, 1977). Care requires to be taken to determine whether previous knowledge or experience with particular drugs at increased pressure exists. Knowledge so far available was collected and published in the recent past by Cox (1982).

Function of ventilators at increased atmospheric pressure

If a ventilator is to be used during the operation or in the postoperative period, then it is important that some provision should be made to test the ventilator chosen before it is used in the pressure chamber. Under normal circumstances, the fluidic type of ventilator will be required to overcome the problems of the use of electricity within the chamber. One of the problems which arises here is that the line pressure of gases normally used in the chamber is different from that normally used to drive the ventilator. Some form of adapter must therefore be provided. Industrial threads for connections to the penetrators in chambers are very often of the left-hand variety and again it may be necessary to provide appropriate adapters for the connection of the ventilator to be used. In addition, the differing physical characteristics of gases at various pressures may mean that the ventilator does not deliver what would be expected from the settings, and the various ventilators often function differently in this respect at different pressures (Ross and Manson, 1979). If the ventilator chosen has not been calibrated, then this is a necessary preliminary to its use at greatly increased atmospheric pressure.

Decompression of underperfused tissue

The various decompression schedules have been designed to take account of the body composition of normally perfused, fit adults. Problems may therefore be caused by locally underperfused areas of tissue, by general states of underperfusion and by dehydration. These problems are of an undefined nature and little work has been undertaken to determine whether this is a major problem or not. The commonest form of decompression sickness takes place in the tendons and ligaments around joints. This is said to be due to the relative underperfusion or the variable perfusion of these areas. Where possible, decompression should therefore not be undertaken in the postoperative period until such factors can be eliminated. If decompression must be undertaken, then this possibility should be borne in mind during that phase of postoperative management of the saturation diver.

Diagnosis of chest and other infections

The postoperative chest must be a considerable hazard to the saturation diver, particularly if decompression is to be undertaken during that phase, since even minor airways obstruction may cause pulmonary barotrauma with the most dangerous or even fatal consequences. The management of the problem is rendered even more difficult by the problems of physical examination in a noisy pressure chamber. To a certain extent this problem has been overcome by the development of techniques for taking X-rays through the ports of pressure chambers, using flexible film passed through the medical lock, and also by the development of the electric stethoscope (Childs, 1979). This allows auscultation of the patient from outside the chamber by means of an electrical penetrator through the hull. In order to avoid such postoperative problems or to minimize them, it may be a reasonable manoeuvre, after the operation has been completed and the patient is stabilized, to transfer him at that stage from the bacteriologically unclean offshore pressure chamber to a large operating chamber such as that owned by the Grampian Health Board in Aberdeen. In order to do this, a system of transfer chambers has been developed by a diving company, International Underwater Contractors, and this system is now owned by a consortium of oil companies and is available to transfer a patient from an offshore saturation chamber to a large, clean, operating facility onshore.

There are thus in existence fairly advanced techniques available to assist in the management of a saturation diver should he develop surgical illness while at work. These have not yet been required to any great extent, which is a tribute to the careful selection and examination of the divers before they are allowed to enter the saturation system and to the development of the safety procedures which have been applied over the years to the North Sea and which have greatly limited the occurrence of traumatic injury in such personnel.

References

ALCOCK, S. R. (1979). Acute otitis externa in divers working in the North Sea: a micro-biological survey of seven saturation dives. In *Hyperbaric Medicine*. Aberdeen; Aberdeen University Press, pp. 434–439

BAILEY, C. P., GREEN, C. J., HALSEY, M. J. and WARDLEY-SMITH, B. (1977). High pressure and intravenous steroid anaesthesia in rats. *J. Appl. Physiol.*, **267**, 46

CHILDS, C. M. (1979). Diagnosis in pressure chambers. In *Hyperbaric Medicine*. Aberdeen; Aberdeen University Press, pp. 440–442

COX, R. A. F. (1982). The use of drugs under pressure. In *Offshore Medicine*. New York; Springer-Verlag, pp. 196–199

LEVER, M. J., MILLER, K. W., PATON, W. D. M., STREET, W. B. and SMITH, E. B. (1971). Pressure reversal of anaesthesia. *Nature,* **231,** 368

NORMAN, J. N. (1981). Medical care in the Antarctic. In *Circumpolar Health 81*. Copenhagen; Nordic Council for Arctic Medical Research, Report Series 33, pp. 74–76

ROBERTS, J. M., HOUSE, A. M. and MCNAMARA, W. C. (1977). Telemedicine at Memorial University of Newfoundland. In *Medinfo 77*. Amsterdam; North-Holland Publishing Company, pp. 869–873

ROSS, J. A. S. and MANSON, H. J. (1979). A resuscitator for use in the hyperbaric environment. In *Hyperbaric Medicine*. Aberdeen; Aberdeen University Press, pp. 453–455

Index